Lourdes Library
Gwynedd-Mercy College
P. O. Box 901
Gwynedd Valley, PA 19437-0901

AF853315

Hyperbaric Nursing
and
Wound Care

BEST PUBLISHING COMPANY

RM
666
.O83
H93
2010

Lourdes Library
Gwynedd-Mercy College
P. O. Box 901
Gwynedd Valley, PA 19437-0901

Hyperbaric Nursing and Wound Care

EDITOR:

Valerie Larson-Lohr, RN

CO-EDITORS:

Helen Norvell, RN

Laura Josefsen, RN

James R. Wilcox, RN

BEST PUBLISHING COMPANY

Editing: Catherine Morris and Linda Locklear

No responsibility is assumed by the Publisher or Editors for any injury and/or damage to persons or property as a matter of product liability, negligence, or otherwise, or from any use or operation of any methods, product, instructions, or ideas contained in the material herein. No suggested test or procedure should be carried out unless, in the reader's judgment, its risk is justified. Because of rapid advances in the medical sciences, we recommend that the independent verification of diagnoses and drug dosages should be made.

All rights reserved. No part of this book may be reproduced, stored in a retrieval system, or transmitted in any form or by any means, electronic, mechanical, photocopying, micro-filming, recording, or otherwise, without written permission from the publisher.

Copyright 2010 by Best Publishing Company

International Standard Book Number: 978-1930536-5-86
Library of Congress catalog card number: 2009910329

For more information contact:
Best Publishing Company
PO Box 30100
Flagstaff, AZ 86003-0100, USA
Telephone: 928.527.1055
Fax: 928.526.0370
E-mail: divebooks@bestpub.com
Website: www.bestpub.com

Table of Contents

Foreword

THE FIELD OF HYPERBARIC MEDICINE, specifically the nursing care of patients undergoing hyperbaric oxygen treatment, has advanced significantly in the eight years following the publication of *Hyperbaric Nursing*. *Hyperbaric Nursing* was a landmark publication, and having undergone extensive revision and update, *Hyperbaric Nursing and Wound Care* is a worthy successor. This book not only addresses changes within the field of hyperbaric medicine, but also how those changes can be integrated into recent advances in nursing practice as a whole.

As the role of hyperbaric oxygen treatment in the management of complex wounds and in support of limb salvage receives further validation, the patients we treat have become increasingly complex with respect to both their medical and nursing care requirements. Add to these patient complexities the emergency and critical care aspects of hyperbaric nursing and the advances in equipment and technology, and the need for a publication like *Hyperbaric Nursing and Wound Care* becomes clear.

The editors and contributors are to be congratulated for providing the knowledge base for hyperbaric nursing practice into the next decade.

Robert A. Warriner III, MD

Preface

It has been nine years since *Hyperbaric Nursing* was published. The field of hyperbaric medicine has grown significantly since then, and with that the role of the hyperbaric nurse. As a result, the editors collaborated to create another, more improved book. We asked ourselves what was great about the first book and what would make a second book better: the result is before you. After a monumental effort from all of the contributing authors, we have produced a new, updated textbook for the hyperbaric nursing community.

We are sincerely grateful to everyone that accepted the task of meeting tough deadlines to complete this book. Our contributors took precious time from their personal schedules to write outstanding chapters for today's hyperbaric nurse, and their efforts have been rewarded with the publication of this book.

Valerie Larson-Lohr, RN

Helen C. Norvell, RN

Laura Josefsen, RN

James R. Wilcox, RN

Author List

Kathy Barr, JD, RN, CPHQ

Richard C. Barry, BBA, CHT

Craig L. Broussard, PhD, CNS, GNP, CWCN, CWS, FAACWS, FAPWCA, CHRNC

Dick Clarke, CHT

Julio R. Garcia, CHT, RN, BSN

Stacy Handley, BSN, ACHRN, CWCN, CHT

Laura Josefsen , RN, ACHRN

Patrick N. Kimbrell, MD, CWSP

Valerie Larson-Lohr, APRN, MS, CWCN, CHRNC, DAPWCA

Susan Mellott, PhD, RN, CPHQ, FNAHQ

JoAnn Mick, PhD, RN, AOCN, NEA-BC

Linda M. Miller, RN, BSN

Helen Norvell, RN, BSN

John S. Peters, MBA, FACHE

E. Patricia Rios, RN, MSN, CHRNC

Monica R. Skarban, MSOLQ, BSN, RN, ACHRN

Robert A. Warriner III, MD, FACA, FCCP, FCCWS, ABPM/UHM

Tricia West, MBA/HCM, BSN, RN, CHN, PHN, LNC

James R. Wilcox, RN, BSN, ACHRN, CWCN, CFCN, CWS, WCC, DAPWCA, FCCWS

W.T. Workman, MS, CAsP, CHT-A, FAsMA

Dedication

THIS BOOK IS DEDICATED TO THE NURSES practicing in the field of hyperbaric nursing worldwide. You have been and are pioneers, entering into a specialty that was unsure if nursing had a role to play, or if nursing could contribute to its advancement. Together, we created a new specialty: that of hyperbaric nursing, where the practice of nursing has proven instrumental to the wellbeing of the patients entrusted to our care. As I look at how far hyperbaric nursing has come in a relatively short time, I feel both proud and humbled. I am proud to be part of a profession that was willing to take a risk to practice in a new and dramatically different setting, to persist in creating a role for nursing, to define standards of nursing practice, and to challenge the traditional role of the nurse. I am humbled by the immense talent, dedication, selflessness, and spirit of the nurses with whom I have had the privilege to share the journey of hyperbaric nursing. Thank you for the adventure.

CHAPTER

1

Hyperbaric History and the Nursing Evolution

STACY HANDLEY AND DICK CLARKE

NURSES ARE AS MUCH A PART OF modern hyperbaric medicine as the chambers themselves. Due to a recent increase in availability of hyperbaric medicine and a broadened scope of clinical indications, the evolution of the role of the hyperbaric nurse since the latter half of the 20th century has been considerable. Historically, staff nurses assessed patients prior to and during each hyperbaric oxygen treatment. They accompanied patients into multiplace chambers and operated monoplace hyperbaric delivery systems. Today's hyperbaric nurses hold key roles in research, education, consulting, surveying and leadership. However, this wasn't always the case. While hyperbaric medicine enjoys a history in excess of 100 years, nurses only became an integral part in the past 50 years of this century of practice.

The British physician and clergyman Henshaw is credited with the first application of an alteration in atmospheric pressure for therapeutic purposes, in 1662. He sealed off a normal room, which he referred to as a "Domicilium." It was driven by pair of organ bellows, with valves to control the flow of air. This sealed room was used to create both hyper- and hypo-baric conditions.

Despite the lack of any scientific basis for his theories, Henshaw believed that patients suffering from acute conditions would benefit from increased air pressure, while those suffering more chronic ailments would profit from a more obscure environment, stating: "In times of good health this domicilium is proposed as a good expedient to help digestion, to promote insensible respiration, to facilitate breathing and expectoration and consequently, of excellent use for prevention of most affections of the lungs."

Introduction of the first purpose-built hyperbaric chamber is attributed to Junod, a French physician.[1] Junod commissioned his chamber in 1834. It was spherical in shape and designed very much along the lines of the steam engine boiler of the day. Constructed of riveted copper, it had an impressive compression capability of 4 ATA and could accommodate several occupants. Air was both the compression gas and the breathing gas. While oxygen had been discovered some 50 years earlier, technologies to separate it from the atmosphere in significant enough volumes, store it in liquid or gaseous forms, and an appreciation of the basis for its therapeutic use were not well understood (Figure 1).

Junod used his chamber under the now-appreciated misguided impression that breathing air under increased ambient pressures would improve tissue perfusion. Certainly, such compressed air environments would result in a modest increase in oxygen delivery, as a function of both Dalton's law of partial pressures and Henry's solubility law. However, Junod did not consider enhanced oxygen delivery to represent a useful therapeutic element. Rather, he was attracted to the potential of raised ambient pressure, per se.

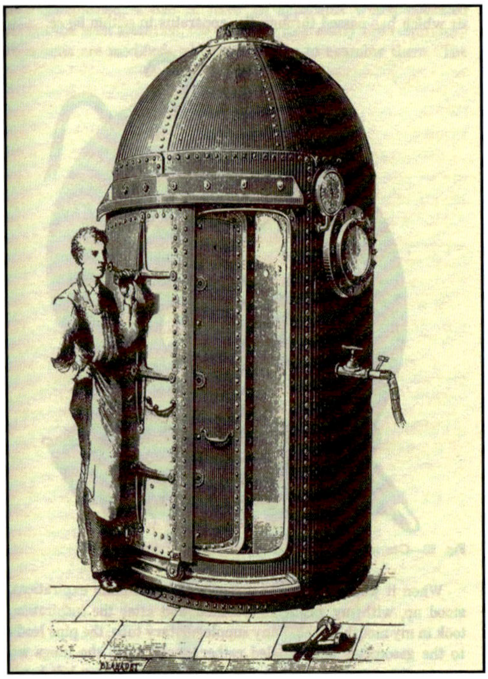

FIGURE 1: ***An artist's representation of Junod's hyperbaric chamber.***

It is highly unlikely that those exposed received any immediate or lasting benefit. This did not deter others, however, as hyperbaric "air baths" quickly found their way into health spas and other non-hospital related settings across much of Western Europe.

Given the relative mechanical complexity of these hyperbaric chambers and their necessary support systems they were almost certainly operated by technicians, under the orders of the prescribing physician. There are no surviving records from this period to suggest that nurses played any sort of supportive role. This might not be too surprising given that the position of a nurse within the health delivery system was also very much in its infancy during this period.

The remainder of the 19th century saw numerous hyperbaric chambers constructed for use in an increasing number of improbable conditions. As quickly as new diseases and illnesses were identified and without obvious cure there were some who suggested that hyperbaric air pressures might prove useful. A review of the conditions being treated during this period and a modern understanding of respective pathophysiologies would suggest that no real benefits were obtained.

As the 19th century transitioned into the 20th century, the first sound therapeutic basis for hyperbaric medicine was identified. It was based upon the mechanical effect of Boyle's law and its essential inverse relationship between pressure and volume. This represented an important resolving effect on intravascular gas bubbles produced as a consequence of decompression from compressed gas exposures. The first patients to benefit from this treatment approach were those caisson and tunnel workers employed in high ambient air pressures.[2] This form of therapy was soon extended to naval diving personnel and resulted in a gradual incorporation of hyperbaric chambers into naval diving operations. These "recompression" chambers were commonly referred to as "iron doctors" and became an essential standard of care for the treatment of decompression sickness, "the bends." Navy divers and technical support personnel operated them; diving medical officers or medical corpsmen accompanied patients under pressure.

The chamber that received the most publicity and was the most actively used at the time was in Kansas City during the 1920's. Dr. Orville J. Cunningham first used his chamber to treat the victims of the Spanish influenza epidemic that swept across the USA during the closing days of the First World War. He claimed to have achieved remarkable improvement in patients who were cyanotic and comatose. However, one night a mechanical failure resulted in a complete loss of compression and all his patients died. He considered this to be proof positive of the chamber's benefit, while a modern analysis would suggest that the chamber's occupants succumbed to decompression illness.

In Cleveland in 1928, Cunningham constructed the largest chamber ever built– five stories high and 64 feet in diameter. Each floor had 12 bedrooms with all the amenities of a good hotel. Dr Cunningham was repeatedly instructed by the Bureau of Investigations of the American Medical Association to document his claims of effectiveness of hyperbaric therapy for his increasing uses. He failed to do so and subsequently had his medical license revoked but he never did so. Cunningham's chamber was dismantled for scrap in 1937.

By the 1930s, commercial diving contractors employed in support of civilian engineering and other underwater projects had likewise evolved their operational practices to include a hyperbaric chamber at the worksite in many instances. This represented the essential practice of hyperbaric (diving) medicine throughout the first half of the 20th century.

It was not until the 1950s that a fundamental shift in the application of hyperbaric medicine occurred which would soon require the nursing discipline's clinical support. Until that point in time, hyperbaric chambers had not been located in hospitals or other comprehensive clinical settings. Rather, they were found at military and civilian diving operation worksites.

The event that evolved hyperbaric medicine into the hospital-based therapeutic technology we appreciate today was the now classic publication "Life Without Blood."[3] Cardiovascular surgeons at the Academic Medical Center in Amsterdam, The Netherlands, had long been frustrated with the very short ischemic times available in the pre-cardiopulmonary bypass era. Under the leadership of Ita Boerema, whole body hypothermia had been introduced in the late 1940s. While this technique did extend the period of ischemia, gains were modest and complications significant. Still not satisfied, they investigated hyperbaric oxygen. At 3 ATA, on 100% oxygen, all of the blood from small pigs was removed by exchange transfusion down to hemoglobin levels of essentially zero. The absence of red blood cells was well tolerated. This finding demonstrated that exceedingly large volumes of oxygen could be carried in physical solution in plasma, sufficient in degree to support basal metabolic needs. Resulting periods of cardiac arrest were now greatly extended. Boerema's group soon began to perform open-heart surgery in a hyperbaric chamber with capabilities greatly enhanced by the much increased ischemic times. These findings were so impressive that many of the world's major medical centers introduced hyperbaric operating rooms. A second hyperbaric therapeutic mechanism had arrived. Boerema often is credited as the father of modern-day hyperbaric medicine (Figure 2).

Nurses first became integrated into the practice of hyperbaric medicine in the late 1950's. All early "hyperbaric" nurses were actually those who were managing patients in the cardiac operating rooms, surgical recovery facilities and the cardiac intensive care. In order for there to be an appropriate continuity of care, select nurses were trained in the procedures necessary to accompany their patients during hyperbaric exposure and safely undergo chamber compression and decompression. These hyperbaric operating rooms were large enough to provide for all of the equipment and staff found in conventional surgical and medical settings (Figure 3).

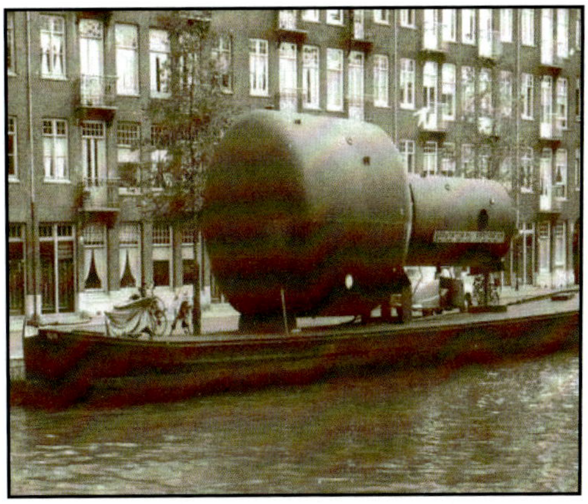

Figure 2: ***Boerema's hyperbaric chamber delivered via an Amsterdam canal to Hospital Wilhelmina Gasthius.***

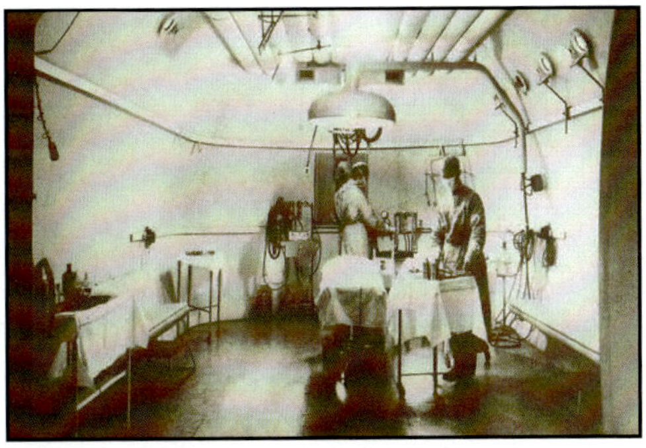

Figure 3: ***Inside Boerema's enormous hyperbaric operating room.***

After the first successful year of cardiac practice under hyperbaric conditions, a colleague of Boerema's, W. H. Brummelkamp, also interested in hyperbaric medicine, discovered in 1959 (and subsequently published in 1961) that anaerobic infections were inhibited by hyperbaric therapy. Boerema's chamber was then introduced to the treatment of surgical infections. A "hopeless case" of gas gangrene, hopeless in that limb amputation was not an option, underwent hyperbaric oxygen therapy. A dramatic arrest of the advancing infection was observed and systemic toxicity soon resolved. Additional compelling clinical experience[4] and laboratory studies[5] eventually produced the third therapeutic basis for HBO therapy, namely its antimicrobial properties. This advancement created a greater demand for eligible nurses to be trained in order to safely care for and remain with their surgical intensive care unit patients during each treatment of hyperbaric oxygenation.

It should be emphasized that these cardiac and surgical nurses were not hyperbaric nurses, per se. Rather, they were simply provided with knowledge sufficient in degree to allow them to competently enter and exit the compressed gas atmosphere without endangering themselves or others. This is in contrast to today's hyperbaric nurse who has undergone formalized training, has access to hyperbaric-specific certification and works in and around hyperbaric chambers in an essential full-time capacity.

By the early 1960s, multiplace chambers were being introduced into the clinical setting on an international scale. As noted above, they were first employed as hyperbaric operating rooms for cardiac surgery. The benefits of hyperbaric medicine were subsequently observed for support of split-thickness skin graft, flap survival and salvage, wound re-epithelization, acute carbon monoxide poisoning, arterial insufficiencies and acute thermal burns. These observations and limited formal study lent some credibility to the therapeutic employment of HBO therapy. This fostered the establishment of scientific organizations such as the International Congress on Hyperbaric Oxygen in 1963 and the Undersea Medical Society (UMS) in 1967, later renamed in 1986 the Undersea and Hyperbaric Medical Society (UHMS) as we know it today. Unfortunately, as the availability of hyperbaric medicine chambers increased, the indiscriminate and inappropriate use of chambers by practitioners searching for a "cure-all" therapy for various medical conditions resulted in something of a backlash from the scientific society, once again tarnishing the credibility of hyperbaric medicine. As a result, and by the late 1970s, the UMS had formulated guidelines for the use of hyperbaric oxygen therapy.

In 1964 an article published in the Canadian Medical Association Journal referred to the safety precautions that were established to protect the nursing staff and other medical attendants serving as tenders inside the multiplace chamber at the Royal Victoria Hospital in Montreal.[6] The perceived 'major dangers' to nursing personnel at that time were decompression sickness, bone infarcts and arterial gas embolism. Measures taken to prevent harm to the nurses included: minimizing each attendant exposure time to depths greater than 2 ATA, adhering to the US Navy decompression tables, tracking the number of dives and performing pulmonary function screenings for staff members to ensure their lungs were suitably fit for pressurizations.

Additionally, a paper published in August of 1969 raised added concerns for nurses entering the field of hyperbaric medicine. Hazards in Hyperbaric Medicine, from the British Medical Journal by Ledingham and Davidson, discussed the incidence of injury to their staff while exposed to the air-pressurized environment of the multiplace chamber. The findings of annual radiological skeletal surveys did not support the growing concern of aseptic bone necrosis or those risks cited in the Canadian paper, as relative work-related risks.[7]

In 1969, Toni Bishop, a registered nurse in the Royal Australian Navy was intrigued with patients she nursed in the sick bay at HMAS Penguin who had received treatment in the hospital's recompression chamber. She requested and attended the training course held at the School of Underwater Medicine at HMAS Penguin in 1969. Hence, the Hyperbaric Technicians and Nurses Association (HTNA) has deemed Toni Bishop the first Hyperbaric Nurse in Australia[8] (Figure 4).

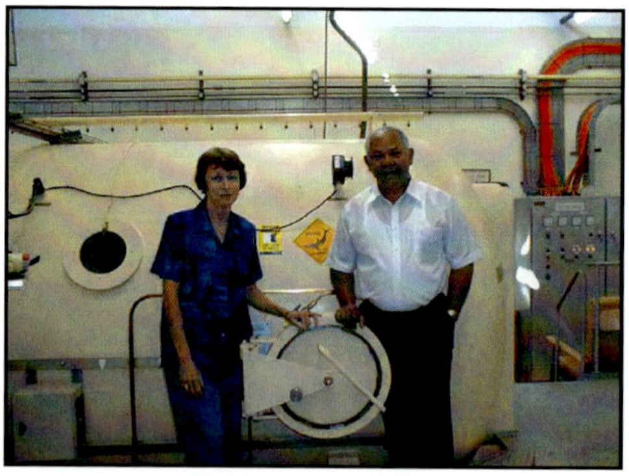

Figure 4: ***Toni Bishop circa 1969.***

The event that consolidated the role of the nurse as a full-time member of the hyperbaric medicine team was the introduction of the acrylic-hulled, single occupant, monoplace hyperbaric chamber. Until this point, all chambers regardless of their principal use were of the multiple occupancy, multiple compartment design. The monoplace chamber, while offering similar therapeutic capability to the multiplace chamber, involved a greatly simplified design, which did not require complex technical and ancillary technologies (air compressors, gas storage containers, fire suppression capabilities and complex control systems) that characterized the multiplace hyperbaric delivery system. Consequently, health care professionals could be quickly and effectively trained to both operate the chamber and manage related patient care. The British-made Vickers hyperbaric chamber (the forerunner to today's monoplace hyperbaric delivery system) was being acquired by civilian hospitals in increasing numbers and the need to train hospital nursing and allied health personnel became very evident. Due to this evolution, the dual capability of the hyperbaric nurse to serve as both caregiver and chamber operator became widely appreciated (Figure 5).

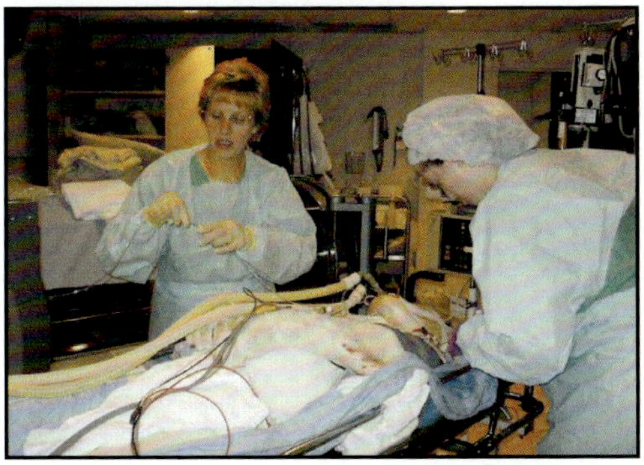

FIGURE 5: *Connie Wilson (left), lead hyperbaric nurse at Nebraska Medical Center, preparing a burn patient for the monoplace chamber with the assistance from a burn nurse.*

One of the first hyperbaric nurses devoted entirely to the practice of hyperbaric medicine, certainly from a U.S. perspective, was Alice LeVeille Gaul. A former U.S. Navy nurse, Alice resigned her commission in 1969 in order to establish a training curriculum for the hyperbaric medicine department at the Long Beach Naval Shipyard in Southern California. Here, medical corpsmen were to become familiar with the operation of multiplace chambers and management of decompression accidents. Alice worked under the direction of Dr. George B. Hart, a hyperbaric pioneer in his own right. Within a year of leaving the navy, her role had been greatly expanded. Alice crisscrossed the country providing weekend instructional courses on behalf of hospitals that were introducing monoplace-based hyperbaric delivery systems. Alice played a key role in the development and early operation of Long Beach Memorial Hospital's monoplace hyperbaric facility. This program became one of the first to introduce formal on-site introductory training, beginning in the late 1970s.

Barely a year after Alice had begun her hyperbaric career, another nurse was to formally train in the emerging field of hyperbaric medicine and likewise proved to be a pioneering force. This nurse, Diane Norkool, had a background in critical care. The installation of a hyperbaric chamber at Virginia Mason Medical Center in Seattle, Washington, in 1970, piqued her interest. The primary purpose of the chamber was to undertake clinical studies with a diving physiology focus. Diane had a long-standing interest in research and saw in this chamber a number of professional opportunities. She volunteered as a subject for several investigations and subsequently became one of the program's researchers. Her resulting publications spanned hyperbaric medicine's uses, with particular focus on carbon monoxide poisoning and late radiation tissue injury. She also published articles on patient management issues relating to pediatric and adult critical care. Her 1976 master's thesis addressed hyperbaric oxygen effects in a rat model of full thickness acute thermal burns. Diane was first author in major peer reviewed medical journals on several occasions.

In 1976, the Undersea and Hyperbaric Medical Society introduced an Associate membership category. Principally a physician and biomedical scientist-based organization, the UHMS had now formally recognized the important team-related contributions of all of those medical and technical personnel who support the practice of undersea medicine and hyperbaric oxygen therapy. Hyperbaric nurses could now become members of the peer international scientific body for their field. It was not too long before some of the Society's nurse members found their way onto various UHMS committees, where they helped to guide and consolidate the professional direction of the Society.

Subsequent hyperbaric nursing notables at Long Beach Memorial Hospital were Diana De Jesus-Greenberg and Valerie Messina. It was during a 1985 joint conference of the UMS and the Tenth Annual Conference on Clinical Application of Hyperbaric Medicine, in Long Beach, where Diana and Valerie, along with 33 other nurses, established the Baromedical Nursing Association (BNA).[9] The BNA would become the professional organization for hyperbaric nursing and would serve to integrate this profession within the international health care delivery system. It was the intent of the BNA to define and implement standards of practice, promote education opportunities for hyperbaric nurses, and support related clinical research. Diana became the BNA's first elected president. By 1988 the BNA served 176 members.

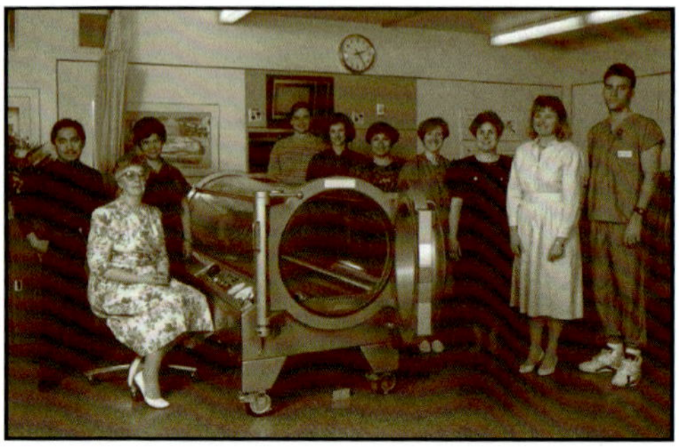

FIGURE 6: ***1987 nursing staff at Long Beach Memorial Hospital. From left: Luis Rivera, Barbara Happe (sitting), Celia Loney, Mitch Goul, Trish Chase, Beth Driscoll, Valerie Messina, Beth Clemenson, Tim Manley.***

During the ensuing years of the BNA, Diane Norkool was very much committed to the education of her peers. She was successful in encouraging the UHMS to incorporate nursing presentations into its annual scientific meetings and she held leadership positions within the BNA and the Society's Pacific Chapter. Along with Valerie Messina, in 1994, Diane authored the hyperbaric nursing chapter in the first edition of the highly regarded Kindwall textbook Hyperbaric Medicine Practice. In 1996, an award in her name and in her honor was introduced by the BNA upon her untimely death at the age of 56. The Diane Norkool Award recognizes those who embody the many qualities that Diane brought to the nursing profession in general and hyperbaric nursing in particular.

In the early 1990s, the BNA began a process that would lead to the introduction of a certification in hyperbaric nursing. A BNA Certification Board was established in 1995 and the first "Certified Hyperbaric Registered Nurse" examination took place that same year. Since then, the certification board has added the categories of Advanced Certified Hyperbaric Registered Nurse (ACHRN), eligible for those with management, teaching or research responsibilities and CHRN-C for nurse clinicians with a master's degree and

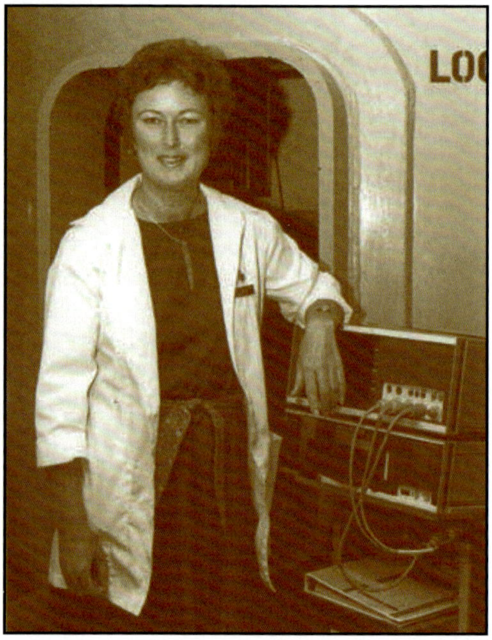

FIGURE 7: ***Diane Norkool, circa 1988.***

five or more years of hyperbaric experience. In recent years the exam underwent a revision by the BNACB. In recognition of the evolving role of the hyperbaric nurse that now frequently serves a dual role as wound nurse exam questions now include wound pathophysiology and management.

By the late 1990s, as a sign of the tremendous clinical growth, as many as six new UHMS approved 40-hour hyperbaric training programs were organized and commonly offered on a monthly basis throughout the U.S. Today this number has more than doubled. Additionally, new programs such as acrylic inspection, safety director, fitness-to-dive and adjunctive wound courses are now being offered as levels of interest and awareness become more robust. In the past decade, a plethora of hyperbaric management companies have contracted with hospitals to help open new programs and to ensure safety and compliance. These new avenues served to further increase hyperbaric nurse opportunities to become knowledgeable experts by way of lecturing on training courses, precepting practicums, and providing on-site consultation to hyperbaric staff.

With the introduction of the UHMS Facility Accreditation program in 2001, certified hyperbaric nurses were sought to train as surveyors. Each survey team consists of a physician, a nurse and a technical representative. The survey team spends two days at the requesting facility where they undertake a detailed and comprehensive assessment of that facility's strengths and areas for improvement. In 2010, the Joint Commission signed an agreement with the UHMS as a Complimentary Accrediting Body. This served to increase public awareness on quality and compliance in the hyperbaric oxygen setting by recognizing the rigorous process to achieve hyperbaric facility accreditation.

During the formative period of the Divers Alert Network (DAN) in the early 1980s, two nurses played key leadership roles and maintained an important long-term presence. DAN, a nonprofit organization, is the leading diving safety, education and research organization in the world and enjoys a global reach[10] Duke University Medical Center hyperbaric nurses Chris Wachholz and Joel Dovenbarger were early DAN employees who were instrumental in the establishment of a world-wide compilation of hyperbaric chambers available to treat injured divers. Both were knowledgeable experts in diving medicine, they served as educators and lecturers. Over the ensuing years each had numerous publications to their credit. Chris worked to grow DAN's supportive network throughout much of the world in order to ensure that those divers who were injured in medically and geographically remote settings could be quickly stabilized and evacuated to appropriate levels of care. Joel manned the emergency hotline at DAN's headquarters for more than a quarter of a century, effectively managing countless medical emergencies.

In 1992, the HTNA was formed in Australia.[11] Membership was open to those technicians and nurses involved in diving and hyperbaric medicine, with most members being residents of Australia and New Zealand. At that point in time, there were less than a dozen chambers, all of multiplace design, in the region. Within the past decade, a growing number of monoplace chambers have been introduced. The HTNA became a vibrant and energetic group and quickly began to convene conferences and develop objectives for training and education courses with some specifically focused on nurses. To their credit, the physicians who worked with the HTNA requested to hold their annual meetings in conjunction with the HTNA meetings. This was agreed to and the Australia and New Zealand Hyperbaric Medicine Group (ANZHMG) has enjoyed a close professional relationship with the HTNA ever since.

One prominent BNA member, and founding president of the HTNA is Christy Pirone. Christy, also a former Diane Norkool Award recipient, was first a hyperbaric nurse in Indianapolis before immigrating to Australia. Christy worked at Royal Adelaide Hospital's hyperbaric medicine service, eventually becoming its nurse manager. During this period she was instrumental in the development and application of HIMS, the Hyperbaric Incident Monitoring Study.[12] HIMS is an anonymous and voluntary method of submitting narrative descriptions of accidents and incidents. It was modeled on a similar project looking at anesthesia related complications and on the Australia Incident Monitoring Study. Christy and her team committed countless hours to mature the project and seek its wider acceptance within the international hyperbaric community. HIMS was eventually translated into five languages and employed in 20 countries. Christy's master's thesis described the genesis, applicability and application of HIMS. The University of Adelaide Health Sciences, Department of Nursing, along with Christy and her nurse colleague Czes Mucha were instrumental in creating the only Graduate Certificate level hyperbaric nursing program (Figure 8).

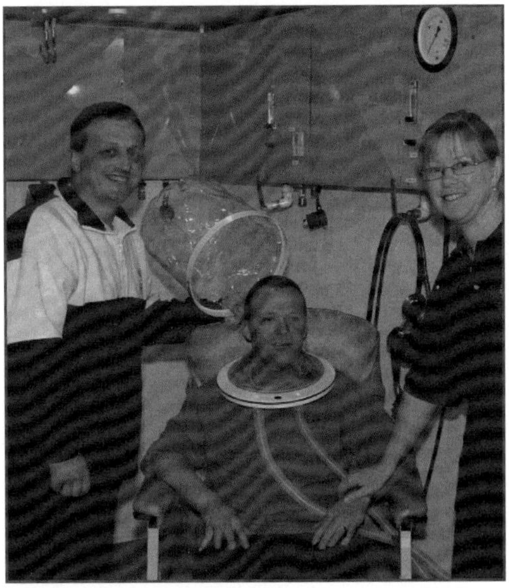

Figure 8: ***From left, hyperbaric nurses Czes Mucha and Christy Pirone (right) caring for a patient in a multiplace chamber.***

A sobering reminder of the potential risks associated with the practice of hyperbaric medicine was brought to bear in 1991. Until then, there had been a number of relatively mild cases of iatrogenic decompression sickness reported in nurses who accompanied patients into multiplace chambers.

While patients would breathe oxygen via personalized delivery systems, nurses breathed the chamber's background air atmosphere. It is considered unsafe for the nurse to breathe pure oxygen due to its increased toxic effects on the central nervous system in those not lying or sitting in a relaxed state. The increased partial pressure of nitrogen in air at elevated pressures places risks of decompression sickness on chamber staff members. The majority of decompression sickness cases are quickly managed by (and seemingly paradoxically) returning the injured nurse to the hyperbaric chamber, this time breathing oxygen under pressure. On July 22, 1991, however, a case of decompression sickness in a hyperbaric nurse proved fatal.[13] The nurse, 52-year-old Joyce Vause, died within two hours after exiting a chamber following the treatment of a recreational SCUBA diver in Panama City, Florida. An analysis of events leading up to this tragic event determined that human error on the part of the chamber operators as well as inadequate training and supervisory oversight led to the nurse being decompressed in a grossly inappropriate manner.

In 1996, another hyperbaric nurse at Los Robles Hospital in Thousand Oaks, California, suffered spinal cord decompression sickness upon exiting an air-filled chamber, resulting in permanent paralysis. The cause of this case was likewise determined to be the result of human error on the part of the chamber's operating and supervisory personnel. She was confined to a wheelchair and died of complications related to her decompression injury a little more than a decade later. These two cases certainly leave no doubt as to importance of comprehensive and formalized training, the need for regular skills updating and a culture of non-complacent safety above all else.

Like all emerging medical fields, research is ongoing and necessary to maintain a basis for evidence based medicine. Hyperbaric oxygen continues to prove to be beneficial in the enhancement of healing in problem wounds that are deficient in tissue oxygen profusion. Studies continue to prove the angiogenic properties of increased oxygen gradients resulting from hyperbaric oxygen therapy. Lower extremity wounds from diabetes, late radiation injuries, and other ischemic wounds have been successfully treated with HBO. Trials and registries involving victims of acute carbon monoxide poisoning in order to identify standards of care in dosing and long term effects continue to be researched. Investigations into hyperbaric treatment for traumatic brain injuries are underway with the U.S. Department of Defense. Prospective blinded randomized trials and well-executed laboratory studies continue to further define the role of hyperbaric therapy in medical therapeutics. The professionals involved in this important research process are a combination of physicians, nurses, technicians, and statisticians. Hyperbaric nurses have been involved in some level of research since as far back as assisting in the operating rooms of Boerema and Brummelkamp.

More recent nurses like Claude Wreford-Brown and Diane Norkool at Virginia Mason Hospital in Seattle, WA have been credited as first and co-authors in various topics of research shared with Dr. Neil Hampson. In Salt Lake City, at LDS Hospital, nurses Valerie Larson-Lohr and Sue Churchill were co-authors of peer-reviewed publications relating to controlled clinical trials headed by Dr. Lindell Weaver. The Duke Center for Hyperbaric Medicine & Environmental Physiology has been involved in research since 1963 with over 1000 publications. The team has investigated a multitude of extreme diving scenarios in hopes of better understanding the clearance of gases from body tissues. Nurses have played supporting roles in these studies, particularly Norma Mann, who began her 30-year hyperbaric career in 1965s. She was Duke's first hyperbaric nurse (Figure 9).

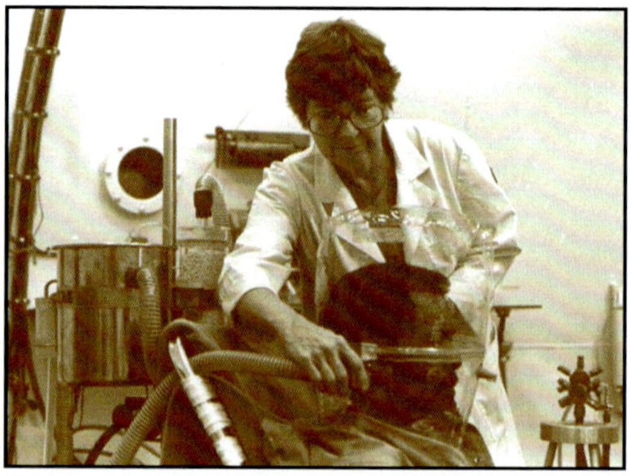

Figure 9: ***Norma Mann, circa 1980, Duke hyperbaric nurse fitting a patient in an oxygen hood for a multiplace chamber treatment.***

In 2002, the first textbook devoted entirely to hyperbaric nursing practice was published. Appropriately titled Hyperbaric Nursing, it was co-edited by nurses Valerie Larson-Lohr and Helen Norvell and included 26 other contributors.[14] This work represented a comprehensive summary of current patient care standards across the spectrum of anticipated states, from the ambulatory outpatient to those critically ill and ventilator dependent. Other sections addressed patient safety, documentation, education, regulatory bodies, professional advancement, clinical research initiatives and urged further efforts that would serve to optimize patient safety and therapeutic effectiveness.

In response to years of requests from troubled nurses and technicians, in 2006, Deborah Sheffield, a hyperbaric nurse practitioner from San Antonio, along with her husband Rob Sheffield, a CHT, published the CHT and CHRN Certification Exam Practice Book. This helpful tool has eased the mind of many nurses as they prepare to sit for this important exam.

The UHMS Associates Recognition Scholarship was established in 2006 with its first recipient being a nurse in 2007. This $2,000 scholarship is intended to stimulate interest among new hyperbaric nurses and technicians, as well as to recognize veteran Associates who have made significant contributions in the field yet have not been afforded the opportunity to attend annual scientific meetings. The requirement is to present an abstract at the annual scientific meeting. In offering this scholarship, the UHMS is helping to foster the professional growth of its colleagues.

Many of today's hyperbaric nurses in the U.S. have become trained and knowledgeable in the care of chronic and refractory wounds. Over the past decade, comprehensive wound healing centers have dominated the practice of hyperbaric oxygen therapy. These centers are commonly outpatient based. Sadly, the emergent life saving and limb sparing hyperbaric cases for which chambers were primarily used, are vanishing in the U.S. Patients may now be required to travel out of state to be treated for decompression illness and carbon monoxide poisoning. The hyperbaric nurse is now encouraged to obtain additional wound certifications when working in outpatient comprehensive wound and hyperbaric centers. Gone are the days of the highly sought after critical care nurse. For every one multiplace chamber in the US, there are approximately 200 monoplace chambers. Of the well over 1000 hyperbaric facilities now in the US, less that 10% offer 24/7 emergency call with the ability to treat the critically ill from which our history came. Indeed times have changed and the evolution of hyperbaric nursing will continue to transform. New opportunities for nurses will continue to blossom.

Established in 1997 by the UHMS Associates, the Paul Baker Award recognizes the outstanding contributions to the advancement of hyperbaric safety. Since that time, three nurses have been recipients: Christy Pirone in 2004, Terry Beard in 2008, and Stacy Handley in 2009.

To help broaden communication and education, hyperbaric nurses write newsletter columns in the HTNA's Offgassing, the BNA's Update and in the Pressure newsletter there is Nursing Notes for the UHMS. Nurses contribute to informational hyperbaric medicine web pages such as Ask-the-Experts on www.MedEdOnline.org. As noted above, hyperbaric nurses have submitted numerous articles to medical and nursing journals and have produced noteworthy textbook chapters in hopes of spreading their knowledge to their colleagues. Nurses engage in Safety Director roles within their departments, participate on the UHMS Accreditation Council and hold a seat on the Executive Council of the NBDHMT. Hyperbaric nurses not only participate on existing UHMS committees such as Publications, Safety, Membership, and Materials Advisory. They also chair them like the newly formed Practice Compliance Committee. Since 2005, nurses have held positions on the Executive Committee of the UHMS Associates. In 2009, the first nurse was appointed to the UHMS Board of Directors as the Corporate Representative. However, July 2010 marks the point in time when the title of Nurse Representative was officially approved for a voting seat on the Board of Directors of the UHMS. Stacy Handley was the first to hold this seat.

In this new era of emerging alternative therapies, hyperbaric medicine has seen scores of freestanding facilities cropping up throughout the US. Critics of hyperbaric medicine continue to question efficacy of even the FDA approved indications largely due to the growing number of "practicing profiteers" looking to take advantage of cash paying patients and their families. Testimonies and promises to cure fatigue, multiple sclerosis, aids, cancer, autism and even aging are examples of the off-label indications being treated at these centers and in some cases without the supervision of a licensed physician. Nursing professionals surely recognize this practice to be very similar to the likes of Dr. Cunningham and even Henshaw. Hyperbaric medicine has a colorful past, however thanks to the improved basic science and controlled clinical research of Brummelkamp, Boerema, Weaver, Hampson and many others we now have evidence-based indications. Hyperbaric oxygen therapy is moving more firmly into mainstream medical practice. Trained and knowledgeable hyperbaric nurses have an obligation to patients to align themselves in established practice patterns that are well researched, proven to have enduring effects, while maintaining safety so to cause no harm to patients. Nurses must stay abreast of emerging research and critically analyze it in order to accurately educate patients on the expectations, risks and benefits of hyperbaric medicine.

In the words of Claude Wreford-Brown "hyperbaric nurses have the rare opportunity to be involved in a field that is still defining itself." The roles of nurses will continue to evolve and grow in this ever-changing specialty in order to fill the niches of hyperbaric medicine.[15]

References

1. Junod VT: Recherches physiologiques et therapeutiques sur les effets de la compression ed de la rarefaction de l'air, tant sur le corps que sur les members isoles. Rev Med Franc Etrange 3:350, 1834
2. Bert P: La Pression Barometrique. 1879. Bert P: Barometric Pressure. Researchers in Experimental Physiology. Hitchcock MA, Hitchcock FA (trans.). Columbus, Ohio, College Book Company, 1943
3. Boerema I, Meyne NG, Brummelkamp WK, et al. Life without Blood (A Study of the Influence of High Atmospheric pressure and Hypothermia on Dilution of the Blood). J Cardiovasc Surg 1:133-146, 1960
4. Brummelkamp WH, Hogendijk J, Boerema I: Treatment of Anaerobic Infections (Clostridial Myositis) by Drenching the Tissues with Oxygen under High Atmospheric Pressure. Surgery 49:299-302, 1961
5. Van Unnik AJM: Inhibition of Toxin Production in Clostridium Perfringens in Vitro by Hyperbaric Oxygen. Antonie Van Leeuwenhoek 31:181-186, 1965
6. Duff JH, Gundel WD, Vignoul HG, et al. The Hyperbaric Chamber at the Royal Victoria Hospital, Montreal. Canadian Med Ass J 91:1051-1055, 1964
7. Lendingham IM, Davidson JK: Hazards in Hyperbaric Medicine. British Medical Journal 3:324-327, 1969
8. Thurston S: HTNA History. Offgassing; Journal of the Hyperbaric Technicians and Nurses Association:18, June 20049.www.hyperbaricnurses.org Baromedical Nurses Association
10. www.diversalertnetwork.org Divers Alert Network
11. www.htna.com.au Hyperbaric Technicians and Nurses Association
12. Pirone C: The hyperbaric incident monitoring study (HIMS): Proceedings; Fifty-second Workshop Undersea and Hyperbaric Medical Society 2002:34-47
13. Hyperbaric chamber nurse dies of decompression sickness; unit gets OK. Hospital Security Safety Management. 1992 Sept; 13(5):3
14. Larson-Lohr V, Norvell HC: Eds. Hyperbaric Nursing; Best Publishing Company 2002: ISBN: 1-930530-00-3
15. Wreford-Brown, C.'Hyperbaric Nursing Research' In Larson-Lohr, V. & Norvell, H.C. (Eds), Hyperbaric Nursing. Best Publishing Company, AZ. 2002:227-239

Notes

CHAPTER

2

Physiology of Hyperbaric Oxygen Treatment

Robert A. Warriner III, MD

Hyperbaric oxygen treatment occurs when a patient breathes 100% oxygen at a pressure greater than one atmosphere absolute (ATA). This requires that the patient be enclosed in a pressure vessel. The FDA defines the treatment pressures meeting the definition of hyperbaric oxygen treatment to be between 1.5 and 3.0 ATA. These treatment pressures fall within the range that can be provided by most monoplace hyperbaric chambers, although higher treatment pressures may be provided in multiplace hyperbaric chambers during the treatment of arterial gas embolism not responsive to compression to 2.8 ATA and complex decompression sickness.

In order to provide safe and effective hyperbaric oxygen treatment, certain basic physical and physiological principles must be understood. This chapter will review these important principles and provide examples of their importance in caring for patients receiving hyperbaric oxygen treatment.

Pressure is force per unit of surface area. Atmospheric pressure is the perpendicular force applied by the weight of the air column from the surface of the earth extending upward to infinity. At sea level this pressure is equal to 14.7 psi (pounds per square inch), or 760 mmHg, one barr, or one atmosphere (ATM). The SI unit for pressure is the Pascal (Pa), equal to one newton per square meter (N/m^2 or $kg{\cdot}m^{-1}{\cdot}s^{-2}$) with 1 ATM of pressure equal to 101 kPa. Since air is compressible, pressure changes are non-linear and are greatest for any distance traveled closer to the earth's surface. Hydrostatic pressure is the additional pressure caused by a water column when a diver submerges below the water surface or gas inside a chamber is compressed. Since water is non-compressible, pressure changes experienced for a given distance traveled underwater (descending or ascending) are much greater in the water column than the air column on the surface of the earth. For each 33 feet of sea water descended or ascended in the water column or the compression chamber, the pressure changes by one additional atmosphere of pressure. Pressures inside the hyperbaric chamber are displayed by a pressure gauge. This is referred to as the gauge pressure, and is the pressure relative to local atmospheric pressure. The letter "g" as in ATMg is often added to the abbreviation for the pressure unit measured in order to distinguish gauge pressure from absolute pressure. These relationships are illustrated in Figure 1.

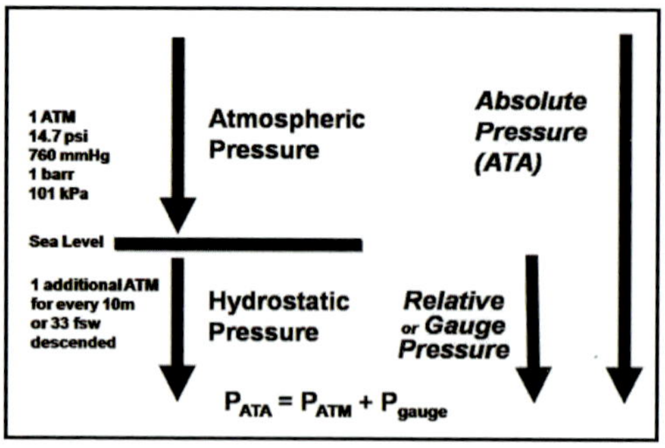

Figure 1: ***Pressure across the continuum of pressure exposure.***

At sea level we are exposed to 1 ATM (atmosphere) of pressure. That pressure decreases as we ascend to altitude and increases as we descend back to our starting point at sea level. We are exposed to an additional 1 ATM (atmosphere) of pressure for each 33 fsw (feet of sea water) descended in the water or compressed in a hyperbaric chamber. This added pressure is measured by a pressure gauge as the relative pressure change from the 1 ATM of pressure at sea level. The total pressure of the 1 ATM from the air column on the surface of the earth and any added pressure by descending below the surface of the water is referred to as total or absolute pressure abbreviated as ATA.

Two other terms require definition. Compression of the hyperbaric chamber occurs any time gas is added to the chamber and the pressure is increased. This is sometimes also referred to as descent, which also occurs as the diver increased his depth in the water. Decompression of the hyperbaric chamber occurs any time gas is removed from the chamber and the pressure is decreased. This is sometimes also referred to as ascent which also occurs as the diver decreases his depth in the water.

The Gas Laws

Now that we have a consistent terminology in which to define pressure and pressure changes, it is important to understand the behavior of gases under the conditions occurring during diving or hyperbaric oxygen treatment. The behavior of gases under these conditions is described by the General Gas Law, which describes the behavior of an "ideal gas" to changes in pressure, volume, and temperature. These relationships can be defined by the following formula.

$$\frac{P_1V_1}{T_1} = \frac{P_2V_2}{T_2}$$

Where P = Pressure (absolute),
V = Volume,
T = Temperature (absolute)

The General Gas Law can be restated emphasizing the relationship of two of the variables while one is held constant as illustrated in Figure 2. Two of these relationships are of particular importance in clinical hyperbaric medicine: Boyle's Law and Gay Lussack's Law. Two other gas laws, Dalton's and Henry's Laws are also important to us and are discussed in the text.

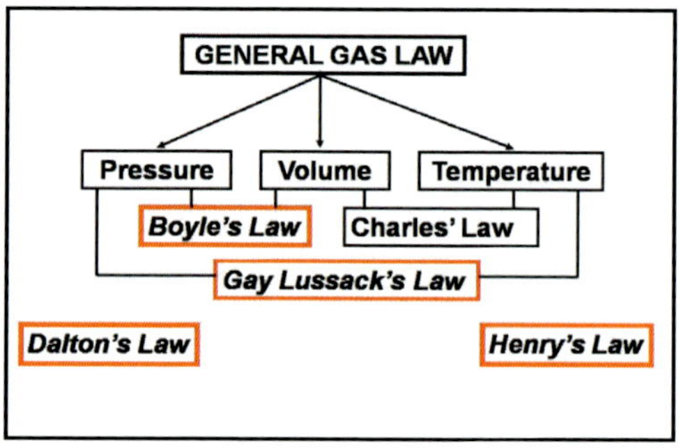

Figure 2: ***The General Gas Law.***

Boyle's Law states that if the temperature remains constant, the volume of a gas is inversely proportional to the pressure applied to the gas. This can be expressed by the following formula:

$$P_1V_1 = P_2V_2$$

Where P = Pressure (absolute), V = Volume

This is the only inverse relationship among the gas laws. As pressure in the hyperbaric chamber increases, the volume of any gas containing space (in the body or in any device inside the chamber) decreases. As pressure in the hyperbaric chamber decreases, the volume of any gas containing space increases. On a day to day basis, Boyle's law is the most important of the gas laws from a clinical perspective. It is the gas law that explains barotrauma, problems associated with gas in medical devices, and the change in the size of intravascular, intratissue, and intracellular bubbles in gas embolism and decompression sickness. Figure 3 shows the relative magnitude of volume changes during compression or decompression. As pressure increases, the volume of any gas bubble decreases. As pressure decreases, the volume of any gas

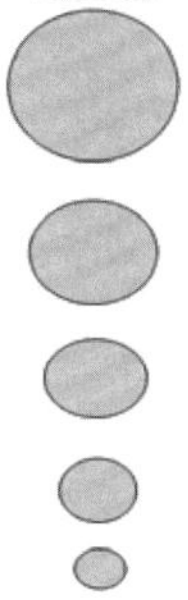

Bubble	Depth	ATA	Relative Volume
	0	1	1
	33	2	.5
	66	3	.333
	99	4	.25
	132	5	.20
	165	6	.166

FIGURE 3: ***Boyle's law effects on bubble size.***

bubble increases. Notice that the relative amount of change is greatest closer to the surface.

For example, as pressure in the hyperbaric chamber is increased during compression, the middle ear space behind the tympanic membrane will undergo a decrease in volume until a sufficient pressure differential is created between the chamber pressure and the middle ear pressure, leading to tympanic membrane rupture. This middle ear barotrauma is prevented by using various methods (Valsalva, Frenzel's maneuver, etc.) to "ventilate" the middle ear space through the Eustachian tube to maintain equal pressures on both sides of the tympanic membrane. Other areas subject to barotrauma include the sinuses, dental caries or spaces between dental appliances (caps, crowns) and the tooth below, the gastrointestinal tract, and the lungs. Pulmonary barotrauma producing a pneumothorax is perhaps the most significant complication during hyperbaric oxygen treatment. It typically occurs when decompression of the chamber occurs at a rate that exceeds the ability of some portion of the lung to ventilate and equilibrate pressure changes resulting in a pneumothorax, with or without arterial gas embolism. By Boyle's Law, once the pneumothorax occurs, with continued decompression of the chamber, the volume of gas in the pleural space will increase, potentially causing a tension pneumothorax, severe pulmonary and cardiac impairment, and an increased risk of arterial gas embolism.

Remember also that as pressure increases, the density of the gas breathed also increases as molecules are packed more closely together. While the increase in gas density usually is not clinically significant within the range of normal hyperbaric oxygen treatment pressures (2.0-3.0 ATA), any significant airway obstruction or neonates, infants, and pediatric patients, especially if breathing through an endotracheal tube, may encounter difficulty in maintaining adequate minute ventilation during hyperbaric oxygen treatment.

Clinical pearl: Because relative volume changes with changes in pressure will be greatest between 1 and 2 ATA, it is important that the chamber operator pay particularly close attention to the patient during this portion of compression or decompression. Barotrauma can be prevented by careful education of the patient in methods to equilibrate middle ear pressure, evaluation of the patient for risks of air trapping and subsequent pulmonary barotrauma, close observation of the patient during compression and decompression, and reducing or slowing the rate of decompression to allow more time for pressure equilibration between gas containing spaces and the chamber environment.

Gay Lussack's Law states that if the volume remains constant, as pressure increases in the chamber, the temperature will also increase and as pressure decreases, the temperature will decrease. This is a direct relationship with pressure and temperature moving in the same direction. This can be expressed by the following formula:

$$\frac{P_1}{T_1} = \frac{P_2}{T_2}$$

Where P = Pressure (absolute), T = Temperature (absolute)

This relationship between pressure and temperature explains why the patient may experience warmth in the chamber during compression or cooling during decompression. It also explains why the pressure in a multiplace chamber could increase to dangerous levels in the event that a fire occurred inside the chamber.

Clinical pearl: Because we make patients aware of the risks of fire in the monoplace chamber, be sure to explain the changes in temperature they will experience during compression and decompression.

The final gas law has little applicability to clinical hyperbaric medicine because chambers have fixed volumes. This is Charles' Law which states that at a constant pressure, the volume of a gas will be directly proportional to the temperature. This can be expressed by the formula below:

$$\frac{V_1}{T_1} = \frac{V_2}{T_2}$$

Where V = Volume, T = Temperature

Charles' Law explains how hot air balloons work. As gas in the bag of the balloon is heated, it expands the balloon, producing lift.

Two additional gas laws as illustrated in Figure 5 play important roles in defining the physiology of the hyperbaric environment, Dalton's Law and Henry's Law.

Dalton's Law states that the total pressure exerted by a mixture of gases is equal to the sum of the partial pressures of each of the different gases making up the mixture with each gas acting independently of the other gases in the mixture, as illustrated in Figure 4. Gas percentages only define the ratios between the numbers of gas molecules in a mixture, and do not define the physiological effects of any gas under pressure. It is the partial pressure of the gas that is responsible for the physiological effects of the individual gas. Gas percentage is important, however, for oxygen in determining the risk of fire. Oxygen concentrations above 23% increase the risk of fire.

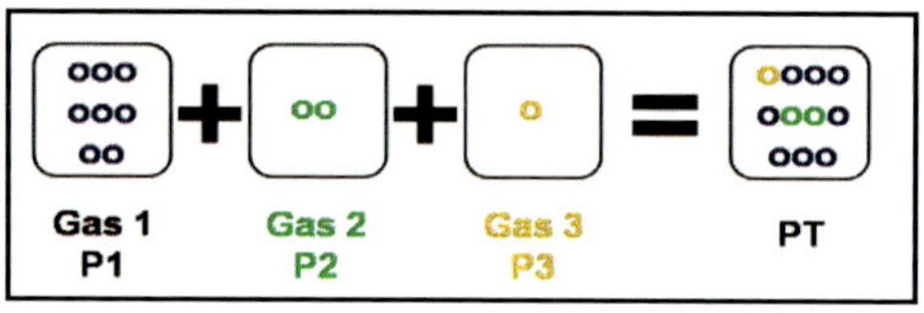

FIGURE 4: ***Dalton's Law.***

Air is a mixture of nitrogen, oxygen, water vapor, and a variety of trace gases that vary in percentage of the mixture slightly, based upon the location of sampling (see Table 1 for a representative distribution gases in air). For the sake of simplicity, consider air to contain 79% nitrogen and 21% oxygen. As air is compressed in a cylinder or in a hyperbaric chamber, the relative percentages of the cases in the mixture does not change, but the partial pressure of those cases increases as the total pressure increases. The specific physiological effects of increasing the partial pressure of nitrogen and oxygen are shown below.

TABLE 1: COMPOSITION OF AIR AT 1 ATA

Nitrogen	78%	593 mmHg
Oxygen	21%	160 mmHg
Carbon Dioxide	0.03%	0.2 mmHg
Other (water vapor, trace gases)	0.97%	6.8 mmHg

(For the sake of simplicity, consider air to contain 79% nitrogen and 21% oxygen.)

Two additional factors influence the actual gas partial pressures in the alveolus where gas exchange occurs between the gas phase (alveolar gas) and the liquid phase (pulmonary capillary blood) across the gas permeable interface of the pulmonary alveolar-capillary membrane. This extremely thin membrane allows, under normal circumstances, almost unrestricted transfer of gas between the gas and liquid phases on either side of the membrane. In order to protect the alveolar membrane lining cells from desiccation on exposure to high gas flows, the upper and mid-level airways humidify inhaled air or oxygen. This is an efficient and effective process at normal ventilatory rates, but can be overwhelmed at very high minute volumes (especially high ventilator rates) and when breathing very dry gases. This humidification adds water vapor to the alveolar gas mixture. Water vapor pressure is determined primarily by body temperature. At a normal body temperature of 37°C or 98.6°F, water vapor pressure is 47mmHg, and will be present regardless of the total pressure to which the diver or patient is exposed. The second is the pulmonary arterial carbon dioxide tension ($PaCO_2$), which is determined by the respiratory quotient (typically 0.8 at normal metabolic rate) and is approximately 40mmHg. As with water vapor, the dilutional effect of carbon dioxide is not affected by the total pressure to which the diver or patient is exposed. These relationships are demonstrated in Figure 5.

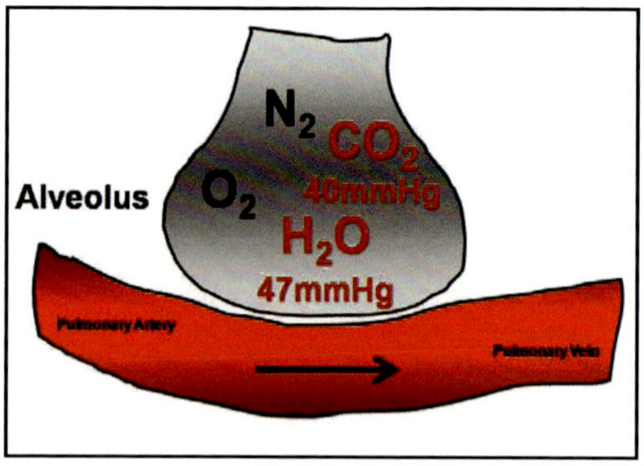

FIGURE 5: ***Alveolar gas composition.***

Henry's Law, illustrated in Figure 6, states that the volume of gas dissolved in a liquid is directly proportional to the partial pressure of the dissolved gas in contact with the liquid. In order to avoid confusion, the partial pressure of the gas in the gas environment is referred to as the gas partial pressure while the gas partial pressure in the tissue or blood is referred to as the gas tension.

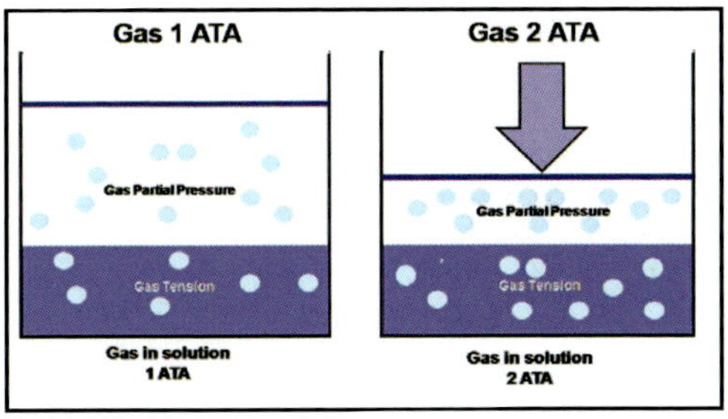

Figure 6: ***Henry's Law.***

On the left of Figure 6 is gas over a liquid at 1 ATA of pressure with equilibrium between the pressures in the gas and liquid phases. In this case, the gas partial pressure and the gas tension are the same, although the number of molecules in each phase is not the same due to the influence of solubility on the actual number of molecules in the liquid. On the right, the transition to a new condition with a higher gas partial pressure leading to an increased gas tension in the liquid below the interface.

At equilibrium when no further movement of gas occurs, the gas partial pressure and the gas tension are equal, although the number of molecules of gas on either side of the gas to liquid or gas to tissue interface may not be equal. That is because the solubility is the second component defining the amount of gas that dissolves in liquids or tissues. Solubility of the gas is a distinct characteristic of each gas, defining its dissolvability in water or fat based liquids and tissues. Temperature is the third component that determines the actual number of gas molecules in the liquid or tissue at a given gas partial pressure above the interface with lower temperature increasing the solubility of all gases. This will be discussed in more detail in the section on decompression physiology below.

P_{total}	Depth (FSW)	Pressure (ATA)	Required O_2	
760 mmHg	Surface	1	21.0%	(160 mmHg)
1,520 mmHg	33	2	10.5%	(160 mmHg)
	66	3	7.0%	
	100	4	5.3%	
	133	5	4.2%	
4.560mmHg	166	6	3.5%	
	200	7	3.0%	
	1000	31	0.6%	
52,440 mmHg	2250	69	0.3%	(160 mmHg)

Figure 7: ***Oxygen partial pressures at various total pressures to maintain normoxia.***

Required oxygen partial pressures at various total pressures to maintain normoxia. You can see in Figure 7 that an alveolar partial pressure of oxygen can be maintained by breathing 21% oxygen at 1 ATA and by breathing only 0.3% oxygen at 69 ATA. It is the partial pressure, not the percentage of a gas, that determines its physiological properties.

Finally, pressure has direct effects on physiological systems including cell membrane performance, receptor activation and function, and enzymatic function.[1] There do appear to be barosensitive cells in the central nervous system whose rate of firing increases as barometric pressure increases.[2] This increase in firing rate appears to be greatest between 1 and 5 ATA (helium was the inert gas in the atmosphere tested to avoid the potential effects of decreased membrane potential conductance seen with the narcotic effects of nitrogen, discussed below). High pressure nervous syndrome was first described in 1965 during oxygen and helium compression to pressures of 600 and 800 fsw when the test divers showed changes in motor and cognitive performance associated with prominent tremors of the extremities and torso, also accompanied by nausea, vomiting, and dizziness.[3] The clinical presentation was associated with specific EEG abnormalities that included increased theta and decreased fast alpha and beta wave frequencies. The mechanisms ultimately responsible for high pressure nervous syndrome are not fully understood, but are likely related to direct compression of neuronal junctions decreasing intermembrane transport distance for neurotransmitters and increased sensitivity to monoamine based neurotransmitters.

Clinical pearl: While not relevant to the pressures to which patients are exposed in clinical hyperbaric medicine, it is important for us to remember that pressure has significant physical and physiological effects.

The Effects of the Increased Partial Pressure of Gases

Nitrogen is a colorless, odorless, and tasteless inert gas (other inert gases that have been used in deep diving include helium, argon, and xenon) that makes up approximately 79% of the gas molecules in air. Inert refers to the lack of any metabolic action or consumption during normal physiology. However, nitrogen is soluble in blood, other body fluids, and tissues and can produce a number of effects when ambient pressures are elevated. These effects include central nervous system depression (nitrogen narcosis) and decompression sickness. In routine clinical hyperbaric medicine, these effects are relatively unimportant because the ambient environment is 100% oxygen and the patient is never exposed to increased PN_2 except during very brief air breaks, if provided. However, in the air filled multiplace chamber, inside attendants are breathing air at increased ambient pressure for periods of time long enough and at pressures high enough to potentially experience some degree of central nervous system depression, and are at risk for decompression sickness during some patient treatment profiles.

The two effects of increased PN_2 important in clinical hyperbaric medicine are 1) decompression sickness, and 2) nitrogen narcosis.

Decompression and decompression sickness: While a full discussion of decompression physiology and decompression sickness is beyond the scope of this chapter and is provided elsewhere,[4] it is important to understand the basic principles of nitrogen (or other inert gas) uptake and distribution when managing patient and inside observer care in the multiplace hyperbaric oxygen treatment environment, or when treating divers with decompression sickness. Standing on the surface of the earth at sea level, we are all saturated with nitrogen at a total pressure of 1 ATA. How much nitrogen is contained in our blood and tissues is dependent upon 1) the partial pressure of nitrogen at 1 ATA, 2) the perfusion or blood flow to each tissue in our bodies, 3) the diffusion rates for nitrogen from blood to each individual tissue type and between adjacent tissue types, and 4) the solubility of nitrogen in each tissue. We have already discussed the calculation of the nitrogen partial pressure in the alveolus and thus in the pulmonary venous and systemic arterial blood. Diffusion of nitrogen from the alveolus to the pulmonary capillary is influenced by the surface area of the pulmonary alveolar and capillary membranes, and the thickness of the membrane that acts as a diffusion barrier. Anything that thickens the membrane barrier impairs the diffusion of nitrogen and oxygen as well. Finally, the amount of nitrogen contained in blood or in any tissue is also a function of the unique solubility of nitrogen in each circumstance. Solubility is different for each inert gas based upon the specific chemical qualities of the gas with solubility differentiated in terms of water solubility and lipid or fat solubility. Nitrogen is, for example, more soluble in lipids of fat than helium, accounting for some of its additional properties discussed below. Solubility is also dependent upon ambient temperature with all gases more soluble at colder temperatures. Therefore, the final amount of an inert gas "stored" or contained in any tissue will depend upon 1) the partial pressure of the gas, 2) the specific solubility characteristics of the gas, 3) the type of tissue (lipid vs. water content), and 4) the temperature of the tissue.

Each tissue has a unique capacity to "store" nitrogen (or any inert gas) based upon the characteristics mentioned above and the rate of change of the ambient pressure of nitrogen over the tissue. Saturation is defined as the maximum amount of gas that a tissue can hold, keeping all gas in solution within the tissue for a given partial pressure of gas in the ambient environment. Supersaturation is defined as a transient state in which the tissue can hold an amount of gas in solution slightly greater than that contained at saturation. This allows for short periods of time when tissues can hold amounts of gas in solution (gas tension) greater than the ambient pressure. Different tissues handle varying degrees of supersaturation differently, and a number of factors can cause nitrogen to rapidly leave solution and transition to the gas phase, forming bubbles within blood or tissues. These factors include sudden changes in temperature, ambient pressure, or adding energy to the system. The classic example of supersaturation we encounter in daily life is the carbonated soda can or bottle. Sodas are supersaturated with carbon dioxide. When we pop the top on the bottle or can the sudden increase in pressure differential (gas tension of carbon dioxide now significantly greater than ambient pressure) causes gas bubbles to form rapidly in the soda. The same transition of carbon dioxide from solution to gas phase occurs if we shake the bottle (adding energy) even without popping the top and decreasing the ambient pressure. These relationships are demonstrated in Figures 8 and 9.

At the surface breathing air, an equilibrium state exists where the partial pressure of nitrogen in alveolar air and the gas tension of nitrogen in the blood and tissues are equal. This does not mean that the number of gas molecules are the same, as that will be determined by perfusion, diffusion, and solubility of the gas, but the pressures will be equal. With compression or descent, the gradient for movement of gas is from the alveolus to the blood and tissues leading to a progressive increase in gas tensions until, at a stable pressure or depth, a new equilibrium is reached.

If on the ascent the ambient pressure reduction is sufficiently slow, bubble formation can be avoided by permitting gradual inert gas elimination without exceeding a state of critical supersaturation. If the ascent is too rapid, the critical saturation of a tissue may be exceeded and result in bubble formation, or PHASE SEPARATION. Once any bubbles form in blood or tissues, if ambient pressure continues to decrease, the bubbles will grow by Boyle's law. There are other factors that contribute to bubble growth, such as counter diffusion of different inert gases, but Boyle's law is the primary determinate of bubble growth under most circumstances.

Thus, the goal of decompression is to ascend at a rate sufficiently slow to avoid exceeding the safe supersaturation limits for blood or any tissue.

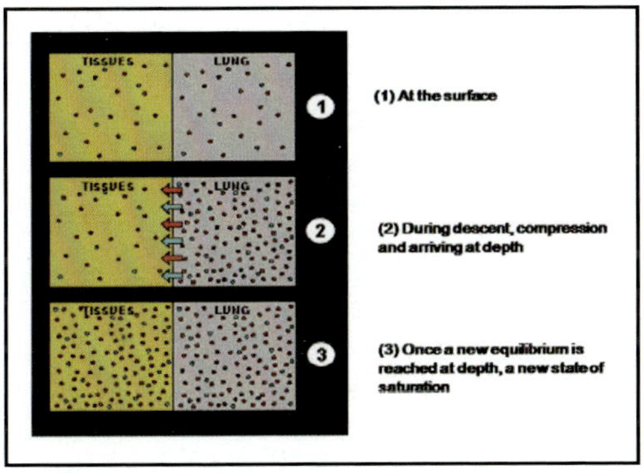

Figure 8: *Equilibrium gas tension with partial pressure during compression.*

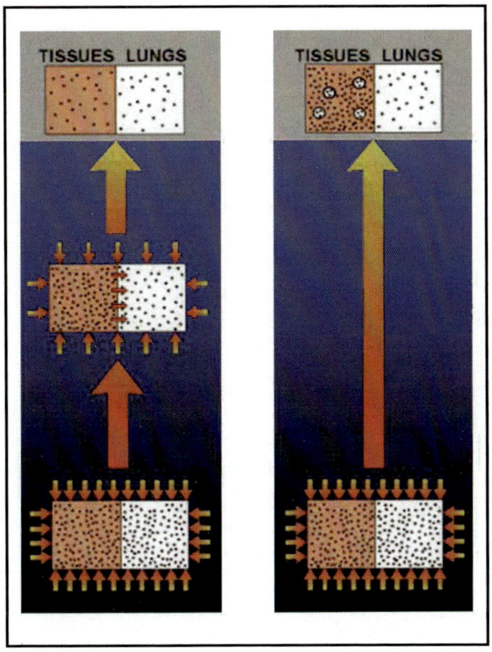

Figure 9: *Getting back to the surface.*

Decompression tables are designed to provide guidance as to the allowable safe rates of decompression or ascent from increased ambient pressure or depth. The first workable decompression tables were developed by John Scott Haldane and published in the Journal of Hygiene in Cambridge, in 1908. The Haldane model of decompression has been used for over 100 years as a practical way to approach decompression table development. While there are non-Haldane models, for the sake of simplicity, the Haldane model will be the focus for this discussion. Haldane recognized that tissues take up and release nitrogen at different rates based upon the difference between the ambient pressure (partial pressure) and tissue pressure (gas tension) and the unique solubility characteristics of the individual tissue that could be described as tissue half-times. A half-time is the time required for 50% uptake or elimination of a substance. Six half-times are required for 98.5% uptake or elimination of a substance (Figure 10).

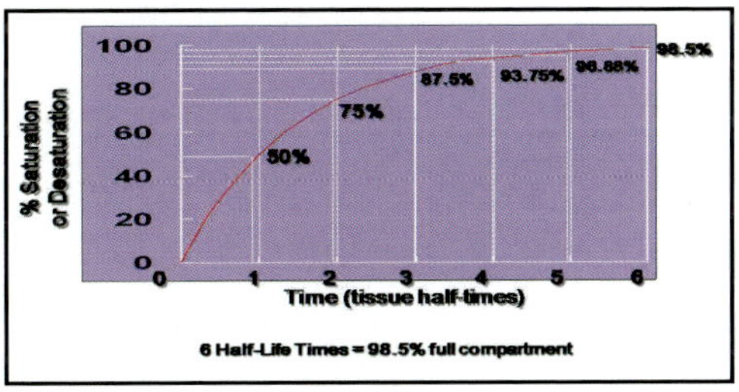

Figure 10: *Concept of half-times.*

A half-time is the time required for a 50% uptake or elimination of a substance from a tissue, and is determined by the tissue itself and the pharmacokinetics of the substance itself.

While Haldane did not attach specific organs or tissue types to his half-time model, he did develop a series of tissue half-times to describe the uptake and elimination characteristics of different tissue "types" for nitrogen, as shown in Figure 11. He referred to tissues with rapid equilibration with changes in ambient pressure as "fast" or short half-time tissues, while tissues with longer equilibration times as "slow" or long half-times.

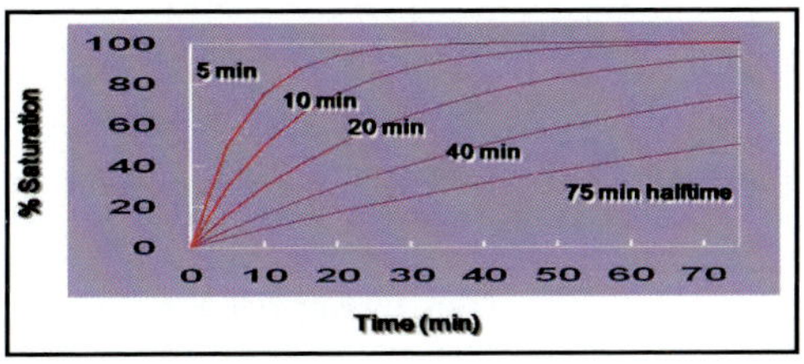

Figure 11: *Haldane's tissue half-times.*

Haldane assumed tissue half-times for nitrogen uptake and elimination of 5, 10, 20, 40 and 75 minutes. He referred to the shorter half-time tissues in the model as "fast" tissues and the long half-time tissues in the model as "slow" tissues. Unfortunately, he underestimated the longest half-time which is probably significantly greater than 75 minutes, in part explaining why the Haldane model doesn't work well at greater pressures or deeper depths.

Haldane developed a series of workable decompression tables by testing his half-time model by compressing goats to depth and then decompressing them based on schedules derived from looking at the "permissible" pressure changes that did not exceed "safe" supersaturation limits for each tissue half-time compartment. He tested both linear and staged decompression models.

Linear decompression shown on the left of Figure 12 has a constant decompression rate with no decompression stops while staged decompression involves periods of constant decompression separated by brief periods of equilibration (decompression stops).

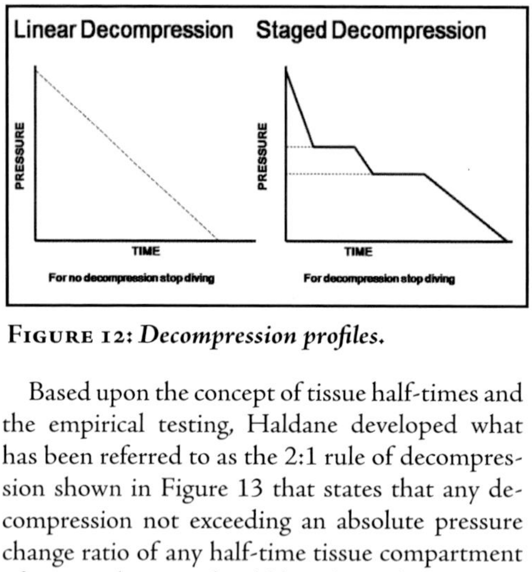

FIGURE 12: ***Decompression profiles.***

Based upon the concept of tissue half-times and the empirical testing, Haldane developed what has been referred to as the 2:1 rule of decompression shown in Figure 13 that states that any decompression not exceeding an absolute pressure change ratio of any half-time tissue compartment of greater than 2:1 should be tolerated.

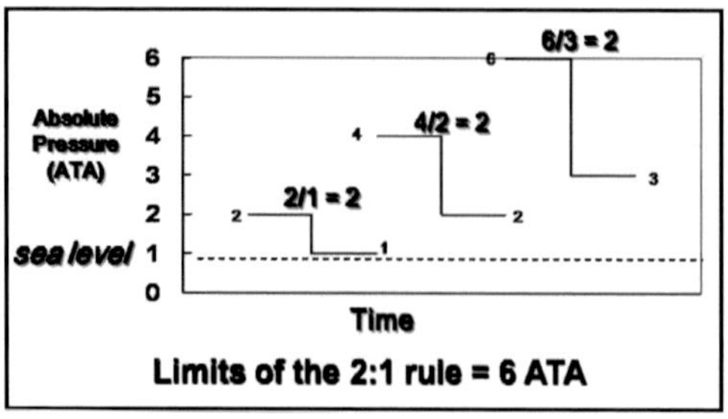

FIGURE 13: ***The Haldane 2:1 rule.***

The Haldane 2:1 rule. defines a safe decompression as one that does not exceed the 2:1 ratio in any half-time tissue compartment. Unfortunately, the Haldane model doesn't work well at depths greater than 6 ATA, probably because Haldane underestimated the longest tissue compartment half-time.

Clinical pearls: Understanding the core principles in inert gas decompression is important in multiplace hyperbaric chamber operations in preventing inside attendant decompression sickness (standard wound care treatment profiles can exceed the air breathing no-decompression limits), and in evaluating the adequacy of decompression provided in dive profiles for divers presenting with possible decompression sickness. In most circumstances today, the U. S. Navy Air Decompression Tables (Rev 6)[5] are used. Typical decompression in monoplace hyperbaric chamber operation is a linear profile at a rate of 1.5 psi (0.1 ATA/min). Decompression rates can be slowed in patients at risk for pulmonary air trapping to decrease the risk of pulmonary barotrauma.

Nitrogen narcosis: In 1935,[6] Behnke demonstrated that compressed air breathing at depths greater than 3 ATA (66 fsw) produced a narcotic-like effect initially manifested by a euphoric state, but with continued exposure at greater pressures resulted in impairment of cognitive function and neuro-muscular coordination. Up to pressures of 4 ATA (99 fsw), these effects can to some extent be reduced by increasing effort. However, as pressure increases, compensation no longer occurs and progressive narcosis with impaired cognitive and motor performance leads to loss of consciousness in almost all divers by 300 fsw. Individual response varies from day to day, as does the response from one individual to another.

Lipid solubility appears to be linked to the narcotic potential of gases with nitrogen greater than helium, but less than argon, krypton, and xenon. Factors can influence, including carbon dioxide retention. A much more detailed discussion of nitrogen narcosis can be found elsewhere.[7]

Carbon dioxide also is colorless, odorless, and tasteless, and is the natural metabolic product of oxidative metabolism and the oxidation occurring during combustion of most materials. The gas tension of carbon dioxide in the blood, whether the result of inhaling increased carbon dioxide from the environment or due to increased carbon dioxide in the body or decreased elimination from the body, plays an important role in regulating pulmonary ventilation (respiratory rate and tidal volume). Increasing arterial $PaCO_2$ tensions stimulate the respiratory control centers of the medulla oblongata in the brain stem. Relatively small changes in $PaCO_2$ tensions can produce significant changes in minute ventilation (the product of respiratory rate and tidal volume) and act as the primary control mechanism for ventilation until arterial $PaCO_2$ tensions reach the high 60-70 mmHg range, where the hypoxic ventilator drive takes over until elevated $PaCO_2$ tensions produce central nervous system depression and eventual respiratory arrest. Increases in $PaCO_2$ tension also causes cerebral vasodilatation that can increase the risk of oxygen toxicity during hyperbaric oxygen treatment as discussed below.

Clinical pearl: Circumstances that lead to increased CO_2 production (fever, increased metabolic states) or CO_2 retention, as can occur in patients with obstructive sleep apnea, may lead to an increased risk of oxygen toxicity seizures.

Oxygen is also a colorless, odorless, tasteless gas, but differs from nitrogen and the other inert gases in that it is essential for cellular metabolism in its role in supporting mitochondrial electron transport in oxidative metabolism, which is the major pathway for cellular energy production. It makes up about 21% of the composition of air and has a relatively narrow spectrum of toxicity on both the low and high ends of exposure. Symptoms of systemic hypoxia with central nervous system dysfunction and other end organ failure begin to occur at partial pressures below 0.16 ATA (Figure 14), while pulmonary oxygen toxicity begins to develop at partial pressures above 0.5 ATA and central nervous system toxicity at partial pressures above 1.8 ATA (Figure 14).

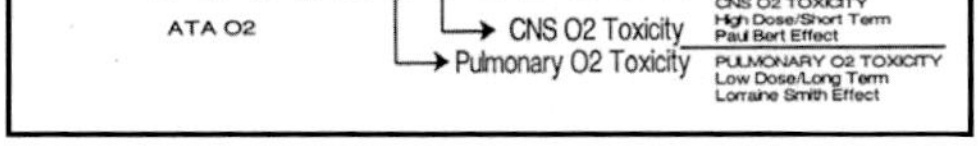

Figure 14: ***U.S. Navy recommended limits for oxygen exposure in life support systems.***

Symptoms of systemic hypoxia with central nervous system dysfunction and other end organ failure begin to occur at partial pressures below 0.16 ATA, while pulmonary oxygen toxicity begins to develop at partial pressures above 0.5 ATA and central nervous system toxicity at partial pressures above 1.8 ATA.

Oxygen is transported to the tissues by two mechanisms. The first and most important mechanism for oxygen transport under normal physiological conditions is by chemical binding to hemoglobin. The hemoglobin molecule contains four oxygen binding sites, two each on an alpha and beta chain. Oxygen binds preferentially to the binding sites with one oxygen molecule to each binding site. Because this is a chemical binding, hemoglobin cannot take up or bind any more oxygen molecules regardless of the amount of oxygen available, so hemoglobin cannot be supersaturated. The amount of oxygen that can be transported in this manner is represented by the following formula:

1.36 ml of oxygen/gram Hb x [Hb] x Hb-Saturation

The two most important determinants of oxygen transport bound to hemoglobin are the hemoglobin (Hb) concentration (grams of Hb) and the saturation of hemoglobin (Hb-Saturation). Hemoglobin saturation is influenced by a number of factors and is described by the oxygen-hemoglobin association or dissociation curve shown in Figure 15. Things that shift the curve to the left cause increased affinity of hemoglobin for oxygen, decreasing the amount of oxygen released to the tissues. These include decreased temperature, decreased 2,3-diphosphoglycerate (2-3 DPG), decreased pH (acidosis), and carbon monoxide. Things that shift the curve to the right reduce oxygen affinity to hemoglobin favoring increased oxygen release to the tissues. These include increased temperature, increased 2,3-diphosphoglycerate (2-3 DPG), and alkalosis.

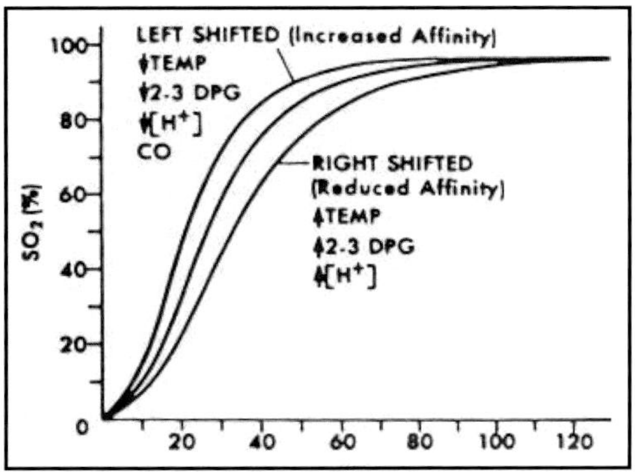

Figure 15: ***The oxy-hemoglobin association or dissociation curve.***

The second mechanism for oxygen transport is oxygen dissolved in plasma. The amount of oxygen dissolved in plasma is shown in the following formula:

$$0.0031 \text{ ml/dl (per mmHg } PaO_2) \text{ x } paO_2$$

While this is a much smaller amount of oxygen transported while breathing air at 1 ATA, all oxygen that ultimately reaches the mitochondrial oxygen transport system must separate from hemoglobin, be dissolved in the plasma, and then diffuse across the capillary endothelial membrane, through the interstitial space, and finally across cell and mitochondrial membranes. While hemoglobin transport of oxygen is limited by chemical binding and hemoglobin concentration, transport of oxygen dissolved in plasma is limited only by the partial pressure of oxygen in the alveoli which is determined by the partial pressure of oxygen in the inspired gas and the efficiency of ventilation. Figure 16 shows the contribution of each mechanism of oxygen transport to available oxygen under normobaric and hyperbaric conditions when breathing 100% oxygen.

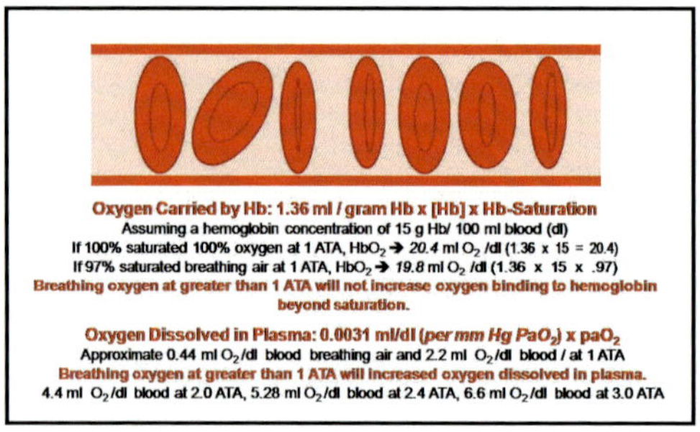

FIGURE 16: ***Oxygen transport by hemoglobin and plasma.***

THE EFFECTS OF THE INCREASED PARTIAL PRESSURE OF OXYGEN

During hyperbaric oxygen treatment, three fundamental physical events occur:

By Boyle's law, any gas bubbles, as might occur in decompression sickness or gas embolism, will compress. As bubble volume decreases, bubbles will more quickly be reabsorbed and obstruction of the microcirculation will be reduced. This effect has been previously discussed in detail and will not be further developed here.

By Henry's law, the gas tension of oxygen in blood and tissues will increase as the partial pressure of oxygen increases in the alveoli. This will lead to increased oxygen availability through increased oxygen transport dissolved in the plasma and ultimately in the tissues. This is the core rationale in maintaining tissue oxygen delivery during acute, severe anemia when hemoglobin is bound by oxygen competing molecules such as carbon monoxide.

By simple physics, the distance that oxygen diffuses from any perfused capillaries will increase in direct proportion to the capillary PO_2 (Figure 17). This enables maintenance of at least improved, if not normal, cellular oxygen delivery between adjacent perfused capillaries in situations in which capillary density is decreased (microvascular occlusion), capillary endothelial gas transfer membrane thickening (endothelial abnormalities, glycosylation of basement membrane proteins as seen in diabetes mellitus), and increased intercapillary distance (acute interstitial edema).

Oxygen diffusion distance increases almost 4 fold on the arterial end of a model capillary with the increased PaO2 from breathing air at 1 ATA and 100% oxygen at 3 ATA.

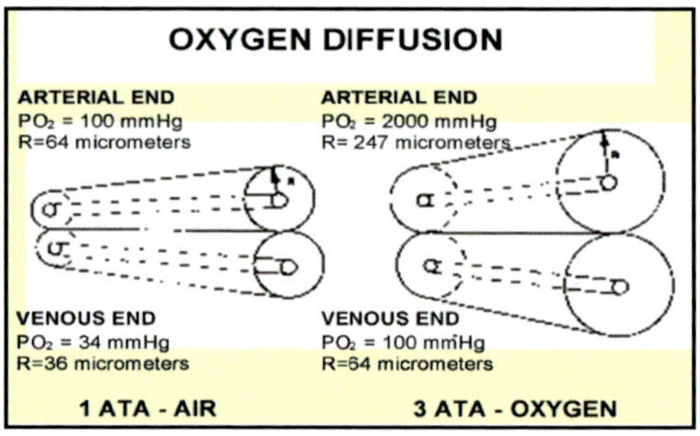

FIGURE 17: ***Oxygen diffusion distance during HBO.***

These 3 physical effects of hyperbaric oxygenation were the original drivers for the original clinical applications of hyperbaric oxygen treatment (HBOT) including the treatment of decompression sickness, necrotizing soft tissue infections, surgical flaps and grafts compromised by ischemia, traumatic ischemic wound injuries, and carbon monoxide poisoning based upon the temporary increase of plasma and tissue PO_2 during treatment. These temporary benefits include:

- Improved local tissue oxygenation leading to improved cellular energy metabolism[8]
- Increased collagen and other extracellular matrix protein deposition, epithelialization[9]

Table 2. Indications for HBOT Linked to Likely Predominant Mechanism(s) Providing Benefit

UHMS Indication for HBOT*	Likely Predominant Mechanism(s) Providing Benefit
Air or gas embolism	1. By *Boyle's Law*, compression of gas bubbles 2. By *Henry's Law*, increased oxygen tension and transport to tissues with improved cellular energy metabolism and function 3. Increased oxygen diffusion distance 4. Alteration in WBC ß-integrin receptor sensitivity. 5. Reduced inflammation.
Carbon monoxide poisoning (with/without cyanide poisoning)	1. By *Henry's Law*, increased oxygen tension and transport to tissues with improved cellular energy metabolism and function 2. Displacement of CO, CN from hemoglobin, myoglobin, and mitochrondrial electron transport chain 3. Increased oxygen diffusion distance 4. Alteration in WBC ß-integrin receptor sensitivity. 5. Reduced inflammation.
Clostridial myositis and Myonecrosis	1. By *Henry's Law*, increased oxygen tension and transport to tissues 2. Increased oxygen diffusion distance with improved cellular energy metabolism and function 3. Decreased local tissue edema due to vasoconstriction of vessels in non-ischemic tissues 4. Improved leukocyte-bacterial-killing (adequate leukocyte count critical for benefit) 5. Suppression of exotoxin production 6. Increased effectiveness of antibiotics which require oxygen for active transport across microbial cell membranes
Crush injury, compartment syndrome, other acute traumatic ischemias	1. By *Boyle's Law*, compression of gas bubbles 2. By *Henry's Law*, increased oxygen tension and transport to tissues with improved cellular energy metabolism and function 3. Increased oxygen diffusion distance 4. Alteration in WBC ß-integrin receptor sensitivity. 5. Reduced inflammation.
Decompression sickness	1. By *Boyle's Law*, compression of gas bubbles 2. By *Henry's Law*, increased oxygen tension and transport to tissues with improved cellular energy metabolism and function 3. Increased oxygen diffusion distance 4. Alteration in WBC ß-integrin receptor sensitivity. 5. Reduced inflammation. 6. Reduced apoptosis.
Arterial insufficiencies: central retinal artery occlusion	1. By *Henry's Law*, increased oxygen tension and transport to tissues with improved cellular energy metabolism and function 2. Increased oxygen diffusion distance
Arterial insufficiencies: enhancement of healing in selected problem wounds	1. By *Henry's Law*, increased oxygen tension and transport to tissues with improved cellular energy metabolism and function 2. Increased oxygen diffusion distance 3. Increased collagen and other extracellular matrix protein deposition 4. Decreased local tissue edema due to vasoconstriction of vessels in non-ischemic tissues 5. Improved leukocyte-bacterial-killing (adequate leukocyte count critical for benefit) 6. Increased effectiveness of antibiotics which require oxygen for active transport across microbial cell membranes 7. Enhanced production of growth factors and receptors (PDGF, VEGF). 8. Reduced inflammation. 9. Reduced apoptosis. 10. Activated stem cell mobilization. 11. Increased angiogenesis through stimulation of VEGF production.
Severe anemia	1. By *Henry's Law*, increased oxygen tension and transport to tissues with improved cellular energy metabolism and function 2. Increased oxygen diffusion distance
Intracranial abscess	1. By *Henry's Law*, increased oxygen tension and transport to tissues with improved cellular energy metabolism and function 2. Increased oxygen diffusion distance 3. Increased collagen and other extracellular matrix protein deposition 4. Decreased local tissue edema due to vasoconstriction of vessels in non-ischemic tissues 5. Improved leukocyte-bacterial-killing (adequate leukocyte count critical for benefit) 6. Increased effectiveness of antibiotics which require oxygen for active transport across microbial cell membranes
Necrotizing soft tissue infections	1. By *Henry's Law*, increased oxygen tension and transport to tissues with improved cellular energy metabolism and function
	2. Increased oxygen diffusion distance 3. Increased collagen and other extracellular matrix protein deposition 4. Decreased local tissue edema due to vasoconstriction of vessels in non-ischemic tissues 5. Improved leukocyte-bacterial-killing (adequate leukocyte count critical for benefit) 6. Suppression of exotoxin production 7. Increased effectiveness of antibiotics which require oxygen for active transport across microbial cell membranes
Osteomyelitis (refractory)	1. By *Henry's Law*, increased oxygen tension and transport to tissues with improved cellular energy metabolism and function 2. Increased oxygen diffusion distance 3. Increased collagen and other extracellular matrix protein deposition 4. Decreased local tissue edema due to vasoconstriction of vessels in non-ischemic tissues 5. Improved leukocyte-bacterial-killing (adequate leukocyte count critical for benefit) 6. Increased effectiveness of antibiotics which require oxygen for active transport across microbial cell membranes

Delayed radiation injury (soft tissue and bony necrosis)	1. By *Henry's Law*, increased oxygen tension and transport to tissues with improved cellular energy metabolism and function 2. Increased oxygen diffusion distance 3. Increased collagen and other extracellular matrix protein deposition 4. Enhanced production of growth factors and receptors (PDGF, VEGF). 5. Reduced inflammation. 6. Reduced apoptosis. 7. Activated stem cell mobilization. 8. Increased angiogenesis through stimulation of VEGF production.
Compromised grafts and flaps	1. By *Henry's Law*, increased oxygen tension and transport to tissues with improved cellular energy metabolism and function 2. Increased oxygen diffusion distance 3. Enhanced production of growth factors and receptors (PDGF, VEGF). 4. Reduced inflammation. 5. Reduced apoptosis. 6. Increased angiogenesis through stimulation of VEGF production.
Acute thermal injury	1. By *Henry's Law*, increased oxygen tension and transport to tissues with improved cellular energy metabolism and function 2. Increased oxygen diffusion distance 3. Decreased local tissue edema due to vasoconstriction of vessels in non-ischemic tissues 4. Improved leukocyte-bacterial-killing (adequate leukocyte count critical for benefit) 5. Increased effectiveness of antibiotics which require oxygen for active transport across microbial cell membranes 6. Reduced inflammation. 7. Increased angiogenesis through stimulation of VEGF production.

*Gesell LB, Chair and Editor. Hyperbaric Oxygen Therapy Indications. 12th Edition. The Hyperbaric Oxygen Therapy Committee Report. Durham, ND: Undersea and Hyperbaric Medical Society.

- More rapid elimination of hemoglobin bound toxins such as carbon monoxide[10, 11]
- Decreased local tissue edema due to vaso constriction of vessels in non-ischemic tis sues[12]
- Improved leukocyte-bacterial-killing (ad equate leukocyte count critical for benefit)[13-18]
- Suppression of exotoxin production [19]
- Increased effectiveness of antibiotics which require oxygen for active transport across microbial cell membranes[20-22]

These effects are largely limited to the time during which the patient is exposed to hyperbaric oxygen, with the exception of suppression of exotoxin production, which may last several hours following the return to 1 ATA air breathing, and were the primary drivers for the application of HBOT for nearly 30 years. Although these were important and well established mechanisms of action of HBOT often seen in the setting of improved wound healing, they were insufficient explanations for wound healing benefits that appeared to extend beyond the period of reversal of tissue hypoxia.

What has been demonstrated through research in the past 15 years is that a number of other effects, best described as pharmacological effects rather than physiological effects, appear to take place when tissue oxygen gas tensions exceed about 200 mmHg.[23-28] The pharmacological effects that do not appear to be significant effects of oxygen in the normal range of tissue gas tensions include:

1. Enhanced production of growth factors and receptors (PDGF, VEGF). It has long been observed that restoration of the normal gradient seen in healing acute wounds in the setting of hypoxic chronic wound failure increases the rate of angiogenesis and subsequent wound healing.[24] The observed angiogenic response is due in part to increased VEGF (vascular endothelial growth factor) production[25] and increased PDGF (platelet derived growth factor) receptor induction.[26]

2. Alteration in WBC ß-integrin receptor sensitivity. Hyperbaric oxygenation inhibits polymorphonuclear leukocytes adherence to vascular endothelial basement membrane $ß_2$ integrin glycoproteins (specifically CD11 and CD18) by impairing cGMP (cyclic guanosine mono phosphate) production by leukocytes activated during periods of ischemia-reperfusion injury.[27, 28] This nitric oxide mediated response to hyperbaric oxygenation may explain the observed clinical value of HBOT in reducing downstream ischemia-reperfusion injury by reducing a range of inflammatory responses and preventing post capillary venular vasoconstriction occurring in a variety of settings.[29, 30]

3. Reduced inflammation. A number of animal model studies have demonstrated addition anti-inflammatory effects of HBOT beyond those observed in ischemia-reperfusion injury. Down regulation of a number of pro-inflammatory markers has been observed in an ischemic flap model in rats[31] in which HIF-1alpha and subsequent target gene expression were down regulated with resultant reduction of inflammation. Other anti-inflammatory models including experimental colitis, Crohn's disease,[32 33] and zymosan-induced SIR (systemic inflammatory response).[34] What is particularly interesting is that hyperbaric oxygenation also has pro-inflammatory responses enhancing leukocyte cell migration and bacterial killing. The timing and extent of pro and anti-inflammatory effects of HBOT may be determined by the presenting state of the wound at the time of initial treatment.[35]

4. Reduced apoptosis. Hyperbaric oxygenation reduces apoptosis (programmed cell involutional death) in an ischemic flap model in rats.[36] Apoptosis is a frequent occurrence in chronic wounds due to ischemia and inflammation.

5. Activated stem cell mobilization. HBOT has been demonstrated to mobilize bone marrow-derived activated (capable of colony formation in vitro) CD34 cells in patients receiving 20 HBOTs for prophylactic treatment for osteoradionecrosis prevention.[37,38] CD34 cell counts increased eight-fold following 20 treatments at 2.0 ATA. The elevation in colony forming cells were all in the CD34 category, but activation was present only in samples obtained immediately post treatment and expressed receptors for VEGF-2 and stromal-derived growth factor. In a mouse model, HBOT increased circulating stem cells by 50%. A similar effect has been observed in patients being treated for diabetic foot ulcers, although down regulation of SDF-1*a* production in the diabetic foot ulcer impairs mobilized CD34 cell homing to the diabetic foot ulcer.[39]

6. Increased angiogenesis through stimulation of VEGF production. Both VEGF to stimulate vascular endothelial cell migration and PDGF to stimulate smooth muscle cell migration alongside budding capillary loops are required for effective angiogenesis in wound healing.

Many of the beneficial pharmacological effects of hyperbaric oxygen treatment are the result of hyperbaric oxygenation driven stimulation of eNOS production, which is decreased in diabetic ulcers.[40] eNOS is selectively expressed by vascular endothelial cells or surrounding stromal cells and plays a critical role in proliferation of endothelial cells and as a modulator of other endothelial growth stimulators.

Clinical pearl. Understanding the mechanisms of oxygen at different gas tensions and the resulting physiological and pharmacological effects of HBOT can assist the clinician in making rational patient selection and treatment decisions. Table 2 links the UHMS approved indications for HBOT to the most likely mechanisms of action, providing benefit in each circumstance.

Unfortunately, short and long term exposures to hyperbaric oxygen can produce a number of unwanted side effects. All tissues are subject to adverse effects of non-physiologic oxygen exposures. The common biochemical mechanisms behind the interaction of high oxidant tissue injury and the action of antioxidant defenses have been well described.[41]

Reactive oxygen species are a normal by-product of cellular metabolism whose rate of production is increased in the presence of increased oxygen availability, as occurs during hyperbaric oxygen exposure.[42] Not only primary, but also secondary generation of reactive oxygen intermediate molecules add to oxidant injury. Neutrophil oxidant production has also been implicated in this process. While the body's defenses against reactive oxygen species is highly effective, it can be overcome with prolonged exposure to high oxygen gas tensions as occurs during hyperbaric oxygen treatment.

1. Central nervous system (CNS). CNS oxygen toxicity is typically manifested by prodromal signs and symptoms including twitching, apprehension, changes in behavior, visual symptoms, auditory symptoms, abdominal discomfort and nausea leading to seizures. The seizure is usually self-limited and terminates with transition to air breathing without sequelae. Typically, the risk of CNS oxygen toxicity begins with exposure to oxygen partial pressures of 1.6 ATA and greater. Individual sensitivity to oxygen varies from day to day and is increased by hypercarbia and certain drugs which may act as cerebrovasodilators or in other ways increase CNS oxygen sensitivity.

Clinical pearl: CNS oxygen toxicity risk is reduced by providing air breaks of short duration (typically 5 minutes duration) in patients considered to be at increased risk and any time treatment pressure is greater than 2.0 ATA.[43]

2. Pulmonary. Pulmonary oxygen toxicity has a slower rate of onset than CNS oxygen toxicity but has a lower threshold of oxygen pressure exposure. Typically the risk of pulmonary oxygen toxicity begins with exposures to an oxygen partial pressure of 0.5 ATA after 12 hours of continuous exposure. Signs and symptoms include substernal chest pain, dyspnea, and cough with a progressive decrease in FVC on pulmonary function testing, bronchitis, interstitial fibrosis, and eventually pulmonary edema.[44,45] Oxygen dosing risk of developing pulmonary oxygen toxicity can be defined and predicted using the concept of monitoring UPTDs (unit pulmonary toxic dose), which represents the number of minutes of 100% oxygen breathing at 1 ATA and links the exposure to a predicted decrease in FVC. At least in the early stages, pulmonary changes are reversible. Underlying pulmonary disease may increase the risk of oxygen toxicity, and certain drugs such as bleomycin and amiodarone have been associated with accelerated development of pulmonary oxygen toxicity with exposures to increased oxygen partial pressures.

Clinical pearl: In clinical hyperbaric medicine, pulmonary oxygen toxicity is most likely to occur when treating acute blood loss anemia, clostridial myonecrosis, and necrotizing soft tissue infections where multiple treatments are administered in a relatively short period of time. Pulmonary oxygen toxicity can also occur in both the diver treated with an extended U.S. Navy Treatment (Table 6) and in the inside attendant in a multiplace setting during prolonged tables to treat serious decompression sickness.

3. Ophthalmic. Ophthalmic complications (and indications) of hyperbaric oxygen treatment have been recently thoroughly reviewed.[46] The most common complication is the occurrence of a significant myopic shift, predominantly in phakic eyes, suggesting a lenticular etiology of refractive change.[47,48] In addition, prolonged HBO has been associated with progression of pre-existing nuclear cataracts. New cataracts have been reported in one series of 7 of 15 patients receiving daily treatments to a total of 130-150 treatments at 2.0-2.5 ATA. These cataracts do not resolve following termination of treatment. There is also a case report of de novo cataract formation following a standard course of HBOT.[49] Extensive experience suggests no appreciable risk with series of 20-50 treatments.

Clinical pearl: All patients undergoing hyperbaric oxygen treatment should receive a pre treatment evaluation including visual acuity. High risk patients (progressive cataracts, diabetic retinopathy, recent ocular surgery) should undergo a fundoscopic examination and an ophthalmology consult. The risk of transient myopia and progression of existing lenticular cataracts should be discussed with all patients, especially those with diabetes mellitus. Patients should be informed not to change contact lenses or glasses prescription until at least 10 weeks following completion of treatment. Any ocular symptom should be promptly evaluated, and post-treatment visual acuity and any residual visual complaint at the completion of treatment should be documented and referred for further evaluation when indicated.

4. Cardiovascular. Hyperbaric oxygen exposure can produce significant hemodynamic changes. An increase in systemic afterload due to hyperoxic vasoconstriction in well perfused tissues can lead to a decrease in left ventricular function and a decrease in ejection fraction in some patients. When this decrease in left ventricular function occurs in the setting of pulmonary arterial vasodilatation due to improved alveolar oxygenation with increased left atrial and left ventricular filling, acute left ventricular dysfunction and pulmonary edema can result.[50] Cases have been reported in patients with a history of pulmonary edema or low left ventricular ejection fractions or in patients with sudden fluid shifts from volume overload.[51] Acute pulmonary edema appears to be more common in monoplace than multiplace treatment settings, perhaps because of the requirement for patients to be in a more supine position in the monoplace chamber rather than the sitting position with legs dependent available in the multiplace chamber.

Clinical pearl: Many patients receiving hyperbaric oxygen treatment have severe peripheral arterial disease or diabetes mellitus. These patients are at increased risk for coronary artery disease and occult left ventricular dysfunction. Have a high index of suspicion for prior episodes which could represent congestive heart failure, especially in patients with renal failure, on dialysis, who may be prone to rapid changes in fluid volume. Obtain an echocardiogram in any patient with a history of congestive heart failure, and when abnormal, refer these patients for evaluation and optimization by a cardiologist. While an absolute safe cutoff for left ventricular ejection fraction cannot be defined, patients with ejection fractions of less than 30% should be considered at very high risk for HBOT induced acute pulmonary edema. Weigh renal failure patients daily before HBOT to determine if excessive fluid retention is present. Monitor these patients observationally closely, and have a low threshold to abort treatment at the first sign of respiratory distress.

Table 3. Critical Events Occurring During a Diver or a Treatment in a Monoplace Hyperbaric Chamber

	Air Breathing Diver in the Water	Oxygen Breathing Patient in Monoplace Chamber
Compression	Absolute pressure increases...the volume of gas containing spaces with flexible boundaries decreases (*Boyle's Law*) 1. Middle ear and sinus barotrauma 2. Mask squeeze 3. Decrease in volume of wet suit, and buoyancy compensator 4. Breathing gas density increases, work of breathing increases 5. Number of gas molecules consumed with each breath increases	Absolute pressure increases...the volume of gas containing spaces with flexible boundaries decreases (*Boyle's Law*) 1. Middle ear and sinus barotrauma 2. Volume of gas containing medical implants or within medical devices decreases, can affect equipment function 3. Breathing gas density increases, work of breathing increases 4. Number of gas molecules consumed with each breath increases
	Partial pressure of gases increases leading to increased gas tensions in blood and tissues...inert gas and oxygen (*Dalton's Law*) 1. Inert gas narcosis 2. Oxygen toxicity 3. Carbon dioxide retention in ambient environment	Partial pressure of gases increases leading to increased gas tensions in blood and tissues...oxygen (*Dalton's Law*) 1. Pharmacophysiologic effects of hyperoxygenation of blood and tissue 2. Oxygen toxicity 3. Carbon dioxide retention in ambient environment
		Pharmacophysiologic effects of hyperoxygenation of blood and tissue 1. Improved oxygen dependent cellular metabolism 2. Antimicrobial effects 3. Protection against ischemia reperfusion injury 4. Tissue regenerative effects (angiogenesis, tissue growth) 5. Anti-inflammatory effects 6. Anti-apoptotic effects 7. Activated stem cell mobilization
	Increased inert gas volume in solution (*Henry's Law*) defined by partial pressure of ambient gas, solubility of gas in water and lipid, gas diffusion	Increased oxygen volume in solution (*Henry's Law*) defined by partial pressure of ambient gas, solubility of gas in water and lipid, gas diffusion
		Ambient temperature increases in the chamber (*Gay-Lussac's Law*)
Decompression	Absolute pressure decreases...the volume of gas containing spaces with flexible boundaries increases (*Boyle's Law*) 1. Middle ear and sinus barotrauma 2. Pulmonary barotrauma, pneumothorax 3. Breathing gas density decreases, work of breathing decreases 4. Number of gas molecules consumed with each breath decreases 5. Any inert gas or oxygen bubbles forming during decompression (phase separation) will increase in size as ambient pressure decreases	Absolute pressure decreases...the volume of gas containing spaces with flexible boundaries increases (*Boyle's Law*) 1. Middle ear and sinus barotrauma 2. Pulmonary barotrauma, pneumothorax 3. Breathing gas density decreases, work of breathing decreases 4. Number of gas molecules consumed with each breath decreases 6. Any inert gas or oxygen bubbles forming during decompression (phase separation) will increase in size as ambient pressure decreases
	Partial pressure of gases decreases leading to decreased gas tensions in blood and tissues...inert gas and oxygen (*Dalton's Law*) 1. Recovery from inert gas narcosis 2. Hypoxia	Partial pressure of gases decreases leading to decreased gas tensions in blood and tissues...inert gas and oxygen (*Dalton's Law*) 1. Blood and tissue oxygen gas tensions decrease but hypoxia cannot occur with normal lungs as patient always breathing 100% oxygen even on return to 1 ATA at surface
	Decreased inert gas volume in solution (*Henry's Law*) defined by partial pressure of ambient gas, solubility of gas in water and lipid, gas diffusion 1. Inert gas decompression sickness	Decreased oxygen gas volume in solution (*Henry's Law*) defined by partial pressure of ambient gas, solubility of gas in water and lipid, gas diffusion 1. Oxygen decompression sickness could occur but would be very short lived due to rapid re-absorption of oxygen as it is metabolically consumed
		Ambient temperature decreases in the chamber (*Gay-Lussac's Law*)

In summary, Table 3 describes the critical events that occur during a dive in the water and during a hyperbaric oxygen treatment and should serve as a reminder of factors to consider in preparing patients for and managing them during hyperbaric oxygen treatment.

References:

1. Daniels S, Grossman Y. 9.1 Biological Effects of Pressure, in Bennett and Elliott's Physiology and Medicine of Diving, 5th ed (AO Brubakk, TS Neuman eds), Saunders, Edenburg, 2003; p265-299. (a good review of the general principles of direct pressure effects on physiological systems)
2. Mulkey DK, Henderson III RA, Putnam RW, et al: Pressure (<4ATA) increases membrane conductance and firing rate in the rat solitary complex. J Appl Physiol 203; 95:922-930.
3. Bennett PB, Rostain JC. 9.3 The High Pressure Nervous Syndrome. in Bennett and Elliott's Physiology and Medicine of Diving, 5th ed (AO Brubakk, TS Neuman eds), Saunders, Edenburg, 2003; p323-357 (a good general review of high pressure nervous syndrome)
4. Tikuisis P, Gerth WA. 10.1 Decompression Theory. in Bennett and Elliott's Physiology and Medicine of Diving, 5th ed (AO Brubakk, TS Neuman eds), Saunders, Edenburg, 2003; p419-454
5. Chapter 9-Air Decompression. U. S. Navy Diving Manual Revision 6, Vol 2, SS521-AG-PRO-010. P 9-63-84.
6. Behnke AR, Thomas RM, Motley EP. The psychologic effects from breathing air at 4 atmospheres pressure. Am J Physiol 1935; 112; 554-558.
7. Bennett PB, Rostain JC. 9.2 Inert Gas Narcosis. in Bennett and Elliott's Physiology and Medi-cine of Diving, 5th ed (AO Brubakk, TS Neuman eds), Saunders, Edenburg, 2003; p300-332.
8. Hunt TK, Pai MP. The effect of varying ambient oxygen tensions on wound metabolism and collagen synthesis. Surg Gynecol Obstet 1972; 135: 561-567.
9. Hunt TK, Pai MP. The effect of varying ambient oxygen tensions on wound metabolism and collagen synthesis. Surg Gynecol Obstet 1972; 135: 561-567.
10. Pace N, Strajman E, Walken EL. Acceleration of carbon monoxide elimination in man by high pressure oxygen. Science 1950; 111: 652-654.
11. Weaver LK, Hopkins RO, Chan, KJ, et al. Hyperbaric oxygen for acute carbon monoxide poisoning, N Engl J Med 2002; 347: 1057-1067.
12. Nylander G, Lewis D, Nordstrom H, et al. Reduction of postischemic edema with hyperbaric oxygen. Plast Reconstr Surg 1985; 76: 596-603.
13. Knighton DR, Fiegel VD, Halverson T, et al. Oxygen as an antibiotic: the effect of inspired oxygen on bacterial on bacterial clearance. Arch Surg 1990; 125: 97-100.
14. Knighton DR, Halliday B, Hunt TK. Oxygen as an antibiotic: a comparison of the effects on inspired oxygen concentration and antibiotic administration on in vivo bacterial clearance. Arch Surg 1986; 121: 191-195.
15. Knighton DR, Halliday B, Hunt TK. Oxygen as an antibiotic: the effect of inspired oxygen on infection. Arch Surg 1984; 119: 199-204.
16. Mader JT, Brown GL,Guckian JC, et al. A mechanism for the amelioration by hyperbaric oxygen of experimental staphylococcal osteomyelitis in rabbits. J Infect Dis 1980; 142: 915-922.
17. Mader JT. Phagocytic killing and hyperbaric oxygen: antibacterial mechanisms. HBO Rev. 1981; 2: 37-49.
18. Bakker D. Pure and mixed aerobic and anaerobic soft tissue infections. HBO Rev 1985; : 65-96.
19. Van Unnik AJM. Inhibition of toxin production in Clostridium perfringens in vitro by hyperbaric oxygen. Antonie van Leeuwenhoek 1965; 31: 181-186.
20. Mader JT, Adams KR, Couch LA, et al. Potentiation of tobramycin by hyperbaric oxygen in experimental Pseudomonas aeruginosa osteomyelitis. Presented at the 27th Interscience Conference on Antimicrobial Agents and Chemotherapy, 1987, New York.
21. Mendel V, Simanowski HJ, Scholz HC. Synergy of HBO2 and a local antibiotic carrier for experi-mental osteomyelitis due to Staphylococcus aureus in rats. Undersea Hyperb Med 2004; 31: 407-416.

22. Adams K, Mader J. Aminoglycoside potentiation with adjunctive hyperbaric oxygen therapy in experimental Pseudomonas aeruginosa osteomyelitis. Undersea Hyperbaric Medical Society Annual Scientific Meeting, Baltimore 1987; Abstract 69.
23. Fife CE, Buyukcakir C, Otto GH, et al. The predictive value of transcutaneous oxygen tension measurement in diabetic lower extremity ulcers treated with hyperbaric oxygen therapy. A retrospective analysis of 1,144 patients. Wound Rep Regen2002; 10: 198-207
24. Knighton, DR, Silver IA, Hunt TK. Regulation of wound healing angiogenesis—effect of oxygen gradients and inspired oxygen concentrations. Surgery 1981; 90: 262-270.
25. Sheikh AY, Gibson JJ, Rollins MD, et al. Effect of hyperoxia on vascular endothelial growth factor levels in a wound model. Arch Surg 2000; 135: 1293-1297.
26. Bonomo SR, Davidson JD, Yu Y, et al. Hyperbaric oxygen as a signal transducer: upregulation of platelet derived growth factor-beta receptor in the presence of HBO_2 and PDGF. Undersea Hyperb Med 1998; 25: 211-216.
27. Thom SR. Function inhibition of leukocyte ß$_2$ integrins by hyperbaric oxygen in carbon monoxide-mediated brain injury in rats. Toxicol Appl Pharmacol 1993; 123: 248-256.
28. Ghom SR, Mendiguren I, Hardy KR, et al. Inhibition of human neutrophil ß$_2$ integrin-dependent adherence by hyperbaric oxygen. Am J Physiol Cell Physiol 1997; 272: C770-C777.
29. Buras J. Basic mechanisms of hyperbaric oxygen in the treatment of ischemia-repefusion injury. Int Anesthesiol Clin 2000; 38: 91-109.
30. Zamboni WA, Roth AC, Russell RC, et al. Morphological analysis of the microcirculation during reperfusion of ischemic skeletal muscle and the effect of hyperbaric oxygen. Plast Reconstr Surg 1993; 91: 1110-1123.
31. Zhang Q, Chang Z, Cos RA, et al. Hyperbaric oxygen attenuates apoptosis and decreases inflammation in an ischemic wound model. J Invest Dermatol 2008; 128(8): 2102-2112.
32. Akin ML, Gulluoglu BM, Uluutku H, et al. Hyperbaric oxygen improves healing in experimental rat colitis. Undersea Hyper Med 2002; 29: 279-285.
33. Rachmilewitz D, Karmeli F, Okon E, et al. Hyperbaric oxygen: a novel modality to ameliorate experimental colitis. Gut 1998; 43: 512-518.
34. Luongo C, Imperatore F, Cuzzocrea S, et al. Effects of hyperbaric oxygen exposure on a zymosan-induced shock model. Crit Care Med 1998; 26: 1972-1986.
35. Nathan C. Oxygen and the inflammatory cell Nature 2003; 17: 675-676.
36. Zhang Q, Chang Z, Cos RA, et al. Hyperbaric oxygen attenuates apoptosis and decreases inflammation in an ischemic wound model. J Invest Dermatol 2008; 128(8): 2102-2112.
37. Thom SR, Bhopale VM, Velazquez OC, et al. Stem cell mobilization by hyperbaric oxygen. Am J Physiol Heart Circ Physiol 2006; 290: H1378-H1386.
38. Milovanova TN, Bhopale VM, Sorokina EM. Hyperbaric oxygen stimulates vasculogenic stem cell growth and differentiation in vivo. J Appl Physiol 2009; 106: 711-728.
39. Gallagher KA, Liu A-J, Xiao M, et al. Diabetic impairments in NO-mediated endothelial progenitor cell mobilization and homing are reversed by hyperoxia and SDF-1⊠. J Clinical Invest 2007; 117(5): 1249-1259.
40. Lui Z-H, Velazquez OC. Hyperoxia, endothelial progenitor cell mobilization, and diabetic wound healing. Antioxid Redox Signal 2008; 10(1): 1869-1882.
41. Clark JM. The toxicity of oxygen. Am Rev Resp Dis 1974; 11-: 40-50.
42. McCord JM, Firdovich I. The biology and pathology of oxygen radicals. Ann Intern Med 1978; 89: 122-127.
43. A mini-forum on air breaks and O_2 toxicity in clinical HBO_2 therapy. Undersea Hyperb Med 2004; 31(2): 185-202.
44. Clark JM, Lambertsen CJ. Pulmonary oxygen toxicity: A review. Pharmacol Rev 1971; 23: 37-133.

45. Demchenko IT, Welty-Wolf KE, Allen BW, Piantadosi CA. Similar but not the same: normobaric and hyperbaric pulmonary oxygen toxicity, the role of nitric oxide. Am J Physiol Lung Cell Mol Physiol 2007; L229-L238.
46. Butler, Jr FK, Hagan C, Murphy-Lavoie H. Hyperbaric oxygen therapy and the eye. Undersea Hyperb Med 2008; 35(5): 327-381.
47. Schaal, S, Beiran H, Rubinstein I, et al. Lenticular oxygen toxicity. Invest Opthal Visual Science 2003; 44(8): 3476-3484.
48. Evanger K, Haugen OH, Irgens A, et al. Ocular refractive changes in patients receiving hyperbaric oxygen administered by oronasal mask or hood. Acta Ophthalmol Scand 2004; 82: 449-453.
49. Gesell LB, Trott A. De novo cataract development following a standard course of hyperbaric oxygen therapy. Undersea Hyperb Med 2007; 34(6): 389-392.
50. Holenat F, Boussuges, A, Grandfond A, et al. Haemodynamic effects of hyperbaric hyperoxia in healthy volunteers: an echocardiographic and Doppler study. Clinical Science 2004; 106: 389-395.
51. Weaver LK, Churchill S. Pulmonary edema associated with hyperbaric oxygen therapy. Chest 2001; 120(4) 1407-1409.

Notes

CHAPTER

3

Prescribing HBO for Wound Healing: *A Question of Pressure and Time*

JAMES R. WILCOX, RN

TWO BASIC BUT PERPLEXING QUESTIONS face any hyperbaric practitioner treating wound care patients with hyperbaric oxygen: What treatment pressure should be used, and how long should the treatment last? Before looking at these common but difficult questions, one must review the training, guidelines, and reference materials available to physicians making these challenging decisions.

It appears that an overwhelming majority of the evidence supports a treatment pressure of 2.4 ATA for 90 minutes. Leaders in the field tend to either work at 2.4 ATA or use $PtcO_2$ as a treatment pressure selection guide. Oxygen toxicity should not be a determining factor. Pulmonary and neurologic manifestations of oxygen poisoning are often cited as major concerns. Oxygen tolerance limits that avoid these manifestations are well defined.[15 16] Pulmonary symptoms are not produced by daily exposures to 2.5 ATA for 2 hours.[15 16] The incidence of oxygen convulsions for similar exposures is approximately 1.3 per 10,000 patients.[1 2 3] Oxygen convulsions have been proven to be a completely unpredictable event, and even when oxygen convulsions do occur, it is well documented that there are no residual effects. [26,27,34] A preponderance of evidence supports the safety of hyperbaric oxygen therapy at 2.0 or 2.5 ATA, for durations up to 2 hours without air breaks in healthy humans. When intermittent air breaks are provided, the safety factor is increased exponentially.[24]

The following is a discussion of the history and evidence of hyperbaric medicine used to justify these conclusions.

The Undersea and Hyperbaric Medical Society (UHMS) has established standards and guidelines on the use of hyperbaric oxygen therapy. UHMS currently recognizes 14 pathologic entities for which hyperbaric oxygen has substantial scientific support, demonstrating therapeutic benefit. These disorders are not only considered an appropriate use of hyperbaric oxygen (HBO), but are covered by Medicare and most third party insurances.

In 1976, the Executive Committee of the UHMS established the Hyperbaric Oxygen Therapy Committee. This Committee was charged with the responsibility of continuously reviewing research and clinical data and rendering recommendations regarding clinical efficacy and safety, along with establishing guidelines for use. Approximately every 7 years an updated version of the UHMS Hyperbaric Oxygen Therapy Committee Report is published; the last was in 2008.

The UHMS has also set standards within the hyperbaric community on the level of training required for physicians who practice hyperbaric medicine. Physicians who practice hyperbaric medicine should attend a 40 hour UHMS approved course. UHMS guidelines require that the majority of the training be focused on diving medicine. The guidelines for diving medicine are clear, direct, well proven, and leave little room for misunderstanding. Over half of the indications approved for HBO are related to wound care, but these guidelines lack the same level of direct guidance. This may have added to some of the confusion seen within clinical hyperbarics, related to selection of treatment pressures and duration.

There are only a limited number of textbooks or manuals on clinical hyperbaric medicine available, with the most recognized of these being Hyperbaric Medicine Practice, edited by Dr. Eric Kindwall. This text is regarded as the gold standard in hyperbaric textbooks, followed by Hyperbaric Medicine Procedures, also edited by Kindwall. Physiology and Medicine of Hyperbaric Oxygen Therapy, edited by Dr. Tom Neuman and Dr. Stephen Thom, is the newest textbook available (2008) and is quickly becoming the new standard. These three textbooks/manuals are recommended and used by most HBO courses within the United States. Kindwall was also the editor and committee chairman of the first Hyperbaric Oxygen Therapy Committee Report published by the UHMS in 1977.

Once the decision to use hyperbaric oxygen therapy has been made, two questions must be answered: "Should the patient be treated at 2.0 or 2.5 ATA?" and "How long should the treatment last, 90 or 120 minutes?" These two questions seem to have very straightforward answers if you have a multiplace chamber or even a monoplace chamber equipped for air breaks. But the answers are anything but straightforward and can quickly become convoluted, especially for those using a monoplace that is not equipped for air breaks. Then the question becomes: What duration at 2.0 ATA?

When using the "Hyperbaric Oxygen Therapy Committee Report: Hyperbaric Oxygen 2008" as a reference, one will find it difficult, at best, to find an answer. Basically, the UHMS guidelines state the following for all hyperbaric treatments related to wound care/healing: "Hyperbaric oxygen treatments are performed at 2.0 to 2.4/2.5 ATA for 120 to 90 minutes, respectively." This answer suggests that a few options are available. But which combination offers the most benefit and least risk? Looking back to the early 1960s when clinical hyperbarics was gaining a foothold in modern medicine, early monoplace chambers did not have the capacity to allow air breaks. Hence, most of the research and books from that time recommended 2.0 ATA for 120 minutes in the monoplace chamber and 2.4/2.5 ATA for 90 minutes in the multiplace chamber.

Before answering the question of time, one must understand the difference between 2.4 ATA and 2.5 ATA. Again this question seems somewhat simple, but like many things in hyperbaric medicine, it requires an understanding of past history.

The first systematic studies to define the physiological effects of HBO on humans were conducted at Harvard in the early 1930s.[43] The first clinical use of HBO was by the U.S. Navy in 1943. The Navy (1943) published the procedures for the treatment of decompression sickness at 2.8 ATA.[44] By mid 1960s, the treatment of decompression sickness at 2.8 ATA with 100% oxygen had become the world standard.[44] In 1960, Dr. Boerema and Dr. Brummelkamp reported treating the first patient with an anaerobic infection with hyperbaric oxygen at 3.0 ATA.[25 45 48] Since 1962, the positive effects of hyperbaric oxygen on anaerobic and aerobic wound infections and on wound healing have been demonstrated in both animal and human studies at both 2.4 and 3.0 ATA.[25, 46, 47] In 1974, Colonel Jefferson C. Davis and his staff at the United States Air Force (USAF) Hyperbaric Center at Brooks Air Force Base were tasked with selecting a safe hyperbaric treatment pressure and duration for enhanced problem wound healing. At the time, the USAF was only using multiplace hyperbaric chambers, pressurized with air, and patients received 100% oxygen by fitted aviators' masks.[45] After reviewing the risks and benefits, Davis and his team implemented a treatment protocol for the enhancement of problem wound healing that consisted of intermittent oxygen administered by mask at 2.36 ATA (45 fsw) for 90 minutes. The 90-minute duration was chosen based on the original work of Dr. Boerema who used 90 minutes of HBO at 3 ATA for treating gas gangrene.[25] It is important to know that Boerema treatment pressure and time limits were based on Dr. Behnke's work at Harvard from the 1930s.[43] However, Boerema's Gas Gangrene Protocol was ruled out for wound healing because of the risk of CNS toxicity. Although acceptable for life threatening gas gangrene, it was considered too risky for patients undergoing a 30-day course of hyperbaric for wound healing.[6]

Tightly fitted aviator masks delivered oxygen to the patients undergoing therapy in USAF multiplace chambers. These aviator masks were found to be very efficient for most patients, but if the mask was improperly fitted or oversized it delivered less than 80% oxygen to the patient.[1] Davis felt that there was a possibility that the patient's mask might not get a perfect seal, so a pressure above 2 ATA was selected. To ensure that the patient received oxygen at least an equivalent to 100% oxygen at 2.0 ATA, he initially chose 2.5 ATA (49.5fws) but desired to stay within the 50-fws decompression tables. He then backed off to 45 fsw because of concern that the chamber operator might overshoot the 49.5 fsw level, which would have required inside tenders to be decompressed on a 60 foot table with a decompression stop at 10 foot. Also, the 45 fsw depth was an easy mark on the gauge for the technician to maintain.[4]

It appears that over time the Davis 2.36 ATA Wound Healing Protocol may have been rounded off to 2.4 ATA when used in monoplace chambers, as these chambers operated on 100% oxygen and did not have inside tenders.

In 1977, Dr. Paul Sheffield, who worked with Dr. Davis, published a paper on the effectiveness of oxygen masks used for patients undergoing hyperbaric oxygen therapy.[5] Although this paper was directed at patients in multiplace chambers receiving oxygen through an aviator's mask, its application was quickly used to supply air breaks in monoplace chambers. The following year a number of physicians reported using monoplace chambers at pressures greater than 2.0 ATA, thanks to the introduction of the aviator's mask for air breaks.

When the UHMS released the first edition of "Hyperbaric Oxygen Therapy Committee Report" in 1977, the committee recommended 2.0 ATA for 120 minutes in the monoplace chamber and 2.4 ATA for 90 minutes in the multiplace chamber. This is the same statement found in "Hyperbaric Medicine Procedures," which was also edited by Kindwall, a year earlier.

18years later, in the first edition of Kindwall's Hyperbaric Medicine Practice, one can still find the same statement throughout the textbook. One can also find the treatment pressure of 2.36 ATA, 2.4 ATA, and 2.5 ATA used interchangeably throughout this text. The only difference between these 3 treatment pressures, other than the 0.15 ATA of oxygen, is a safety concern for the inside tender when using the multiplace chamber.

A few years later, when Kindwall was no longer editing the "Hyperbaric Oxygen Therapy Committee Report" for the UHMS and new authors were assigned this task, the recommendations were abruptly changed to "2.0 - 2.5 ATA for 90 to 120 minutes of oxygen breathing" with no explanation, and this is still the standard language used today.

One can now see that the original intent was to treat patients at 2.0 ATA for 120 minutes in the monoplace and 90 minutes at 2.5 ATA in the multiplace chamber. These 2 treatment tables were chosen to provide the safest treatment schedule possible for the patient and tender with the lowest possible risk and greatest benefit. The 2.0 ATA for 120 minutes was based on monoplace chambers not having an air break capacity, making them unable to treat patients safely at 2.5 ATA. In the multiplace chamber, the 2.36 ATA for 90 minutes table did not require decompression stops, while the 2.5 ATA for 90 minutes did.

Davis understood that one of the greatest risks in clinical hyperbarics was oxygen toxicity. A review of oxygen toxicity reveals a long complicated history. Many have added to the volumes of knowledge that exist, but a few stand out.

Paul Bert (1878) made enormous strides in our knowledge of the effects of varying oxygen tensions. He showed that oxygen at increased pressure was highly poisonous and that no living matter was exempt. Bert demonstrated that oxygen tension was the decisive factor in any mixture of nitrogen and oxygen at pressure. He suspected that convulsions were caused by the action of oxygen on the central nervous system. Bert went on to demonstrate that oxygen was a general poison and that the central nervous system was the first body system to be grossly affected by it, and that it could cause violent convulsions and death before changes could be found in other organs systems.[6]

A few years later, Lorrain Smith (1899) demonstrated for the first time that animals breathing oxygen at moderately low tensions over prolonged periods suffered pulmonary damage. Higher oxygen tensions caused the onset of these events to be much faster. Smith also noted a reversibility of the lung damage when the high level of oxygen was removed and returned to normal levels. He found that mice had a remarkable power of recovery from the effects of high oxygen tensions, and that the same was probably true for man. He went on to demonstrate that alternating between ordinary atmosphere levels and elevated levels of oxygen was much less dangerous than in an exposure which was continuously high.[7, 8]

The rate of development of pulmonary toxicity is roughly proportional to the tension of oxygen breathed. This can be calculated by using the unit pulmonary toxic dose (UPTD) formula developed by Bardin and Lambertsen in 1970, which allows for comparison of pulmonary effects of oxygen at the various pressures used in clinical hyperbarics.[11] This has caused some confusion in the past, as 120 minutes at 2.0 ATA and 90 minutes at 2.5 ATA are both approximately 300 UPTD and well within the safe limits established by the U.S. Navy and the University of Pennsylvania. It is important to remember that UPTD is a tool used to predict the onset of pulmonary oxygen toxicity and has nothing to do with its therapeutic treatment levels.[11 12]

The next major studies on oxygen toxicity were undertaken in 1942 by Dr. Kenneth Donald. At the time, the Royal Navy was conducting oxygen diving for various covert operations on a large scale with a high number of fatal incidents. The Royal Navy tasked Commander Donald with finding a comprehensive and accurate picture of the reaction of human subjects to high oxygen tensions. Donald completed over two thousand experiments during the next few years. One of his early experiments was to determine the oxygen tolerance of a group of 37 healthy subjects at a fixed oxygen tension of 3.71 ATA in a dry environment at rest. These test subjects were timed to the development of symptoms necessitating their removal from oxygen. The most striking finding was the enormous variation in oxygen tolerance among test subjects, as the onset of symptoms varied from 6 to 96 minutes. Donald found that the tolerance of each subject was unpredictable. He also found that physical fitness, athleticism, smoking, ingestion of alcohol, psychological health, and age did not influence tolerance levels. He also established that oxygen convulsions are not inherently harmful.[26, 27] Donald noted that oxygen tolerance in a wet diver was markedly less than that of a diver resting in a dry environment. He went on to set the safe wet working limits of oxygen at 25 fsw for 120 minutes in 1945. This may have played a part in selecting 120 minutes as a safe dose of oxygen at 2.0 ATA years later.[9] In 1947, the United States Navy Experimental Diving Unit confirmed all of Donald's findings and adopted his original warning list for signs and symptoms of CNS toxicity that is still in use today.[26]

In 1947, Captain Yarbrough and Behnke, both physicians at the U.S. Navy Experimental Diving Unit, published "Symptoms of Oxygen Poisoning and Limits of Tolerance at Rest and at Work." They established that oxygen was safe and well tolerated at 3 ATA for 2 hours by resting divers in a dry environment.[10]

Dr. J. M. Clark and Dr. C. J. Lambertsen, both from the University of Pennsylvania, are considered the world's leading experts on oxygen toxicity today. They developed a graph that is considered the gold standard on oxygen tolerance predictions (see below). It is important to recognize that the curves represent an average response to a toxic stress for which individual responses are known to vary widely. In addition, the curves shown were

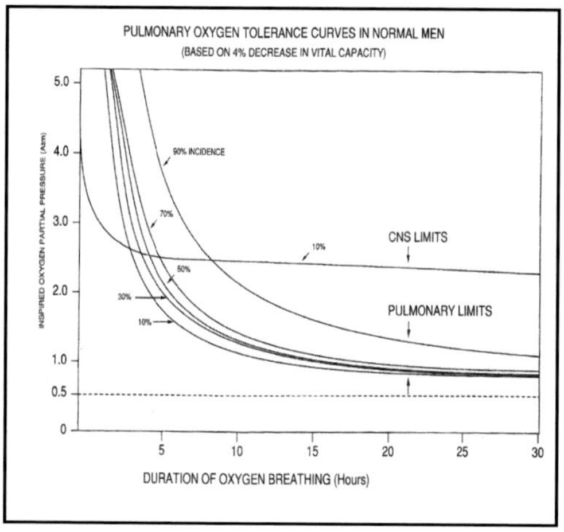

Figure 1: ***Pulmonary oxygen tolerance curves in normal men.***

derived from data obtained during continuous oxygen exposure and therefore do not reflect the beneficial effects of intermittent periods of air breathing under pressure. Intermittent air breathing periods under pressure extended the use of oxygen at 3.0 ATA to approximately 5 hours, at which time the limiting factor becomes pulmonary toxicity.[24] It is also important to know that the University of Pennsylvania no longer studies oxygen toxicity at 2.0 ATA because of the difficulty of invoking a CNS response in healthy test subjects before symptoms of pulmonary toxicity are developed (approximately 6 hours). Clark also states that hyperbaric oxygen therapy has a favorable risk-to-benefit ratio when it is used appropriately and recommends staying to the left of the curve as much as possible while achieving the desired therapeutic effect needed. [17] Below, one can also clearly see that 2.0 to 2.5 ATA at 90 and

120 minutes are not only to the left but also below the 10% curve (4% decrease in vital capacity) for both CNS and pulmonary toxicity.[11, 12]

The incidence of CNS oxygen toxicity resulting in convulsions was reported to be approximately 1.3 per 10,000 in the early 1990's.[1, 2, 3] Dr. Welslau reported in 1996 that out of a population of 107,264 patients, the overall incidence of CNS toxicity was 1 in 6,704.[13] In 2003, Dr. Hampson from the Center for Hyperbaric Medicine at Virgina Mason Medical Center in Seattle, Washington, reported an incidence rate of 1 per 3,388 treatments. Dr. Hampson treated a total of 20,328 patients from 1992 to 2001, of which 6 patients experienced seizure activity. All of Hampson's patients were treated on the Davis 2.36 ATA problem wound healing profile. In 2004, Doctor Yildiz, Dr. Ay, and Dr. Qyrdedi from the military hospital in Istanbul, Turkey, reported a seizure rate of 1 per 12,166 patients treated over a 7-year period; a total of 36,500 treatments were completed during this time.[14] This seizure rate is very close to the rate reported by Davis, Stone, and Hart during the 1990s. In 2005, Dr. R. Warriner completed a retrospective analysis of 48,060 well validated and controlled hyperbaric treatments and reported a seizure rate of 0.039% at 2.0 ATA and 0.168% at 2.5 ATA.[52] Although Warriner reported a significant increase in seizure activity between 2.0 and 2.5 ATA, it is a significant increase in a very, very small number. All of these reports had different treatment pressure and exposure times and applied different protocols for air breaks. One thing that did stand out was that Davis used a 10 minute air break for every 30 minutes on oxygen, while Hampson used 5 minutes.[29]

As for long term effects of hyperbaric oxygen, Davis completed long term follow-up study of 563 patients who had a number of daily treatments using his 2.36 ATA protocol and no chronic or late effects due to hyperbaric oxygen were found.[1]

What is the ideal treatment pressure for chronic wounds? Is it 2.0 ATA or 2.5 ATA? Does one provide for more improved wound healing over the other? Is there evidence that supports the use of one over the other? These are also difficult questions that do not have direct answers and require a review of the present evidence to make an informed decision.

One of the earliest papers presented on the effects of oxygen on wound healing was presented by Dr. T. K. Hunt in 1972. This research paper did not look at increased pressure of oxygen, but did look at varying degrees of oxygen at 1 ATA. This was one of the first papers describing the effect of oxygen on collagen synthesis, demonstrated that collagen accumulation was roughly proportional to arterial oxygen levels, and laid the groundwork for other researchers.

Dr. W. J. Ehler, Dr. R. E. Marx and Dr. M. J. Pelepo presented a paper at the UHMS 1993 Annual Scientific Meeting, titled "Oxygen as a Drug: A Dose Response Curve for Radiation Necrosis." These researchers were able to prove that angiogenesis is directly proportional to the oxygen pressure in the hyperbaric environment. Their results demonstrated in irradiated tissue increased vascularity when exposed to daily 2.4 ATA HBO treatments, but not with 1 ATA treatments.[18, 49] This

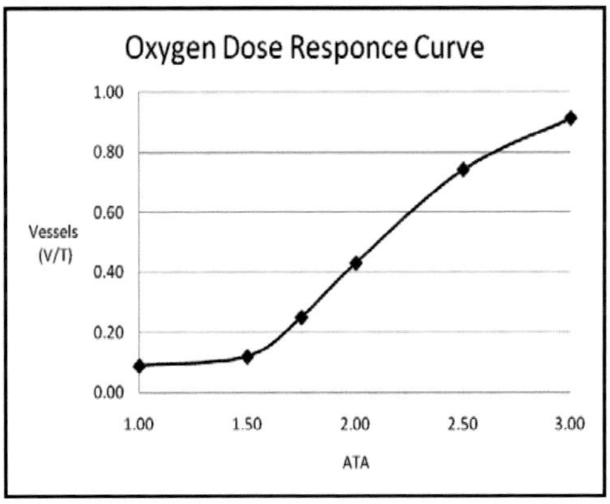

FIGURE 2: ***"The curve of V/T (vessels per tissue area) versus ATA shows a minimal and only gradual increase to 2.0 ATA. At 2.5 ATA, a sharp increase in angiogenesis is noted. This strongly implies a greatly reduced response at treatment depth of 2.0 ATA as compared to 2.5 ATA and to 3.0 ATA."*** [18]

research is consistent with the oxygen gradient concept proposed by Knighton and Hunt in non-irradiated surgical wounds in the early 1980s, suggesting that this information applies to all hypoxic chronic wounds.[50, 51]

In 1993, Dr. S. Thom demonstrated a linear relationship between B-2 integrin inhibition, inhibition of intravascular neutrophil adhesion, and the level of hyperbaric oxygenation.[30] Maximum inhibition of activated neutrophil-endothelial adhesions appears to be observed at about 2.8 ATA. At 2.5 ATA, an 80% reduction in adhesions was observed in human in vitro studies. Significant inhibition of cellular adhesion was observed for up to 8 hours after hyperbaric oxygenation was ended.[31]

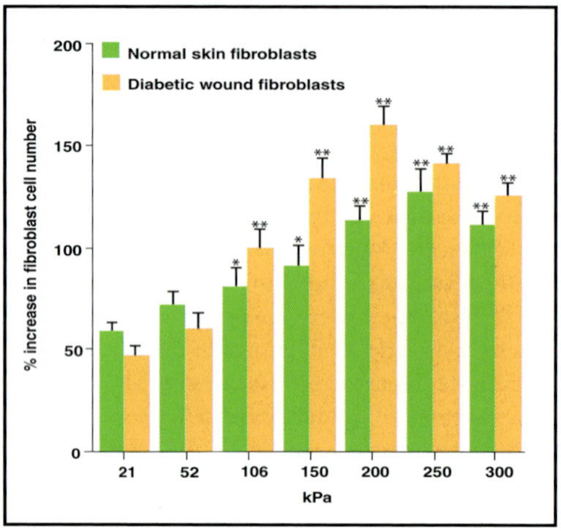

Figure 3: *Hehenberger et al.[19] (The second column represents the diabetic wound fibroblast.)*

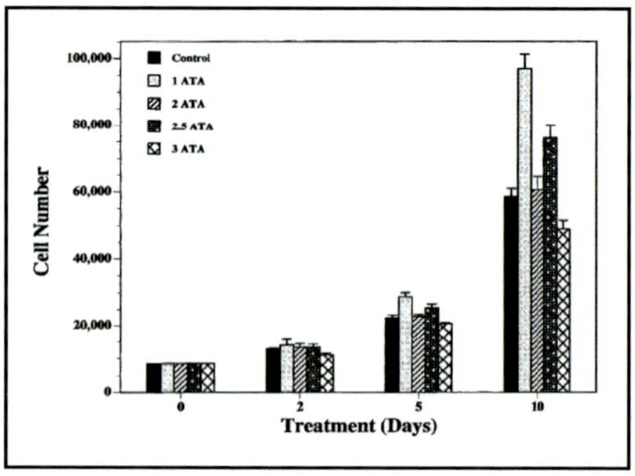

Figure 4: *Effect of hyperbaric oxygen treatment on the proliferation of normal human fibroblast. HBO at the indicated pressures was applied for 90 minutes each day.[22]*

In 1997, Hehenberger published "Dose-Dependent Hyperbaric Oxygen Stimulation of Human Fibroblast Proliferation." These researchers noted that diabetic wounds were characterized by a prolonged wound healing process with insufficient formation of granulation tissue. They also noted that HBO has been observed to improve healing of these wounds. They studied the in vitro effects of HBO on proliferation of human fibroblasts from normal skin and from chronic foot wounds in diabetics with non-insulin dependent diabetes. They found that the stimulatory effect was dose dependent, with peak increases in cell proliferation occurring at approximately 2.5 ATA.[19]

A second paper in 1997 by Dr. P.C. Tompach, et al., found that cellular activity during wound healing is related to tissue oxygen levels. Tompach's data demonstrated that HBO treatments at 2.4 ATA effectively stimulated cell proliferation. One thing that stands out in this study was that fibroblasts require 120 minutes of HBO to produce a response. He also found that 120 minutes of HBO exposure stimulated fibroblast proliferation for 72 hours after the exposure.[21]

In vitro studies conducted by Reenstra, et al., (1998) on human dermal fibroblast proliferation and expression of growth factor receptors noticed that fibroblast from older adults (>60 years) proliferate at a slower rate than those from young adults (20-40). Reenstra noticed that the decreased proliferation rate in older adult fibroblasts was coupled with fewer epidermal growth factor receptor sites (EGFR). A 90-minute HBO treatment at 2.5 ATA significantly increased the proliferation rates and upregulated the number of fibroblast, EGFR, and platelet derived growth factors (PDGF) receptors when measured 24 hours post exposure. The author also found that the HBO response on proliferation was largest in the fibroblast from the older adult where the number of EGFR tripled.[32, 33]

In 1999, Dimitrijevich, et al. noted that the effect of increased growth of cultured fibroblasts seen after daily HBO treatments at 1 and 2.5 ATA was not observed with 3 ATA treatments. These results show that a significant ($p < 0.05$) increase in cell number after 5 days of treatment becomes even more pronounced after day 10. Dimitrijevich noted that consistent stimulation of cell proliferation was observed at 1 and 2.5 ATA of 100% oxygen, whereas treatment at 3 ATA was consistently nonstimulating and perhaps even marginally antimitotic.[22]

A 2005 paper from Dr. Harriet Hopf titled "Hyperoxia and Angiogenesis" concluded that angiogenesis requires oxygen and that angiogenic response is dose dependent. They found that angiogenesis was significantly increased at 2.5 ATA with a p value of <0.05 and significantly decreased in the hypoxic group ($p = 0.001$). Hopf noted that the angiogenesis increases with increasing pressure until 2.5 ATA when it begins to decline.[20]

Below is a treatment table of common usage from leaders in the field of hyperbarics today. Dr. Weaver states that he treats patients at 2.0 ATA to avoid attendant decompression due to the fact that his starting and returning pressure is at altitude. Dr. Fife stated that she treated a significant number of patients in her DFU outcomes study

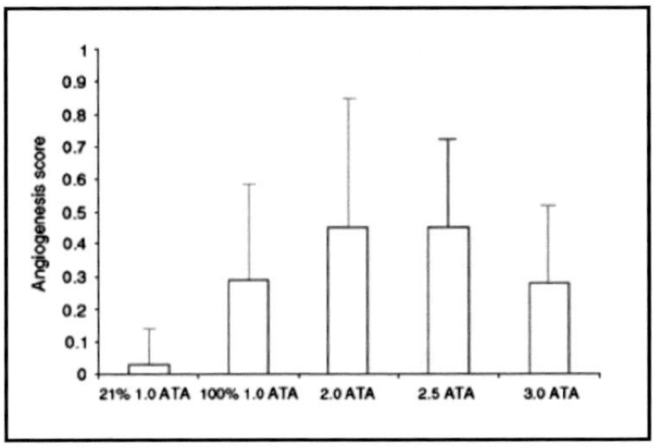

Figure 5: Bar graph of the mean angiogenesis score at various pressure and oxygen levels.[20]

at 2.0 ATA, but has now gone back to 2.4 ATA.

A large number of reported case series and clinical trials on hyperbarics can be found. The critical issue is that most evidence is based upon 2.4 ATA treatments for 90 minutes. Leaders in the field tend to either work at 2.4 ATA (altitude issues in Salt Lake City notwithstanding) or use $PtcO_2$ as a treatment pressure selection guide.

Edema, whatever the cause, is always detrimental to wound healing and infection control.[36, 37] Edema always contributes to hypoxia, as it increases the distance oxygen must diffuse from the capillaries.[35, 40] Diffusion distances of oxygen from the capillary to the cell through tissue fluid is proportional to the square root of the oxygen content in the capillary.[38] Consequently, oxygen diffusion through edema is decreased by approximately a factor of 3, because edema increases the distance from the capillary to the cell.[38] As interstitial pressure increases around the capillaries from edema, it quickly exceeds capillary perfusion pressure, the capillary bed collapses, and flow to the microcirculation ceases.[39] Because of this, ischemia and edema contribute to each other's progression and a vicious cycle is established. A number of researchers have observed that hyperbaric oxygen results in vasoconstriction with reduction of blood flow by approximately 20%, as a protective reaction to hyperoxia, resulting in a corresponding reduction in edema.[39-42] Volumes of research have been conducted on this subject, and a majority of this research was conducted at 2.5 ATA. The immediate effect of HBO therapy is hyperoxygenation resulting in increased amounts of physically dissolved oxygen in plasma, which is directly proportional to the partial pressure of oxygen.[42] As the partial pressure of oxygen increases, so does the amount of dissolved oxygen in the blood, resulting in increased diffusion distances and increased vasoconstriction which further reduces edema.[42] Therefore, 2.5 ATA would have to be superior to 2.0 ATA.

Hyperbaric oxygen affects living tissue by increasing partial pressure of oxygen within it. Placing a patient under 2.5 ATA with 100% oxygen increases the percent of oxygen dissolved in the plasma approximately 20 fold. The overall effect is that the hemoglobin is still fully saturated in the blood returning to the heart.[28] Thus, the body's tissues develop a high PO_2. This effect has been proven in wounds and has proven to be beneficial in collagen deposition, angiogenesis, and the upregulation of growth factors and their receptor sites. A great number of case studies support hyperbaric oxygen therapy at 2.0 ATA, but none compare results to 2.5 ATA. There is also a number of interesting research articles on cellular activity at 2.0 ATA, but again none are compared to 2.5 ATA. The evidence supports the safe use of hyperbaric oxygen therapy at 2.4 ATA for duration up to 90 minutes. When intermittent air breaks are provided, the safety factor is increased exponentially. Forty years later, it would be difficult to improve on Colonel Jefferson C. Davis' statement, "With all of these variables, the highest dose of oxygen that is safe for a given patient should be used."

Table 1: ***Weaver, Fife, and Hampson Treatment Table***

Indication	Mono wound	Multi wound	Mono radiation	Multi radiation
Weaver	2.0 ATA 90 mins 5 min air breaks each 30 mins	2.0 ATA 90 mins 5 min air breaks each 30 mins	2.0 ATA 90 mins 5 min air breaks each 30 mins	2.0 ATA 90 mins 5 min air breaks each 30 mins
Fife	NA	2.4ATA 90 mins 2 5 min air breaks each 30 mins	NA	2.4ATA 90 mins 2 5min air breaks each 30 mins
Hampson	NA	2.4 ATA 90 mins 5 min air breaks each 30 mins	NA	2.4 ATA 90 mins 5 min air breaks each 30 mins

Table 2: ***Case Studies/Clinical Trials on HBO***

Author Year, Country	Study Design	N	Condition	Results
Doctor [87] 1992 India	RCT	30 (15 HBO, 15 control)	Hospitalized DFU	Above ankle amputations: HBO 2/15, Control: 7/15 $P<0.05$; Minor amputations NS Number of + cultures decreased in HBO group $P<0.05$
Faglia[88] 1996 Italy	RCT	70 (35 HBO, 33 control, 2 lost to follow-up)	Severe, infected, ischemic DFU	Major amputations: HBO 3/35 (8.6%) Control 11/33 (33.3%) P=0.016 2.5 ATA 90 mins treatment 1, 2.4 ATA 90 mins all subsequent treatments (multiplace)
Abidia[89] 2003 UK	RCT, double-blind, sham	18 (8 HBO, 8 control; 2 lost to follow-up)	Ischemic DFU, 1-10 mm diameter,	Healing at 12 week follow up point:: HBO: 5/8, Control: 1/8; 2.4 ATA 90 mins (mult iplace)
Kalani[90] 2002 Sweden	RCT + CT	38 (17 HBO, 21 control)	DFU	Healing at 3 year follow-up point: HBO: 13/17 (76%), Control 10/21 (48%); Amputations: HBO: 2/17 (12%), Control 7/21 (33%) Treatment profile not stated
Kessler 2003	RCT	28	Wagner 1-3 DFU	HBO: wounds smaller at 2 and 4 weeks, more healed at 2 weeks 2.5 ATA 90 mins (multiplace)
Zamboni 1997 USA	CT	10 (5 HBO, 5 control)	DFU	HBO with standard wound care reduced wound size compared to standard wound care alone $P<0.05$ At 4-6 months HBO group had higher rate of complete healing (4/5 compared to controls 1/5) 2.0 ATA 120 mins (monoplace)
Baroni 1987 Italy	CT	28 (18 HBO,10 control)	DFU	Healing: HBO: 16/18 (89%), Control: 1/10 (10%) P=0.001 Amputations: HBO: 2/18, Control: 4/10 2.4 ATA 90 mins (multiplace)
Davis 1987 USA	Retro review	168 HBO	DFU	118/168 (70%) patients healed at a level providing for bipedal ambulation, 50/168 (30%) required a BKA or AKA, failures in patients with non bypassable arterial disease at or above ankle 2.4 ATA 90 mins (multiplace)
Oriani 1990 Italy	Retro comp	80 (62 HBO, 18 control)	DFU	"Recovery": HBO: 59/62 (96%), Control: 12/18 (67%); Amputation: HBO: 3/62 (5%), 6/18 (33%) $P<0.001$ 2.4 ATA 90 mins (multiplace)
Wattel 1991 France	Retro consecutive review	59 HBO	DFU	52/59 (88%) healed without major amputation, 7/59 (12%) required major amputation, significantly higher PtcO2 values achieved during HBO (786 +-258mmHg vs 323 +-214) in success compared to failures

Oriani 1992 Italy	Retro consecutive review uncontrolled	151 HBO (may include patients from 1990 series)	DFU	130/151, 86% healed with HBO, 21/15, 14% failed with HBO 2.4 ATA 90 mins (multiplace)
Stone 1995 USA	Retro review Abstract	469 (87 HBO,382 control)	DFU	Limb salvage: HBO: 72%, Control: 53% P<0.002 2.4 ATA 90 mins (multiplace)
Faglia 1998 Italy	Compare		115 (51 HBO, 64 control)	DFU
Fife91 2007 USA	Retro review	1144 HBO	DFU	Overall 75% of patients improved with HBO, mean 34 treatments; By Wagner score: I: 100% (n=3), II: 83.1% (N=130), III: 77.2% (n=465), IV: 64.5% (n=64.5%), V: 29.7% (n=37) 2.4 ATA 90 mins most, some treated at 2.0 ATA 90 mins (multiplace)
Marx 1983 USA	RCT		ORN	2.4 ATA 90 mins (multiplace)
Clarke 2008 multinational	RCT		SRN radiation proctitis	2.0 ATA 90 mins (monoplace)
Hampson 2003	Retro review		SRN radiation cystitis	2.4 ATA 90 mins (multiplace)

References

1. Davis JC, Dunn JM, Heimbach RD. Hyperbaric medicine: Patient selection, treatment procedures, and side effects. In: Davis JC, Hunt TK, eds. Problem wounds: The role of oxygen. New York: Elsevier, 988: 225-235.
2. Stone JA, Loar H, Rudge FW. An eleven year review of hyperbaric oxygenation in a military clinical setting. Undersea Biomed Res 1991: 18 (suppl): 80.
3. Hart GB, Strauss MB. Central nervous system oxygen toxicity in a clinical setting. In: Bove AA, Bachrach AJ, Greenbaum LJ, Eds. Undersea and hyperbaric physiology IX. Proceeding of the ninth international symposium on underwater and hyperbaric physiology. Bethesda, MD: Undersea and Hyperbaric Medical Society, 1987: 695-699.
4. Sheffield PJ. How the Davis 2.36 ATA wound healing enhancement treatment table was established-Undersea Hyperbaric Medical 2004; 31 (1): 193-194.
5. Sheffield P, Stork R, Morgan T. Efficient oxygen mask for patients undergoing hyperbaric oxygen therapy. Aviat. Space Enviro Med. 1977; 48 (2): 132-137.
6. Bert, P. (1943). Barometric pressure. (Fred A. Hitchcock & Mary Alice Hitchcock, Trans.). Ohio: College Book Company. (Original work published 1878).
7. Smith, Lorrain J. (1899). The pathological effects due to increase of oxygen tension in air breathed. Journal of Physiology. 24; 19-35.
8. Smith Lorrain J. The influence of pathological conditions on active absorption of oxygen by the lungs. Lecture on Pathology, Queen's Collage, Belfast published in Journal of Physiology. Date unknown.
9. Donald, K. (1992). Oxygen and the diver. Worcs: The SPA Ltd.
10. Yarbrough O, Welham W, Brinton E, Behnke A. Symptoms of oxygen poisoning and limits of tolerance at rest and at work. Experimental Diving Unit, Naval Gun Factory. Project X-337 (Sub. No. 62) January, 1947 Washington, D.C.
11. Bardin H, Lambertsen CJ. A quantitative method for calculating cumulative pulmonary oxygen toxicity: Use of the unit pulmonary toxicity dose (UPTD). Philadelphia, University of Pennsylvania, Institute for Environmental Medicine Report, 1970.
12. Wright WB. Use of the University of Pennsylvania Institute for Environmental Medicine procedure for calculation of cumulative pulmonary oxygen toxicity: U.S. Navy Experimental Diving Unit Report 2-72. Washington, DC, 1972.
13. Welslau W, Almeling M. Incidence of oxygen intoxication to central nerve system in Hyperbaric Oxygen Therapy. In: Marroni A, Oriani G, Wattel F. Proceedings of the International Joint Meeting on Hyperbaric and Undersea Medicine. Malan 1966: 211-216.
14. Yildiz S, Ay H, Qyrdedi T. Central nervous system oxygen toxicity during routine hyperbaric oxygen therapy. Undersea Hyperbaric Medical 2004; 31 (1): 193-194.
15. Clark JM. Oxygen toxicity. In: Bennett PB, Elliott DH, Eds. The Physiology and Medicine of Div ing, 3rd ed. London: Bailliere, Tindall & Cox, 1982: 200-238.
16. Lambertsen CJ. Effects of hyperoxia on organs and their tissue. In: Robin E. (Ed.) Extrapulmonary manifestation of respiratory disease. New York: Marcel Dekker, 1978: 239-303.
17. Clark JM. Oxygen toxicity. In: Neuman, TS and Thom SR, (eds.) Physiology and medicine of hyperbaric oxygen therapy. Philadelphia: Saunders Elsevier. 2008: 527-563.
18. Ehler WJ, Marx RE, and Pelepo MJ. Oxygen as a drug: a dose response curve for radiation necrosis. SPUMS Journal. 1995: 25; 2 86-87.
19. Hehenberger K, Brismar K, Folke L, Gunnar K. Dose-dependent hyperbaric oxygen stimulation of human fibroblast proliferation. Wound Rep Reg 1997; 5: 147-150.
20. Hopf HW, Gibson JJ, Angeles AP, Constant JS, Feng JJ, Rollins MD, Hussain MZ, and Hunt TK. Hyperoxia and angiogenesis. Wound Rep Reg 2005; 13: 558-564.
21. Tompach PC, Lew D, and Stoll JL. Cell response to hyperbaric oxygen treatment. Int. J. Oral Maxillofac. Surg. 1997; 26: 82-86.
22. Dimitrijevich SD, Paranjape S, Wilson JR, Gracy RW, Mills JG. Effects of hyperbaric oxygen on human skin cells in culture and in human dermal and skin equivalents. Wound Rep Reg 1999; 7: 53-64.

23. Davis JC, Hunt TK. (1988). Problem wounds the role of oxygen. New York: Elsevier.
24. Clark JM, Fisher AB. (1977). Oxygen toxicity and extension of tolerance in oxygen therapy. In: Davis JC, Hunt TK, (Ed.) Hyperbaric Oxygen Therapy. (1977). Bethesda: Undersea Medical Society.
25. Bakker DJ. (1984). The use of hyperbaric oxygen in the treatment of certain infectious diseases especially gas gangrene and acute dermal gangrene. (Thesis). Drukkerij: Wageningen.
26. Donald Kenneth W: Oxygen Poisoning in Man Part I. British Medical Journal May 17, 1947; 667-672.
27. Donald Kenneth W: Oxygen Poisoning in Man Part II. British Medical Journal May 24, 1947; 712-717.
28. Hammarlund C. (1994). The physiologic effects of hyperbaric oxygen. In: Hyperbaric Medicine Practice. EP Kindwall. (Ed.) Best Publishing Co.: Flagstaff, Arizona, pp. 17-32.
29. Hampson NB: CNS O_2 toxicity: Dr. Hampson's response. Letter to the Editor. Undersea Hyperbaric Medical 2004: 31 (2): 191.
30. Thom SR. Function inhibition of leukocyte B2 integrins by hyperbaric oxygen in carbon monoxide-mediated brain injury in rats. Toxicol Appl Pharmacol. 1993;123: 248-256.
31. Thom SR, Mendiguren II, Nebolon M, Campbell D, et al. Temporary inhibition of human neutrophil B2 integrin function by hyperbaric oxygen (HBO). Clinical Research 1994;42:130A.
32. Reenstra WR, Bursa JA, Svoboda KS. Hyperbaric oxygen increases human dermal fibroblast proliferation, growth factor receptor number and in vitro wound closure. Undersea & Hyperbaric Medical Society Annual Meeting, abstract 1998; 25:53.
33. Reenstra WR, Bursa JA, Svoboda KS. Hyperbaric oxygen increases human dermal fibroblast expression of EGF receptors (EGFR). Undersea & Hyperbaric Medical Society Annual Meeting, abstract 1998; 25:54.
34. Lambertsen CJ. Oxygen toxicity. In: Bond, GF. (Ed.). Fundamentals of Hyperbaric Medicine. Washington D.C.: National Academy of Sciences. 1966; 21-32.
35. Strauss MB. Crush injury and other acute traumatic peripheral ischemias. In. Kindwall, EP, (Ed.). (1995). Hyperbaric Medicine Practice. Flagstaff: Best Publishing. pp 525-549.
36. Silver IA. The physiology of wound healing. In: Hunt, T. K., (Ed.). (1980). Wound healing and wound infection: theory and surgical practice. New York: Appleton-Century-Crofts. pp 11-31.
37. Hunt TK. Disorders of repair and their management. In. Hunt, TK, & Dunphy, JE. (Eds.). (1979). Fundamentals of Wound Healing. New York: Appleton-Century-Crofts. pp. 68-169.
38. Peirce EC. II. Pathophysiology, apparatus, and methods, including the special techniques of hypothermia and hyperbaric oxygen. In: Thomas CC. (Ed.) (1969). Extracorporeal Circulation for Open Heart Surgery. Springfield, IL, pp. 84-88.
39. Nylander G, Lewis D, Nordstrom H, Larsson J. Reduction of post ischemic edema with hyperbaric oxygen. Plast Reconstr Surg. 1985; 76: 596
40. Strauss MB, Hargens AR, Gershuni DH, et al. Reduction of skeletal muscle necrosis using intermittent hyperbaric oxygen in a model compartment syndrome. Journal of Bone and Joint Surgery 1983; 65-A (5): 656-662.
41. Bird AD, Telfer ABM. Effect of hyperbaric oxygen on limb circulation. Lancet. 1965;1:355-356.
42. Basset BE, Bennett PB. Introduction to physical and physiological bases of hyperbaric therapy. In: Davis, JC, & Hunt, TK, ed. Hyperbaric Oxygen Therapy. (1977). Bethesda: Undersea Medical Society.
43. Behnke AR, Johnson PS, Poppen JR, Motelt EP. The effect of oxygen on man at pressures from 1 to 4 atmospheres. Am J Physiol 1935; 110: 565-570.
44. Davis JC. Hyperbaric oxygen therapy. J. Intensive Care Med. 1989; 4: 55-57.
45. Davis JC, Dunn JM, Hagood CO, Bassett BE. Hyperbaric Medicine in the US Air Force. JAMA. 1973; 224 (2): 205-209.
46. Hunt TK, Niinikoski J, Zederfeldt BH, Silver IA. Oxygen in wound healing enhancement; cellular effects of oxygen. In: Davis, JC, & Hunt, TK, ed. Hyperbaric Oxygen Therapy. (1977). Bethesda: Undersea Medical Society.
47. Rabkin JM, Hunt TK. Infection and oxygen. In: Davis JC, & Hunt TK, (Ed.) Problem Wounds: the Role of Oxygen. New York: Elsevier, 1988: 1-16.

48. Brummelkamp WH, Hogenduk J, and Boerema I. Treatment of anaerobic infections (clostridial mycositis) by drenching the tissue with oxygen under high atmospheric pressure. Surgery 1961; 49: 299-302.
49. Marx RE, Ehler WJ, Tayapongsak P, Pierce LW. Relationship of oxygen dose to angiogenesis induction in irradiated tissue. The American Journal of Surgery. 1990;160:519-524.
50. Knighton DR, Silver IA, Hunt TK. Regulation of wound healing angiogenesis: effect of oxygen gradients and inspired oxygen concentration. Surgery 1981; 90: 262.
51. Knighton DR, Hunt TK, Schenestuhl H, et al. Oxygen tension regulates the expression of angio genesis factors by microphages. Science 1983; 221:1283-1287.
52. Beard T, Warriner R III, Pasceri PP, Fife C, Otto G. Adverse events during hyperbaric oxygen therapy (HBOT) a retrospective analysis from 25 centers. UHMS. 2005; 32 (4): 313.

CHAPTER

4

Make or Buy: *A Critical Look at Outsourcing*

John S. Peters, MBA and Scott A. Filgo

There are as many as 7 million Americans suffering from chronic wounds annually. Chronic wound care costs the U.S. $20 to $25 billion annually, and another $7 to $10 billion for acute and traumatic wound care, according to Richard Ikeda, PhD of the National Institute of General Medicine Services in January 2008.

Wound care is a burgeoning business in the U.S. due in large part to the rapid rise of diabetes. The CDC reported in 2007 that nearly 24 million Americans or 8% of the U.S. population suffered with the malady, and that 95% of those with diabetes are Type 2 or insulin dependent.[1] Of those over age 60, 23% or 12.2 million have diabetes. The number of cases of diabetes has increased by 3 million in the past 2 years and an estimated 57 million people are to be in a pre diabetic stage, according to the Jeff Levine with HHS HealthBeat, a publication of the Department of Health and Human Services (December 1, 2009).

Diabetes was the seventh leading cause of death in the U.S. in 2006, and the overall risk for death in the diabetic is twice that of a non-diabetic of the same age. 60% of non-traumatic amputations occur in people with diabetes.

According to the Ontario Ministry of Health and Long-Term Care, Canada also experiences a rate of diabetes close to the U.S. with 7% of the population having the disease. Globally, diabetes is an even larger problem with 80% of all new cases expected to appear in developing countries, according the World Health Organization (WHO). 230 million people or 6% of the world's adult population have the disease, and this number is expected to grow to over 350 million in 20 years or by 2030. India, for example, has the highest diabetes population in the world.

Current Healthcare Environment

National health expenditures in the U.S. have been rising at an average of 6.5% per year and are expected to grow at the rate of 7.1% per year between 2003 and 2014.[2] As a percentage of U.S. GDP, health expenditures have gone from 13% in 2000 to 16.2% in 2007,[2] and CMS projects that by 2016 healthcare spending will be over $4.1 trillion or 19.6% of GDP.[3]

Add this unsustainable growth to the most severe recession, both in the depth and length of the contraction (chartoftheday.com) the U.S. has experienced in over 70 years; reductions in public health insurance payments to hospitals, particularly state Medicaid plans; and skyrocketing unemployment leading to more bad debt and a reduction in the amount of credit available to hospitals,[4] and it is understandable why hospitals are struggling to keep their doors open. These factors have led to a continued decline in hospitals from 5,747 in 2006 to 5,708 in 2007.[5] The credit crunch as a result of the collapse of many banking institutions around the world has hit hospitals particularly hard, as hospitals borrow for everything including expansions, equipment, supplies and payroll. Deloitte reports that hospitals with less than pristine credit will have to delay new investments or capital projects, some indefinitely.[6]

With all of the negativity in the healthcare marketplace, hospitals need to focus on reducing costs including reducing payrolls and closing service lines or departments that detract from the overall margin of the operation, while simultaneously increasing focus on the areas which will continue to drive profitability, particularly service lines such as orthopedics, cardiology, some areas of oncology, and (arguably) wound care.[6] One method for achieving a reduction in costs while adding new services or realigning services which are underperforming is to outsource.

THE NEED TO OUTSOURCE

Outsourcing in hospitals is not a new concept for management. Traditionally, outsourcing has been well accepted for departments such as laundry, housekeeping, and food service which were ranked in the top 3 service lines outsourced in 2007, followed by clinical diagnostic equipment maintenance, according to Modern Healthcare's 30th Annual Outsourcing Survey in 2007.

Healthcare organizations are concentrating on reductions in cost by identifying lines that are not in their core competency offering, such as those listed above and thereby focusing resources on delivering better patient care.[7]

VHA, Inc. of Irving, TX is a national healthcare alliance that provides industry-leading supply chain management services for not-for-profit hospitals. They performed a survey of its member hospitals, the seventh in a series of research defining current trends and attitudes of contracting for services. The VHA survey defined the following reasons for contracting services externally. [8]

TABLE 1: ***Reasons for Contracting Services Internally***

Resources are not available internally	74%
Reduce operating costs	51%
Free up resources for other purposes	48%
Function is difficult to manage/out of control	32%
Focus on patient care	29%
Make capital funding available	8%
Provide a cash infusion	6%

The Global Sourcing Group law firm of Morrison and Foerster, who annually produce a report on global outsourcing, has found that outsourcing is actually counter-cyclical to periods of non-recession because many companies use outsourcing as a way to cut short-term costs. "Many companies use outsourcing to increase flexibility of their cost base while at the same time take advantage of specialist resources and greater quality in the delivery of essential services."[9]

A danger health care organizations face when cutting costs is inadvertently weakening current competencies. An example is the significant decline in continuing education expenditure, a 41% per learner reduction in 2008 compared to 2006, according to the Bersin & Associates, 2009 Corporate Learning Factbook: Healthcare Edition. It was noted that high-performing organizations spent almost 200% more on development per employee than under-performing organizations. Not only does this impact employee satisfaction and retention, it directly impacts the service level and potentially the safety and quality of patient care.

Therefore, it is vital that organizations define their competencies before refocusing. Outsourcing should reduce an organization's learning curve and improve performance through best practice standards, implementation knowledge, and resources required for the successful launch of the service line. In a December 2009 interview with Calvin Glidewell, CEO of Imperial Point Medical Center (Fort Lauderdale, FL), Glidewell states that he considers "speed to market" and achieving "competitive advantage" key expectations when partnering with an outsourced firm.

Modern Healthcare's 2009 Survey demonstrated a 16.2% increase in the number of contractors providing services for hospitals between 2007 and 2008. Wound care contracting was buried in the 20th ranking of the "others" category with the likes of hospitalists and supply chain operators. The category experienced an 18% increase in the same period, according to the survey's authors.[10]

Interestingly in the VHA survey, "increasing revenue generation" was not mentioned as a key factor for outsourcing. Also, wound care was not listed among the clinical operations services outsourced, but neither were orthopedics, cardiology, or oncology, which were noted to still be key revenue drivers for hospitals. However, the rankings for clinical outsourced departments ran short of defining any below 29%.

Mr. Glidewell clarified the oversight in the VHA study when asked the question: "Understanding that departments like housekeeping, food services, bio-med, and laundry are common departments to outsource, how does this translate to clinical departments like wound care or rehab, in your opinion?" He responded that he evaluates outsourcing of services based on whether the department is a revenue center or a cost center. "If it's a cost center the decision is simple, we focus on reducing the cost. If the service is a revenue center, can the facility add new sources of revenue, achieve competitive advantage, speed to market, and achieve results faster?" The firm's expertise in the niche market and reputation are also critical in making the decision.

Mr. Glidewell also commented on the outsourcing of wound care, stating that it is an easy product line to outsource because of the long history that firms have in providing the service in the marketplace. He claims that while the hospital could make wound care a core competency, sometimes it is better to outsource when considering resource allocation and other factors mentioned above.

Choosing an Outsourcing Firm

There is a qualitative and quantitative process approach for evaluating which specialists firms are right for the hospital organization. Dan Brown of Dan Brown Consulting (www.danbrownconsulting.com) defines six key points to consider before choosing an outsourcing firm (similarly identified in the VHA 2007 Services Contracting Study).

- Experience and references
- Culture
- Pricing relative to value
- Performance outcomes
- Contracting
- Resources

A quick turnkey solution should reduce the learning curve, accelerate performance, and improve speed to market- a provider with experience in the marketplace is more likely to deliver on the expectations.

The power of testimony is enormous. In the VHA study, 85% of respondents use hospitals or health systems for guidance or referrals. Experience equals results, producing testimonials that should benefit the hospital organizations by picking better specialists firms.

When considering culture, it is important to note that the majority of hospitals do not operate like for-profit businesses, while the vast majority of specialist firms do- this can be the reason the hospital organization chooses to outsource. While change is difficult, hospitals forced to change might look to an outsourced firm to make the difficult decisions. This is represented in the VHA study where 32% of respondents stated they choose outsourcing because the "function is difficult to manage or out of control." According to Mitch Weiner, president of Archer Management Services (212-502-2100/ www.arhermgt.com), many vendors have the experience, quality, and resources to meet the client's needs, but not all of them share the same business philosophies, practices, and ideals as the organization. The importance of this must not be underestimated. Time and time again, companies hire a vendor and are later forced to dissolve the relationship because the partnership simply did not fit. Choosing a vendor is choosing a partner. This fit sustains the partnership.

The outsourcing firm's approach in changing the hospital's operation can also cause tension between the organizations, causing a "culture war."[11] In the VHA study, 32% of respondents defined the organization's unique culture as a barrier or concern of contracting for external services.

A key to success is for the outsourcing firm to take the time to understand the hospital organization's culture and commit to following it. Most often, culture will seep through in its policies, procedures, mission, vision statements, and during the sales process, which is paramount to an interview for both parties. If the local management is employed by the outsourcing firm, they must adapt to the hospital's organizational culture in order for the relationship to succeed.

In the VHA study, 95% of respondents use cost as the main driver when evaluating a supplier of services, while 82% rated value-added as the key driver; however, 42% responded that it is difficult to measure the value of external contracting.

There are fundamental offerings that every niche specialist firm should provide, representing the core value of purchased services. For example, wound care firms should all provide safe, effective, patient-centered, timely, efficient, and equitable services to the patient, hospital organization, government agencies, and providers. These components represent the AAWC (Association for the Advancement of Wound Care) Conceptual Framework of Quality Systems for Wound Care.[12] All other "value-added" offerings by the various firms should exist as a menu of services, which can be negotiated depending on the perception of value by the hospital and the willingness of the specialists firms to allow for carve outs.

All other things being equal, particularly with regard to the AAWC Framework, identifying the right wound care management firm should be as simple as choosing the low cost provider.

Perception of value can be overcome by the specialist firms quantifying the results of contracting services; however, it can be difficult to compare outsourced and insourced departments and competitors side-by-side without appearing biased or degrading during the sales process. The hospital executives often immediately discount pro formas during the sales process as one-sided, and attempt to recreate the pro forma with their own assumptions. This can be prudent from the standpoint of identifying hidden or escalating charges that are not readily visible in the specialists firm's pro formas. Conversely, it can be detrimental because assumptions for growth in the business and corresponding revenues and ancillary services revenues can be discounted to a point where the return is not viable for the hospital to commit to the outsourcing relationship. This might mean the hospital misses the opportunity to correct poor performing departments or benefit from new revenue streams.

When questioned whether he would consider paying more for an outsourced service than if the hospital insourced the function Glidewill responded, "Possibly, it's weighing the benefits to the facility including intangibles like increased reputation by association, heightened performance which translates to additional revenue that is not easily measured, versus the increase in cost over what the facility could provide it."

Performance should be agreed to by both parties and defined in the contract, certainly before the agreement is signed and services are rendered. Outcomes are achieved in the trenches, where the quality of the service delivered and management oversight is critical to outsourcing being effective. Glidewell reiterated that he believes the quality of the onsite manager and the ability to deliver what was promised makes or breaks the contract.

It is vital for the hospital organization to have the ability to hold the specialist firms accountable for their performance standards. John M. Callahan's article in HFMA's September 2005 publication recommends the contracts include the provisions in accordance with: [13]

- Applicable law
- The standards of the hospital's accreditation agencies
- The hospital's policies and procedures
- Industry standards observed by other vendors
- Potential reward/penalty for patient satisfaction scores

He also recommends that if the specialist firm is uncomfortable with signing an agreement with these provisions, the hospital organization should continue its search beyond the firm.

Value does not equal "stickiness." Often, specialist firms believe that it is vital for their best interest to make a contract that is nearly impossible for the hospital organization to extract itself. Hospital organizations should weigh these factors when considering outsourcing.

Callahan stresses that health care organizations should leave themselves an out, particularly in situations where the specialist firm fails to meet its obligations or performs poorly. He lists the following provisions as critical for inclusion in a contract:

- The vendor fails to correct a problem after being notified and given a reasonable period of time to fix it (breach of contract provisions)
- The vendor files for bankruptcy, is excluded from the Medicare program, or is investigated by federal or state authorities for fraud– all events that could have an adverse impact on the hospital or its reputation
- The law changes in any way that calls into question the legality of the hospital vendor relationship ("change of law" provisions)– a situation that most likely arises when the outsourced service is one that could affect either the hospital's Medicare certification or its tax exempt status

- The hospital should have an absolute right to request the removal of individual employees based on violations of the hospital's policies

Identifying the scope of the project and a healthy dose of realism can lead to a successful relationship with the right firm because it aligns costs with services provided. In the article "RX for Healthcare Outsourcing Success: Abandon Tradition Roles," a successful outsourcing case study at Brigham and Women's Hospital was outlined and clearly stated that the size of the specialist firm did matter: "We didn't want a mom-and-pop operation that couldn't match our volume and growth needs."[14]

In addition, before the agreement is executed, it might be relevant to inquire as to what the potential outsourcing partner would not be willing to do. The answer might reveal the firm's determination, drive, flexibility, and character. Weiner believes that a good vendor should be willing to do anything that improves the business. However, quantifying "anything" not listed in a written agreement is more than a little ambiguous and may introduce confusion and misunderstanding in the partner relationship. Applying a cost to "anything" has to be accretive to the outcome. Accretive is defined as growing in size by external addition, according to InvestorWords.com. If the organization asks the partnering firm to help grow the business at the expense of the partnering firm's margin, then the situation potentially becomes a win/lose relationship and the partnering firm will be forced to reduce services, exit prematurely, or drop back to the language of the contract. At this point, the partnership is almost sure to fail. Therefore, all expectations should be defined in a formal agreement and executed by both parties. If a request is made by the organization to the partnering firm, an amendment to the original agreement should be memorialized.

In the VHA study, 94% of respondents ranked "ongoing customer service and support" as key drivers in evaluating a supplier of services. It is important that resource provisions are clearly outlined in the contract, addressing such key points as management coverage for FMLA situations or other leaves of absence. It is not the hospital's responsibility to cover for the management firm when the employee(s) is/are out for training and other specialist firms' activities for extended periods or on a high frequency basis.

Potential Pitfalls of Outsourcing

To recap, healthcare spending in the United States is roughly $2.5 trillion, or about 17.6 percent of the U.S. economy, in 2009. President Barack Obama has signed into law the most comprehensive healthcare package since Lyndon B. Johnson's Medicare bill in 1965, creating the Medicare and Medicaid programs. The Patient Protection and Affordable Care Act of 2010 expands healthcare coverage to millions of Americans currently uninsured, addresses gaps in prescription drugs, and prevents insurance companies from denying coverage for pre-existing conditions. To pay for the bill, there will be increases and new taxes for a multitude of services and $500 billion in Medicare cuts. In addition, the Improper Payments Elimination and Recovery Act of 2010 is in the Senate and expected to pass. The President has already promised to sign it, and it is projected to recapture an additional $2 billion. These are on top of the American Recovery and Reinvestment Act of 2009, which requires providers to adopt certified electronic health record platforms estimated to cost $1 million to $5 million for installation and around $1 million annually for maintenance.[15] All of these new initiatives are intended to benefit the overall healthcare system by expanding coverage and arguably reducing provider's bad debt, providing better care through standardization by quantifying how patients are managed everywhere, and reducing wasteful spending, fraud, and unnecessary treatments.

These mandates will force hospitals to further focus on their core responsibility of providing patient care and cut costs on non-core functions by using specialist firms. Therefore, outsourcing appears to be a viable and growing solution for bridging the gap for hospitals into the next decade, at least.

However, there are potential concerns and pitfalls to outsourcing, particularly with clinical service lines and/or revenue centers as detailed in the HFMA publication "Possibilities and Pitfalls of Outsourcing, October 2005."[16]

Not-for-profit hospitals have been under fire including Provena Covenant Medical Center in Urbana, Illinois, where the facility lost a legal battle in Illinois Supreme Court over its tax-exempt status in part due to the use of for-profit outsourcing.[17,18]

Liability remains a major concern in the provision of care, as does the Stark and Anti Kickback

Act Safe Harbor Act. Callahan states that hospitals should at a minimum evaluate whether state or federal healthcare programs ultimately pay for any of the items or services provided. If they do, the hospital must ensure the agreement complies with the federal anti kick back statute.

From a Medicare fraud and abuse perspective, hospitals should maintain control or monitor utilization rates of procedures billed to providers that are driven by protocols "created" by an outsourcing firm. This is critical, as hospitals cannot delegate risk or liability of a for-profit entity's actions.

A good case example is the Adventist Health System Sunbelt Healthcare Corporation settling two whistleblower lawsuits that stemmed from overbilling Medicare for ambulance transports that were not medically necessary.[19] The Adventist system contracted with an outsourcing firm to operate and manage the ambulance service. According to then-spokesman Kevin Edgerton, "We contracted with an ambulance firm and relied on their expertise and it's evident our oversight was inadequate."

Hazelwood, et al. also list the ethical consideration of informing patients that their information is being outsourced. They also list confidentiality and HIPAA (Health Insurance Portability and Accountability Act of 1996) as big concerns or pitfalls. HIPAA requires entities that provide services to healthcare organizations, such as outsourcing vendors, to keep the information they receive confidential. These entities, which are considered business associates, include vendors such as a management company. HIPAA's privacy regulation requires that contracts with business associates contain specific provisions, such as what disclosures of information and permitted uses of the information the business associate may make. Contracts must also require that the business associate does not further disclose the information unless permitted by law. If a business associate uses a subcontractor, the subcontractor must abide by the same provisions as the original business associate. The contract should also specify that if a breach occurs, the contract will be terminated.

Despite precautions, breaches can occur. In 2003, the University of California, San Francisco Medical Center forwarded a portion of its transcription to its vendor, which has 15 subcontractors nationwide. UCSF had been working with the vendor for more than 2 decades without any problems. In this case, however, the work allegedly was subcontracted twice more, finally going out of the country. A payment dispute among the subcontractors led to a threat (never carried out) to expose patient records. No breach of patient privacy occurred, although the situation illustrates the major risks related to contracting out work without diligence in determining who has access to the information.[16]

From an EMTALA standpoint, what happens if the hospital or management company knowingly, willingly, or negligently violates the EMTALA statute? The Emergency Medical Treatment and Active Labor Act is a statute which governs the emergency evaluation and treatment of patients who present to a hospital campus. EMTALA was passed as part of the Consolidated Omnibus Budget Reconciliation Act of 1986, and it is sometimes referred to as "the COBRA law," or Section 1867(a) of the Social Security Act. It is included as part of the section of the U.S. Code which governs Medicare.

EMTALA applies only to "participating hospitals" i.e., hospitals that have entered into "provider agreements" under which they will accept payment from the Department of Health and Human Services, Centers for Medicare and Medicaid Services (CMS) under the Medicare program for services provided to beneficiaries of that program. In practical terms, this means that it applies to virtually all hospitals in the United States.

Maintaining scope of practice, terminology used by state licensing boards for various professions defines the procedures, actions, and processes that are permitted for the licensed individual. The scope of practice is limited to that which the law allows for specific education, experience, and specific demonstrated competency. Each state has laws, licensing bodies, and regulations that describe requirements for education and training. It is important that the contracted parties agree upon the scope and not work outside of their scope and introduce liability. Each side is held responsible for the other side's actions.

A good case example was when a patient who had been diving in the Gulf of Mexico suffered severe decompression illness and went to the nearest emergency room, which was known to have a hyperbaric unit. Once arrived, he was denied access to the chamber because it was after hours and the chamber was not operated 24/7. By time he was shipped to a facility that could treat him, his condition had deteriorated to the point of paraplegia. In turn, he sued the facility for delay of treatment and was awarded a large settlement mainly due to the fact that the scope of practice did not state they were not a 24/7 operation.[20] Strictly defining a scope of practice and maintaining those guidelines will shield both parties from hours of unnecessary litigation.

Conclusion

The U.S. wound care burden is enormous and there will be continued focus by providers, payers, and government agencies to curb spending while improving the care model. It is also a large business and companies will continue to flow into the marketplace to serve the needs of patients, providers, and in some cases, themselves– buyer beware.

There were approximately 800 organized wound care programs managed by wound care outsourcing firms, and approximately 1200 wound care programs located in hospitals both outsourced and insourced in the U.S. in 2008. This indicates that there is still opportunity in the marketplace for growth, since there were 5,700 hospitals in 2007.

Existing environmental factors will continue to make outsourcing an attractive option for healthcare organizations as they attempt to become more trim and efficient. Both cost reduction and the value of a specialists firm's resources are keys to achieving those goals. Depending on whether the department is a revenue center or cost center will dictate which factor is the primary driver for outsourcing, according to Glidewell.

While the predictions of healthcare outsourcing growth are prevalent in many publications, it is also clear that healthcare institutions will use the current economic environment to realign current outsourced agreements. It is unlikely that hospitals will forego breaches of the service company's obligations.[21,22]

After determining that outsourcing is required, Callahan recommends the following tips for success.

- Compare apples to apples
- Pay attention to the agreements
- Hire a professional
- Hold them accountable
- Watch out for hidden charges
- Don't forget HIPAA
- Remember your employees
- Leave yourself an out
- Keep Uncle Sam happy
- Don't rush it

References

1. http://www.cdc.gov/diabetes/pubs/references07.htm National Diabetes Fact Sheet, Unites States 2007
2. Centers for Medicare and Medicaid Services, Office of the Actuary, National Health Statistics Group; U.S. Department of Commerce, Bureau of Economic Analysis and U.S. Bureau of the Census. NHE Web Tables 1, 2, 6. http://www.cms.hhs.gov/NationalHealthExpend Data/downloads/tables.pdf.
3. The Henry J. Kaiser Family Foundation. Trends in Health Care Costs and Spending Fact Sheet September 2007.
4. Itchue, M. Hospitals Ill From More Bad Debt, Credit troubles, December 28, 2008. http://www.mlive.com/health/index.ssf/2008/12/hospitals_ill_from_more_bad_de.html
5. American Hospital Association, "Hospital Statistics," 2007 & 2009 Editions, Chicago: Health Forum LLC 2008.
6. Deloitte Center for Health Sciences. 2009 Industry Outlook: Health Sciences Challenging Times, Emerging Opportunities. http://www.deloitte.com/view/en_US/us/search/index.htm?searchKeywordsField=hospital+upgrades&searchKeywordsFieldDefault=Search
7. Beggs, B. American Laundry News, 11/14/2008. Survey: Laundry Remains Most-outsourced Hospital Department.
8. VHA inc. 2007 Services Contracting Survey.
9. Global Sourcing Trends in 2009, Morrison and Foerster, LLC. http://www.mofo.com/docs/pdf/GlobalSourcingTrends2009.pdf
10. Modern Healthcare, 2009 Outsourcing Survey – Top 20 Hospital Department Management Categories.
11. DeJohn, P. When Outsourcing Works: Know When Vendor Intervention can be a Benefit or Hindrance. Materials Management in Health Care. www.matmanag.com.
12. Paine, T.G, Milne, C.T., et al. The AAWC Conceptual Framework of Quality Systems for Wound Care. Ostomy Wound Management, Vol 52, Issue 11.
13. Callahan, J.M, 10 practical tips for successful outsourcing: horror stories about vendors keep many hospitals from capitalizing on the benefits of outsourcing unnecessarily. Know how to prepare for contract negotiations can help you optimize those relationships. Healthcare Financial Management, Sept, 2005.
14. Rosenthal, B.E., Editor. RX for Healthcare Outsourcing Success: Abandon Tradition Roles, Outsourcing Journal, September 2007.
15. Wise, P.B. The Meaning of Meaningful Use: Several Technology Applications Are Needed to Qualify, Healthcare Executive Magazine. Vol 25, No 3 May/June 2010. American College of Healthcare Executives, Chicago, IL.
16. Hazelwood, S.E., Hazelwood, A.C., Cook, E.D. HFMA publication of the Possibilities and Pitfalls of Outsourcing, October 2005.
17. Hylak-Reinholtz, J. Provena Covenant Medical Center and Its Unresolved Tax-Exempt Status–It's Time for the Illinois Supreme Court to Revise the MethodistOld People's Home Test, 2008. www.works.bepress.com/cgi/viewcontentcgi?article=1000&context=joseph_hylak_reinholtz
18. Blesch, G. Supreme Court rules against Provena. Modern Healthcare Online Mar 18, 2010.
19. Taylor, M. Transporting trouble; Ambulance contracts give Fla. System a rough ride. Modern Healthcare, April 11, 2005.
20. Delegal, M.K., Gorrie, J., Healthcare Risk Management, Mar 1, 2001 Tallahassee, FL.
21. Millstein, J.S., Roughton, T. Outsourcing and the Economic Crises, Part II:Re-structuring Existing Outsourcings. December 2008. http://www.mofo.com/news/updates/bulletins/15024.html.
22. Tholons Top 10 Trends for Global Outsourcing in 2009. http://www.mmdnewswire.com/tholons-announces-top-10-trends-for-global-outsourcing-in-2009-4388-2.html.

CHAPTER

5

Operational Management of Comprehensive Wound Care and Hyperbaric Centers

Valerie Larson-Lohr, RN and James Strain

Thirty years ago heralded the advent of the first wound centers, and with it recognition that a chronic wound is metabolically different than an acute wound. As the knowledge of chronic wounds grew, so did the number of wound centers, the complexities of treatments, the recognition of comprehensive wound care as a specialty, and the challenges of reimbursement. Today, there are hundreds of comprehensive wound centers in operation serving an ever-growing number of patients with chronic wounds. The majority of the wound centers in operation today are centers that are operated in a partnership between a hospital and one of the many outsourced management companies. Amongst these wound centers, even within the same outsourced management company, there is a broad diversity of success, both clinically and financially. What makes the difference between success and failure? Can we define those aspects and replicate the successful ones? In our experience, the answers are yes, we can define the differences that make a successful center from one that is not, and yes, we have been able to replicate the success.

In this chapter, we are going to discuss those aspects that have been successful and those things to avoid. We hope to trigger a thoughtful process that will lead to success either for a brand new wound center or one that is being reshaped. We challenge you to think outside the box and to identify new aspects to success as this industry of healthcare and chronic wound management grows and changes.

Developmental Considerations for a Wound Care Center

The design considerations given to a potential wound care center (WCC) are paramount and contribute to the overall success of the new WCC. There are many factors that should be evaluated in detail to ensure the optimal balance is achieved between the size, cost, and overall efficiency of a potential center. The preplanning and evaluation prior to construction will produce a center layout that maximizes the overall efficiency in which the wound care staff operates on a daily basis.

Wound Center Site Selection

In the design phase, the first thing to determine is where the wound center should be placed. Will it occupy previously used space that needs to be reconfigured, or will the area be raw space in which to design without previous limitations? In selecting the site, serious attention needs to be paid to the available square footage. For efficient flow of patients, 2500 square feet should be a starting point. This size square footage could easily accommodate 2 to 3 hyperbaric chambers and 6 to 7 treatment rooms. If the vision is for 4 hyperbaric chambers and 9 to 10 rooms, then the needed square footage is in the 5000 square foot range.

The next question in site selection is whether the center will be within a healthcare facility or freestanding. In determining this, 2 questions need to be considered. The first question is, what is the mission of the WCC? Is the mission to only treat chronic wounds, or will the WCC also treat more emergent conditions that require hyperbaric oxygen therapy (such as carbon monoxide poisoning, decompression sickness, acute thermal burns, and gas gangrene)? If the decision is to maintain a mission of only chronic wound management, then either freestanding or within a healthcare facility would be appropriate. If the mission is also to care for emergent hyperbaric conditions, then the WCC is mandated to be within the confines of a healthcare facility.

Another design consideration is where the oxygen farm is currently located and the distance to pipe to the WCC. Hyperbaric chambers receive their oxygen from a high-flow liquid oxygen source. Copper tubing supplies the oxygen from the oxygen farm to the WCC. Long oxygen pipes running in excess of 300 feet should be avoided where possible, given their high initial installation cost. In other words, the greater the distance to the oxygen farm, the greater the cost to supply oxygen for the hyperbaric chambers.

Specific Interior Design Considerations

The design and layout of the WCC is critical to efficient use of staff, flow of patients, and productivity of the center. Local, state, and federal building codes will dictate some of the center design and layout process, but the following are general considerations found to contribute to successful flow and productivity.

In determining the number of patient treatment rooms, look to the vision of where the WCC will be in 1, 2, and 5 years. Don't think, "start slow and see what happens." Plan for the growth and be able to accommodate the patient flow. In addressing specifics of treatment rooms, each patient treatment room should be 120 square feet. This allows space for patients to enter by a variety of transportation modes, such as oversize wheelchairs, motorized wheelchairs, and gurneys. Cabinets selected for treatment rooms should be of adequate width. Cabinets should be at least 4 feet in width and contain a single-sink basin, although a dual-basin sink would be optimal. Each treatment room needs at least one overhead cabinet, typically above the sink area. More overhead space is preferred for stocking of patient treatment supplies, as this improves the overall staff efficiency and can reduce time spent in supply retrieval.

Storage, office space, and ancillary spaces are necessary and can use a large portion of allocated WCC space. Medical supply closets should be located in close proximity to the actual treatment rooms. Clean and dirty utility rooms, laundry, and medical record space should be placed with ease of staff access in mind. Once again, look for features that will increase staff efficiency and improve productivity within the center.

Office space within a WCC should also be strategically located in order to provide ease of access to the clinic and allow managers to monitor the daily activities of the clinic. Typically, a WCC has a Program Director/Manager, RN Clinical Coordinator/Manager, and a Medical Director. For WCC staff to manage the demanding need of their primary and ancillary job responsibilities, it is optimal for each to have a dedicated office space. The typical office for the Program Director/Manager would be approximately 120 square feet, allowing for a small conference table to be placed in the room for staff meetings. The Medical Director and Clinical Coordinator offices should also be located close to the clinical treatment rooms and typically would be 75 square feet or larger, depending on available space.

Hyperbaric Chamber Space Considerations

The design consideration for any hyperbaric chamber area will be driven, in part, using the guidance from the National Fire Protection Act

(NFPA) as well as the local, state, and federal agencies, and American Institute of Architects (AIA) guidelines. These agencies govern the mandated requirements and considerations for the safety of the facility, given the space and the type of hyperbaric chambers being used within the facility.

If the hyperbaric chamber to be installed is a multiplace chamber, design features and regulatory requirements are complex and will not be addressed in this section. Monoplace hyperbaric chambers are also regulated, but design features are less complex.

The size of the hyperbaric room will largely be dictated by the number of monoplace hyperbaric chambers. Once again, plan for where you will be down the road and plumb for the number you will need then. You do not have to start with the full complement of chambers, as long as the space has been designed to accommodate the growth. Renovation costs generally prohibit the expansion of the hyperbaric facility, once the initial space is completed.

Technology

Evolving technologies need to be considered in the WCC design. Currently, there is a trend to move towards electronic medical records and imaging technologies that will require computers, terminals, printers, routers, etc. How this is designed and integrated will be dictated by how the center is interfaced with a hospital's Information Technology (IT) department. Technology, infrastructure, and wiring should be planned upon during the design phase to support existing and future infrastructure needs. Each treatment room and office space should, at a minimum, have data and voice capability infrastructure wiring. Possible future needs could include the capability of video-wiring, as well. It is much more cost-effective to set the facility up for any anticipated technology needs at the onset, versus the cost to retrofit a facility once it is in operation.

Finally, do not underestimate the value of materials selected to finish a center. This determines the overall aesthetic appeal. Finishing material can vary greatly in price, so once again careful consideration should be placed on striking a balance between the aesthetic value and the overall cost to complete the center. Some materials will have a higher installation cost; however, some of these finish materials can reduce the overall amount of maintenance cost over the life of the facility.

Creation and Selection of a Physician Panel

Wound centers have had two main physician models: the panel model where coverage of the center is done by a group of physicians based on specialty of primary practice, and the single physician model. The reasons for choosing one model over the other are varied and have engendered a passion for one or the other.

The Multi-Physician Panel

The multi-physician model was pioneered by Curative Wound Centers. It was designed to be a core of specialists that not only served the wound patients referred to the center, but also brought a variety of the physicians' own patients from their private practice into a wound center. Routinely, the panel models would include general, vascular, plastic and orthopedic surgeons, podiatrists, and an internal medicine physician. Physicians would have their own clinics which were either from 0800 to 1200 or 1300 to 1630 once or twice each week. If a patient was evaluated by a plastic surgeon and required an assessment by a vascular surgeon, then the patient would be scheduled into the vascular surgeon's clinic time. The multi-physician model put into practice the concept of being able to come to a single clinic with the ability to see any specialist that was needed to deliver comprehensive wound care. This model has been used both successfully and unsuccessfully over the last 25 years. In order for this model to be successful, practitioners need to have a good understanding of the inherent weaknesses of the model.

Perception of the physicians practicing in this model is that of a vascular, plastic or general surgeon who does wound care. This is a true perception, as the physicians in this model maintain practices in their original specialty. Depending on the professional culture of the practice community, this may or may not hinder referrals into the program.

The next area deals with the complexities of the patients who have chronic, non-healing wounds. These patients can require a great deal of follow-up and coordination of care. With a physician holding only one four-hour clinic per week, another mechanism would need to be in place to compensate. This has frequently been the case management model of nursing.

Program ownership by physicians may be a problem, depending on how the individual clinics are structured, and whether the physicians practicing within the wound center are from the same physician practice group or many groups. This can be reflected in inconsistencies in following established practice guidelines of the clinic, such as arriving late, leaving early for an individual clinic, or canceling a clinic when patients are scheduled, requiring rescheduling of patients, which leads to patient dissatisfaction. Additionally, there can be a deficit in complete physician documentation that can contribute to reimbursement denials.

In order for the multi-physician model to work successfully within a comprehensive wound center, a strategy should be developed prior to implementation that addresses the inherent weaknesses of this model and methodology for excellent communication established.

The Single Physician Model

The majority of time, this does not involve a single physician, but rather two physicians that share coverage. Generally, one physician will work the majority of the time with the second physician as back-up. This model is becoming increasingly common as chronic wound management is coming into its own as a physician specialty. The lead physician's sole practice is the wound center, so they are able to carry the mantle as wound specialist, not a physician who has a weekly wound clinic. This can be an important factor in many communities. If it is a community of specialists, the referral pattern is to use a specialist in wound care. Additionally, depending on the physician density of the area, return of patients to the primary referring physician can be especially important. If the physician's sole practice is chronic wound management, there can be less of a perceived threat of patients not being returned to the referring physician after the wound has healed.

It has been noted in centers that utilize the single physician model that there is more consistency of care, with improved follow up, and the case management model of nursing is not required. Additionally, as it is the physician's sole practice, the single physician model promotes commitment and involvement in all aspect of the wound center operation by the physician.

Recruitment of the Wound Specialist Physician

Over the 25+ year history of outpatient wound centers, a pattern had developed for physician recruitment into the wound center. In the early years, the medical director position was frequently given for political or influence reasons. The hospital administrator may invite a particular physician to be the medical director of the wound center in the belief this physician can bring other physicians on board to use the service, or he/she can bring many of their private patients into the wound center. Or the converse may be true, in that if a particular physician was not invited to be the medical director, they would remove their patients or practice from the hospital. Throughout the mid-1990s into the mid-2000s, surgeons were primarily recruited. The rationale behind this recruitment was twofold; the first is surgeons knew how to debride, and it would not be a problem getting the clinical debridements performed on the patients; and secondly, surgeons already practiced acute wound care, so the transfer to working with chronic wounds should be smooth. The 2000s have also seen a difference in the perspective of the work performed in a wound center. Many practitioners saw chronic wound management as a place to slow down, and possibly a good practice area to become involved in when they retire.

As the industry has been able to look at history and see what works and what doesn't, we now know that the previous methods of physician recruitment were flawed. The physician that leads the wound center today must become the "champion" for the center. While political appointments still exist, the economic environment today requires that the center be financially viable, as well as provide good clinical outcomes. This requires a higher level of commitment and leadership on the part of the physician. The physician leader needs to have the ability to manage the chronic wound patient and the process that is associated with successful outcomes. They have to be team-oriented and able to work closely with both the clinical coordinator and program director on a variety of processes, and be able to understand and manage the business of running a financially viable center. A successful wound center is a physically and mentally demanding practice for a physician. It is not a place to slow down or retire, particularly in the role of medical director. The physician choosing to become the medical director will need to have a full view of the scope of the responsibilities, both in the administrative and the medical arena. This can be achieved through observation and discussion with successful medical directors, through a job description that lays out the scope of responsibilities (see Appendix 1), and open discussions with the hospital administrator and program director.

Education of the Wound Specialists

Today there is an abundance of literature that demonstrates the marked differences in acute wound management and chronic wound management. The previous assumption that a physician who practices acute wound management can freely move to chronic wound management without additional training, both didactic and clinical, is erroneous. Today, any healthcare provider who works in this specialty needs to have specific classroom and clinical practice training in order to understand and become competent in this specialty. The educational course chosen by the physician should be one that is recognized by a national organization that represents and accredits wound care and hyperbaric courses. Generally, these courses are 5 to 6 day training events. This should be followed by a period of clinical practicum. There are a variety of fellowships and mentorships available to physicians who wish to make the transition to chronic wound management.

Staffing of Comprehensive Wound Centers

Selection of Key Center Positions

Today, in a comprehensive wound clinic which offers hyperbaric oxygen therapy, it is generally agreed that the four key positions are the Program Director, Clinical Coordinator, Hyperbaric Safety Director and Medical Director. These four positions must be able to work closely together and form the senior leadership of the wound center.

Over the last 25+ years of outpatient wound center operations, the role of Program Director has been filled by nurses, business majors, healthcare administrators, respiratory therapists, physical therapists, and hyperbaric technicians. Every hospital, center, or management company has been looking for the right mix of characteristics in an individual to fill this role. It has been difficult, as each of the professions previously named have some of the strengths required, but are also lacking in experience in other areas. The individual filling the role of Program Director needs to be able to understand the clinical aspects, understand the business aspects, be able to market and lead a diverse group of professionals working within the center, communicate well at a variety of levels, and excel at multitasking. When you add a management company into the mix, the individual chosen for the position of Program Director will truly understand the meaning of the term "middle management." This is a difficult role to step into for the first time unless the new Program Director has the benefit of a strong, supportive mentoring system. The ideal situation is for the new Program Director to be paired with an experienced Program Director for the first year and learn from an individual practicing in that role.

The Clinical Coordinator is the clinical leader for the staff of the comprehensive wound center. This person must be able to work closely with the Program Director and the Medical Director. The Clinical Coordinator position implements and assures clinical excellence, while assisting the Program Director to assure financial viability. The Clinical Coordinator is a registered nurse who has a background in operating a busy outpatient clinic, management of staff with a variety of skill levels, and experience in chronic wound management. This position is both a direct care and a supervisor position. One of the most difficult aspects of the Clinical Coordinator is to marry clinical care and financial responsibility. Every clinic is exposed to an array of companies offering new innovations to chronic wound management. Many have a valid benefit. Unfortunately, most of these products are also costly, without added reimbursement for their use in the clinic. The temptation is there to give the new items a trial, but care needs to be taken to balance the financial aspects with the clinical benefit.

The Medical Director position is the one position that can either make a successful wound clinic or lead to its demise. Great care should be taken in the selection of the candidate to fill this position. Further discussion on this position can be found in the "Physicians and Physician Panels" section.

The Safety Director is a technician who is experienced in staffing a hyperbaric center and has successfully completed certification for a Hyperbaric Technician, as well as a Safety Director course. The Safety Director works closely with both the program director and medical director to assure the operations of the hyperbaric aspect is in compliance with NFPA, PVHO, and other state/local regulations, plans and implements a hyperbaric oxygen therapy safety program that includes staff education, staff competency, and chamber maintenance. This is a critical position, as it pertains to safety and hyperbaric education of the staff. Unfortunately, there is a current nationwide shortage of personnel trained and experienced in this area. An alternative to experience is a 2 to 4 week training period in an established center with an experienced Safety Director. This training relationship would then move into a mentoring relationship until the new Safety Director is comfortable in the role.

After the key positions are filled, the remainder of the staff is comprised of RNs, LVNs/LPNS, HBO technicians, nurses' aides, unit secretaries, and intake persons. The mix will be dictated by state licensing agencies and patient population. Some comprehensive wound centers are strictly outpatient centers, while others see both inpatients and outpatients. The centers that treat inpatients have a tendency towards higher acuity patients and would need a heavier mix of RNs and LVNs in the staffing ratio.

While previous successful wound center experience is always desired, there is no consensus with selecting individuals without successful wound center experience. Personal experience has lead to selecting nursing staff from busy acute care medical-surgical units or other robust clinic environments. Assessment skills are well developed in these nurses and they are able to handle the pace of a busy wound center. For selection of technical staff, certified nurses' aides have become successful in this role. They are accustomed to working in a facility environment doing patient care. I have not seen the adaptation issues with CNAs as with staff, such as EMTs or paramedics that are used to working in the field making autonomous decisions. While you will find little agreement on the type of experience, individual characteristics leading to success have been identified. Team oriented individuals with the ability to multitask and highly motivated self starters with the willingness to learn will have the greatest opportunity for success and be the most satisfied with their area of employment.

New staff coming into a comprehensive wound environment for the first time will require education in this specialty in order to be successful. Like any specialty, however, a week-long training course will not produce a trained specialist; it will only be the beginning of the journey of learning. The training of hyperbaric personnel can be challenging from a couple perspectives. First, the individual is learning a new language. While experienced hyperbaric staffs easily think in terms of gas laws, psig, fsw, and barotrauma, for the inexperienced staff, they see a jumble of letters with difficult-to-envision relationships. The second challenge is the technical, regulated nature of clinical hyperbaric medicine. While the NFPA, state, and PVHO regulations and codes are part of the everyday life in a wound center with hyperbaric chambers, it can be intimidating and difficult to understand for the new staff. It will take time and mentoring for inexperienced staff to become competent practitioners. Ongoing training and education should be a routine part of comprehensive wound center operations, and certifications in both hyperbaric and chronic wound care should be strongly encouraged. Today in many centers, certifications are used as baseline of staff competency, and when certifying organizations inspect a facility, they are looking for the number of certified staff.

The next question is how to best utilize the staff and the methodology for determining the number of full time employee (FTEs) to staff the wound center. First is utilization. Experience has shown that the most efficient use of staff and to provide thorough coverage of the center, all staff should be cross trained and rotate through the positions. Cross training has the added benefits of building a more cohesive team, allowing the staff to have a more in-depth understanding of the multiple roles within the center and prevents the thought of "it not being my job" to enter into the process. Staff cohesion can be a challenge in comprehensive wound centers that utilize hyperbaric oxygen if staffs are not cross trained and rotate in the different roles. It is not uncommon for the wound care only side to perceive the hyperbaric staff isn't working hard as they glance over and see them sitting at the chamber. It can easily become a "we against them" scenario. Great benefit is demonstrated by having staff walk in each other's shoes on a regular basis.

The next issue with staff utilization occurs when patient volume exceeds the typical 8 hour day. There are a couple different solutions depending on how high the patient volume is and whether it is consistently at this level. If the volume is not consistently outside the 8 hour day, then temporarily lengthening staff's hours may be the easiest solution. It is recommended that what was commonly known as the "hyperbaric waiting list" method not be used, as it puts the patient at risk if hyperbaric therapy is really a needed option, and it can send the message that it is only done at the convenience of the wound center. The other method is to move to 10 hour days. Clinical staff works four 10 hour days per week, allowing them a day off during the week to take care of personal appointments, etc. In our experience, staff morale is much higher, burnout is lower, fewer sick calls are made, and overtime very low. The staffs are positive when they come to work and that is reflected in the care of the patients. It has been a successful methodology for us for the past 10 years.

One of the greatest challenges a director of a comprehensive wound center has is to determine the number of staff to care for a certain number of patients. The majority of other hospital departments have an array of nursing productivity tools that reflect both the acuity of the patients and the work of the staff, translating into the number of FTEs. If you look at the limited tools available to wound centers, the tools look only at productivity and just at the wound care portion, not the hyperbaric oxygen therapy treatments. In 2002, we began an extensive time study/patient acuity project to develop a tool that reflected both acuity and productivity, and to include hyperbaric oxygen treatments as well as wound care. In 2003, we published the first report of the initial tool developed to assess acuity and productivity in wound care and hyperbaric centers. Patient classifications were created to define acuity based on disease and associated procedures. The initial tool had 38 distinct indicators identified for wound care and 22 for hyperbaric oxygen therapy. The tool was further tested in urban and rural wound care centers in 2004. Additional distinct indicators were identified. These indicators were timed and weighted and returned to the field for further testing. The revised tool has over 500 patient acuity days in testing and has been examined for content validity and clinical applicability. The tool was not designed to be used as a daily tool, but as a benchmarking tool to be run on an as needed basis to determine if there had been a change in either patient acuity or FTE requirements1. The tool can be found in Appendix 2.

Developing Marketing Strategies

The marketing aspects of having a financially viable wound center can be underrated, overrated, or entirely forgotten, depending on your professional perspective. For the most part, physicians and nurses in the wound center will not have a marketing strategies focus. Their primary focus is delivering care to the patients and providing positive outcomes for those patients. This is as it should be, for while being successful at their jobs, they are accomplishing the first part of a marketing strategy -- providing a product.

The Product of Comprehensive Wound Care

Often in the development and opening of a new wound center, marketing strategy focuses on selling the product of a comprehensive wound care center when in reality, a complete product frequently isn't present. A new wound center may open with practice guidelines in place, policies and procedures, newly trained nursing and physician staff and equipment, but often the clinical staff is new to chronic wound management and lacks in experience and practical application. This is the dilemma. How do you market a product, such as a comprehensive wound center, when it is too new to exist? You have to choose the staff well, selecting physicians who want to become chronic wound specialists, provide not only classroom education, but intensive hands-on experience for all staff, while acknowledging the new wound center is an incomplete product and will need much support during the first year of operation.

Knowing the Culture

Knowing the culture of your demographic base is essential to a successful marketing strategy. Don't look at the numbers first, look at the culture. While it is easy to see the difference between urban versus rural areas, it will take more insight to see the difference between urban vs. urban and rural vs. rural. Start by tapping into colleagues who have marketed in the area where the comprehensive wound center will open. Learn current referral patterns- not only who refers to whom, but why they refer to that hospital, clinic, or physician. Positive established referral patterns are just as important as the established negative referral patterns. Are there any practice groups, clinics, or hospitals that key groups do not refer to? Always ask why. Can these referral patterns be changed, and where in the mix will the new comprehensive wound center be placed? Are there any "invisible" lines that may divide the area? These 'invisible" lines may not make rational sense to an outsider, but may be born of habit, fear, economic, or racial attitudes. These will be the most difficult to change. Next, learn how the professionals within your catchment area like to receive information and what is effective. While a large group may come for an expensive steak dinner, they may not refer any patients afterwards. What may be most effective is developing ways to keep the referring physicians abreast of what is occurring with their patient(s). This can be through a fax that lets them know an appointment has been scheduled for their patient, communicating plan of care on the day of the visit, updates during their treatment, and a healed letter which indicates the length of time until the wound was healed. This way, it is easy for the referring physician to see results and to see that their patient has been returned to their practice. Third, develop your own network within the community. Examples would be joining the Rotary, Case Manager Society, WOCN, local medical societies, Chamber of Commerce, etc. Be a presence. Be visible at community events, professional meetings, and other events where you will be seen as the wound expert. People are more likely to refer to someone they know rather than someone they do not, and these are opportunities for the community to get to know you.

Evaluate your Resources

Is your comprehensive wound center within the framework of a hospital that already has a track record of successful marketing, or are you in an environment that has limited resources? If you work for a contract service, what resources can they provide to assist your efforts?

If you are working within the framework of a hospital that recognizes and promotes successful marketing strategies, your first step is to become integrated into the team. Take the time to listen, learn, ask questions, and be introduced into the community. This is a powerful mechanism to open doors and enables you to present the product of comprehensive wound care. Remember, you are also a fresh set of eyes on the scene. After you have time to look at the established processes, you may see opportunities that were not previously recognized.

If you work with a contract service that provides marketing and educational material, spend some time reviewing the material and determining what will work in your community and when you should implement the different pieces. There are a few standard pieces that are helpful to have available. Brochures with a general overview of hyperbaric medicine and chronic wound management are the first pieces. One brochure should be designated for providers with brief, referenced statements. Remember to have the direct telephone and fax numbers for the wound center. The second brochure should be patient focused, easy to read, with appropriate contact numbers and a statement on insurances and self referrals. White papers or newsletters that focus on a specific diagnosis, such as osteoradionecrosis, can be an excellent resource for providers who want focused information they can immediately use with their patient population. These white papers or newsletters need to be referenced and clearly written. The third item

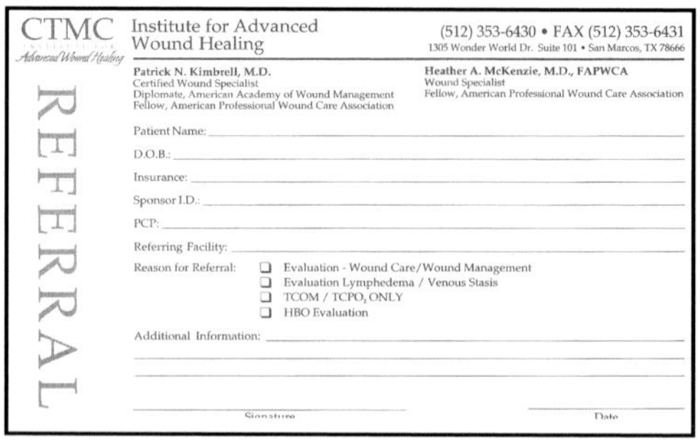
CTMC Institute for Advanced Wound Healing
Institute for Advanced Wound Healing
(512) 353-6430 • FAX (512) 353-6431
1305 Wonder World Dr. Suite 101 • San Marcos, TX 78666

REFERRAL

Patrick N. Kimbrell, M.D.
Certified Wound Specialist
Diplomate, American Academy of Wound Management
Fellow, American Professional Wound Care Association

Heather A. McKenzie, M.D., FAPWCA
Wound Specialist
Fellow, American Professional Wound Care Association

Patient Name: ______
D.O.B.: ______
Insurance: ______
Sponsor I.D.: ______
PCP: ______
Referring Facility: ______
Reason for Referral:
- ❑ Evaluation - Wound Care/Wound Management
- ❑ Evaluation Lymphedema / Venous Stasis
- ❑ TCOM / TCPO, ONLY
- ❑ HBO Evaluation

Additional Information: ______

Signature ______ Date ______

Figure 1: ***Referral.***

considered standard is a referral or prescription pad for the wound center (see an example in Figure 1). The referring provider can quickly fill it out and either fax directly to the wound center or give to the patient to make their appointment. This makes a referral quick and easy. The remainder of your marketing and education selection should be based on what your current target is and how it affects the methodology, and this is for your community.

Strategy: Targeting your Education

There are many different strategies that can be learned from marketing texts and other health-related fields such as the pharmaceutical industry. I approach marketing strategy by first focusing on what I would want as a consumer. What would be important to me if I was either the patient or the referrer? Most basic is excellent customer service. Components of excellent customer service are: an appointment in a reasonable length of time, such as 1-3 days, ease of referring a patient, staff that understands the variety of insurances and could assist the patient and family, friendly professional staff, clean environment, excellent reputation in healing difficult wounds, and a good value for my dollar. What I have just described is the "product" of comprehensive wound care or excellent customer service.

The next step is who we are going to tell about the product. The first logical response is the physicians who have chronic wound patients. This touches just about every medical specialty, along with dentists, oral surgeons, nurse practitioners, physician assistants, and podiatrists. The key to being successful here is to know your product and develop a relationship with the referral coordinator, office manager, nurse, or whoever the gatekeeper is for the office.

The next group is not as clear. One option is to look at service providers that would share common patients. These would be home health, skilled nursing facilities, acute care facilities transitioning inpatients to outpatients, and other care centers. While there may be many patients who could benefit from a wound center, this is where an understanding of the current reimbursement environment is needed. An outpatient wound facility may not be able to receive Medicare payment from a patient in a skilled nursing facility. Know your current reimbursement rules of insurance and Medicare as you determine which service providers to target.

The other option would be the insurance companies and the case managers. This is an underdeveloped target market. What strategies could be used to approach and successfully develop the referral patterns? The first step is to determine what key factors or needs there are for these entities. Generally speaking, insurance companies are looking for excellent outcomes, satisfied customers, good value for the dollar, and return to work as soon as possible. Then analyze your program. Can you provide your outcomes for the different disease classes, such as venous disease, diabetes, etc.? Do you know what your average cost is to heal each category of patients? One focus of insurances is to compare different wound centers. For instance, Center A is able to heal most of the patients in 12 weeks at an average cost of $5000. Center B is able to heal the same group in 8 weeks at the cost of $3000. Both sets of patients are satisfied with their care. Which center do you think the insurance and case managers are going to direct their patients to for their chronic wound care? Before you approach this group of potential referrers, make sure you have a solid track record of positive outcomes and controlled costs (see Table 1).

Finally, the last target group is the general public. Nothing is more powerful than a "word of mouth" referral. Today, through access to the Internet, the general public is well informed and there is an abundance of different websites that provide a "report card" type function. This includes Medicare. Be aware of any websites offering report card features for your wound center and/or hospital. If something is reported in error, inquire as to mechanisms to have a correction done. If you have a negative report, acknowledge it and work to improve. Some of the most powerful actions are accepting responsibility for missing the mark and committing to improve.

When a patient makes it into your wound center, you have several opportunities to make the impression of "WOW". That "WOW" impression is what generates the word of mouth. It is not just doing it right, but really hitting the mark. The opportunities can be as simple as greeting the patient with a smile upon arrival, closing the patient door for privacy, asking if the patient has questions, and then taking the time to teach, and when the healed patient is discharged, asking the patient to refer his friends and family if they should have a wound that doesn't heal. It is the accumulation of the little things that will make the patient remember their experience and speak about it positively.

Table 1: ***Ingredients to Partnering with Payers***

• Cost	Cost per visit $34
• Healing	Demonstrate reliable outcomes over at least 6 months
• Healed	89%, Median Days to Heal 21
• Trust	Build trust with private practices Majority of patients are scheduled during 1st referral call Provide reliable follow-up status reporting
• Workflow	Get all referrals in to see the doctor within 36 hours of the referral call
• Workload	Minimize case manager paperwork/burden: must demonstrate this during due diligence
• Productivity	Patient to have minimal waiting time and good interactions with staff

Setting clinical and operational expectations

As the plans for a comprehensive wound center are developed, clinical and operational expectations need to be established. If the wound center is opened by a management company, most of the established companies have clinical expectations, as well as operational expectations, built into their plans. If the comprehensive wound center is opened independent of a management company, then consideration to setting these expectations should begin in the planning stages.

Clinical Expectations

Clinical expectations can be derived from expert experience, use of national resources, and a focus on the mission of comprehensive wound center practice. Experience in managing chronic wounds and an in-depth understanding of mechanisms that have caused the wound to cease the healing progression are needed in order to logically understand what can be done and where the expectations should be set. There are several national resources, such as WOCN, UHMS, CMS, as well as commissions that publish national standards and expectations on outcomes, median days to heal per specific diagnosis, percent of outliers, etc. The mission of most chronic wound centers is to develop a center of excellence that enables a focused approach to restoring the body's ability to heal wounds which surpasses the general medical community's ability. In combining these three concepts, your clinical expectations will emerge.

Which expectations should be established? First are your outcomes and how you measure and track them. It is important that you are able to communicate to your patients, referrers, and insurances how long it takes, on an average, to heal a specific type of wound that is cared for within the wound center. Patients are more educated today and look for facilities that can provide positive results. The physician or case manager who refers to your center is looking to see if you are able to heal the patients' wounds better than a less expensive community option, and if the patients are satisfied with the care your wound center delivers. Insurance carriers are looking for the satisfied patient, as well as a decrease in cost. The decrease in cost is not necessarily the cheapest care, but can also be a reasonable cost of care, but in a shorter healing time.

What are the other aspects that go hand in hand with clinical outcomes? Measurements that can impact your outcomes are median days to heal, outliers, the number of encounters per patient, and the number of clinical debridements per patient. All of these components are part of what will make outstanding outcomes or can reveal why your outcomes are not where they should be.

Performance improvement, by any of the several methodologies (see Chapter 17) should be an active part of your clinical outcomes. Staff should be encouraged to bring forth ideas for areas needing improvement and be an integral part of the solution. Select those areas that can have the greatest impact on the clinical or operational success and will push the wound center towards excellence. Avoid the trap of selecting an area just for the sake of having a performance improvement project identified because is it required; make it an area that has meaning to your center.

Operational Expectations

Operational expectations are a reflection of the success of the wound center. It starts with planning and examining the demographics for the catchment area for your wound center. Do you have a population with a disease mix that will support a chronic wound center? If yes, then what are the numbers of new patients, encounters, and hyperbaric treatments that can be projected on an annual basis? How are you going to drive business into your center? What marketing approaches will you use, and when will you implement them? The answers to these questions will allow you to begin to build a baseline business expectation to determine your potential for revenue generation.

Next is your cost of doing business. Many of these aspects have been discussed in early sections of this chapter. Included are: your staffing mix, staffing based on productivity and patient acuity, overtime, staff satisfaction and retention, and cost of supplies per patient visit. Determining the methodology to measure, evaluate, and effectively intervene, where appropriate, will aid you in the financial viability of the wound center.

Third is setting up and effectively managing the financial aspects of your center: the charge master, how patients are registered, co-pays collected, insurance verified, coding and billing of charges, and how denial of claims are handled. Most healthcare systems have a methodology in place for the majority of these aspects. What is needed is a focused person to shepherd the process and assure each step is in place and working properly. Frequently, if chronic wound management is a new service line to the healthcare system, education will be needed on CPT and ICD-9 coding, documentation to support the coding, how to bill these procedures, and what local coverage determinations (LCDs) are issued by the Medicare Intermediary that apply to this new service. Setting up a system so close attention is paid to any reimbursement denials and subsequent appeals, is key to maintaining successful operation of the wound center.

Conclusion

This chapter has been written from our successful experiences in operating comprehensive wound centers in a variety of settings. Our centers have been from urban to rural, in long term acute care, rehabilitation, and acute care hospitals, freestanding, and immediately adjacent to a facility. Some of the sections of this chapter in and of themselves could have formed the basis for an entire book. We have tried to highlight the "pearls" of success. It takes a strong, committed team to truly excel in the operations of a comprehensive wound center. Remember to develop your "product" before you market it and to always think outside the box.

References

1. Larson-Lohr, V. Productivity and Acuity Tool for Wound Care and Hyperbaric Medicine Centers. UHMS 2003;30(4): 271-75.

CHAPTER

6

Accreditation and Regulation in Hyperbaric and Wound Centers

Wilbur T. Workman

The regulatory community that directly impacts the practice of hyperbaric medicine is reasonably well-defined. However, it suffers from a lack of effective awareness, coordination, and implementation among the various organizations that have responsibilities, specifically to the practice of hyperbaric medicine, and more generally to wound care.

The concept of clinical hyperbaric facility accreditation is just slightly over a decade old. First introduced publicly at the 1999 meeting of the Gulf Coast Chapter of the Undersea and Hyperbaric Medical Society in Atlanta, Georgia, it has now become the industry gold standard for defining quality of care and safety for the hyperbaric patient.

Regulation and accreditation are directly related, in that a large portion of the accreditation process is an assessment of compliance, not only to industry standards of practice, but to public law, codes, and standards as well. While this chapter will not be an exhaustive coverage of regulatory issues, it will be sufficiently detailed so the reader can gain an understanding of at least the most basic regulations. This will transition into a broad discussion of how clinical hyperbaric facility accreditation supports the regulatory process, and how it hopefully leads to improved compliance to this process by serving as a measure of improved outcomes, patient safety, and risk management.

Regulatory Environment

Before the regulatory environment is described, it is important to understand some basic definitions. First, a law is a rule that, when not adhered to, some form of punishment will follow. Laws are generally enforced by a governmental agency. Second, a code is a compliance document that contains only mandatory provisions using words like "shall", etc., to indicate requirements. Codes are generally written in a form that is suitable for adoption into law with virtually no change to its content. Third, a standard is a compliance document that is similar to a code in that it also contains mandatory provisions using words like "shall", etc., to indicate requirements, but also includes non-mandatory provisions using terms like "should", etc. Non-mandatory provisions are usually found in an annex or appendix. Fourth, a recommended practice is a document that is similar in content and structure to a code or standard, but uses only non-mandatory language in the text to indicate recommendations. Last, a guideline is a document that contains information that is advisory or informative in nature and contains only non-mandatory provisions. Figure 1 represents the hierarchy of authority of these concepts, progressing from guidelines, which form the foundation, to the pinnacle of law.

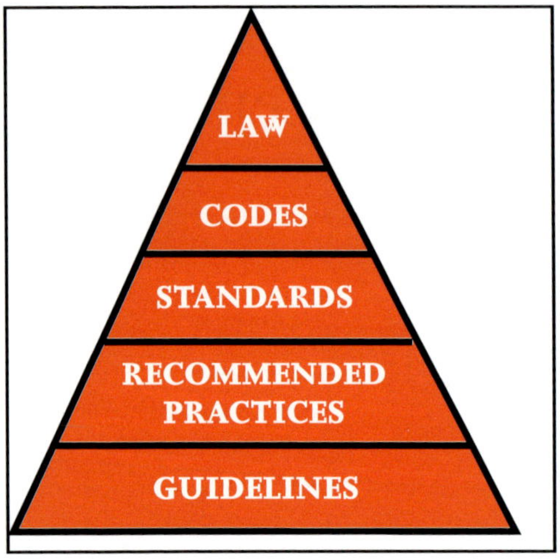

Figure 1: *Hierarchy.*

At the present time, there are at least 18 different organizations that influence, to varying degrees, the practice of hyperbaric medicine and the safe operation of hyperbaric facilities. It is important to understand that throughout this chapter, the focus will be primarily on hyperbaric facilities that are independent from or part of a comprehensive wound care program, not specifically on wound care centers that do not provide hyperbaric medicine services. Very few of the 18 organizations actually have regulatory authority. The vast majority are simply responsible for setting codes, standards, and professional guidelines.

Organizations with Authority

There are three general types of authoritative groups: federal, state, and local. Those with federal authority are the Centers for Medicare and Medicaid Services (CMS) and the Food and Drug Administration (FDA). State and local agencies include Authorities Having Jurisdiction (AHJs) such as state departments of health, state and local fire marshals, code compliance offices, etc.

Centers for Medicare and Medicaid Services

The primary hyperbaric authority of CMS is to establish national coverage policy defining physician supervision of therapy and reimbursement criteria of selected indications amenable to hyperbaric oxygen therapy. CMS administers their authority through a select number of Medicare Area Contractors (MACS). While CMS bases its reimbursement criteria on recommendations from the Undersea & Hyperbaric Medical Society (UHMS), they are not bound to adopt the Society's recommendations entirely. As matter of fact, they have proven in the past to be selective. An example of this selectivity is that CMS does not currently reimburse for exceptional blood loss anemia, thermal burns, or intracranial abscess, even though these conditions are recognized by the UHMS.

Food and Drug Administration

It should be well-understood by all that the FDA does not regulate the practice of medicine. Instead, they regulate the safety, effectiveness, marketing, and use of drugs and devices. Beginning with the Medical Device Amendments to the Food, Drug and Cosmetic Act of 1976, hyperbaric chambers were classified as a Class II medical device.[1] This Act and its subsequent amendments (the Safe Medical Device Act of 1990 and the Food and Drug Administration Modernization Act of 1997)[2] further set the requirement that hyperbaric chambers not be used for medical purposes unless treatment is supported by a prescription issued by a licensed practitioner. It also established the requirement that hyperbaric chamber manufacturers obtain marketing clearance for their device via the Premarket Notification submittal process before the chamber can be legally marketed. This process is commonly referred to as the 510k clearance.

In 1978, the FDA formally recognized the treatment recommendations of the Undersea & Hyperbaric Medical Society (UHMS). Since 1996, they have been mandated.[3] These recommendations remain the basis of establishing the indications of use for a hyperbaric chamber. They are:

1. Air or gas embolism
2. Carbon monoxide poisoning and carbon monoxide poisoning complicated by cyanide poisoning
3. Clostridial myositis and myonecrosis
4. Crush injury, compartment syndrome, and other acute traumatic ischemias

5. Decompression sickness
6. Enhanced healing of selected problem wounds
7. Exceptional blood loss anemia
8. Necrotizing soft tissue infections
9. Osteomyelitis (refractory)
10. Delayed radiation injury (soft tissue and bony necrosis)
11. Skin grafts and flaps (compromised)
12. Thermal burns
13. Intracranial abscess

Authorities Having Jurisdiction (State and Local)

At the state level, there are several different classifications for AHJs: fire safety and prevention, boiler and pressure vessel regulators, and state departments of health.

The one AHJ that has the most impact is the state Fire Marshal in those states for which the National Fire Protection Association's (NFPA) NFPA 99, Health Care Facilities or NFPA 101, Life Safety Code is mandated by state law. It is a common belief that NFPA 99, which contains safety code requirements for hyperbaric facilities, is mandatory in all 50 states. This is not correct, as it is not a universal requirement. One must assess if NFPA 99 applies in their state of operation.

Whereas NFPA 99 is not a national mandate, NFPA 101 is more widely recognized. The link between NFPA 99 and NFPA 101 is that the Life Safety Code invokes compliance to NFPA 99 (the chapter specific to hyperbaric facilities). Therefore, in those jurisdictions that have adopted the Life Safety Code, any hyperbaric facility must also comply with the hyperbaric facility-specific requirements of NFPA 99.

There are 11 states, 3 cities, and 5 Canadian provinces/territories in which the Boiler and Pressure Vessel Inspector has jurisdiction over the installation, use, and inspection of pressure vessels for human occupancy (hyperbaric chambers).[4] They are:

States:

Arkansas
California
Delaware
Georgia
Hawaii
Minnesota
North Carolina
Oregon
Tennessee
Washington
Wisconsin

Cities:

Denver
Seattle
District of Columbia

Canadian Provinces/Territories:

Alberta
British Columbia
New Brunswick
Nova Scotia
Ontario

In the locations listed above, each year the state Boiler and Pressure Vessel Inspector is to inspect any pressure vessel for human occupancy (PVHO) designed for an operational pressure of 30 psi or greater. Until recently, this annual inspection had not been occurring. However, recent events in Delaware and North Carolina related to exhausting chamber pressure relief valves have focused more attention from state regulators on clinical hyperbaric chambers. Due to a lack of state resources, the actual inspections are frequently conducted under contract by agencies such as the Zurich and Hartford insurance companies. An increase in awareness and involvement by this segment of the regulatory community should be anticipated.

The degree of involvement of state departments of health varies by state; therefore, a state-by-state comparison is beyond the scope of this chapter and will not be attempted. Some states, such as Florida, North Carolina, and Texas have facility design and construction requirements that are specific to hyperbaric facilities. Once these requirements have been met, the departments generally do not exert direct operational oversight.

At the local level, the AHJ with the most direct influence over the installation and operation of a clinical hyperbaric facility is the local Fire Marshal. This person has the authority to issue certificates of occupancy after an assessment of compliance to code requirements identified in the hyperbaric-specific chapter of NFPA 99 has been made. While not well understood, their authority even extends to compliance to daily operational safety procedures as set forth in the standard. Generally, local Fire Marshals have not exercised this aspect of their authority.

Organizations With No Authority

It is another common misconception that organizations that develop codes and standards have authority. This is not the case. The two most recognized organizations of this type in the hyperbaric community are the American Society of Mechanical Engineers (ASME) and the National Fire Protection Association. The codes and standards developed by either of these organizations do not have force until they are formally adopted by a federal, state, or local governmental body as law in their jurisdiction. Without a governmental mandate, they are little more than a comprehensive set of engineering and operational principles.

Codes and standards developed under criteria set by the American National Standards Institute (ANSI) are more amenable to adoption into law than those that do not follow its criteria. ANSI is a private, non-profit organization that administers and coordinates the voluntary standardization and conformity assessment system in the United States. They were established in 1918 by a coordinated group of engineering societies and government agencies. There are over 200 organizations that develop standards in accordance with their criteria which are listed below. There are now more than 10,000 ANSI standards in print.[5]

ANSI essential requirements are:

- Openness (public review and comment)
- Balance (no one industry can dominate the process)
- Consensus
- Due process (right for differing opinions to be expressed with rights to appeal)

As stated above, ASME has no regulatory authority. In this case, the code developed by ASME for the design, fabrication, and testing of hyperbaric chambers for human occupancy (ASME PVHO-1) is only mandatory in those jurisdictions that have invoked compliance through legislative action. Enforcement is performed by the State Boiler and Pressure Vessel Inspector or designated agent. It is important to know that the scope of ASME PVHO-1 covers any PVHO designed for a pressure differential of 2 psi or greater across the pressure boundary. While it is not a mandatory requirement, the FDA looks for compliance to ASME PVHO-1 for 510k clearance as discussed above.

Just like ASME, the NFPA has no authority except as provided by legislative action. Whereas ASME authority resides at the state level, NFPA's authority related to healthcare facilities resides at both the state and local level.

The NFPA definition of a healthcare facility is very clear. According to NFPA 99, Health Care Facilities, 2005 Edition, a healthcare facility is a "Building or portions of buildings in which medical, psychiatric, obstetrical or surgical care are provided."[6] (NFPA 99, 3.3.68*) Information in the annex provides additional clarification. *A.3.3.68 states, "Health care facilities include, but are not limited to, hospitals, nursing homes, limited care facilities, clinics, medical and dental offices, and ambulatory health care centers, whether permanent or movable."[7]

While the scope of ASME PVHO covers any hyperbaric chamber with an operational design pressure of 2 psi or greater, the scope of NFPA covers any hyperbaric chamber designed with a pressure differential of 0 psi to 100 psi across the pressure boundary. Its scope also pertains to any hyperbaric chamber used for treatment or research purposes in a healthcare facility and requires compliance to ASME PVHO-1. A large portion of NFPA 99's hyperbaric chapter is devoted to building construction standards and engineering performance standards for hyperbaric systems (such as wall-rating requirements, fire suppression, electrical systems, etc.). However, for the users of hyperbaric chambers, most of the construction and engineering requirements are the responsibility of the architect, building contractor and hyperbaric systems engineer. User responsibilities are focused on the comprehensive operational requirements set forth in the standard. Of key importance is the requirement for a locally designated Safety Director and the defined responsibilities of the individual assuming this role. A detailed discussion of daily operational requirements and responsibilities of the Safety Director is beyond the scope of this chapter. For additional guidance, review the relative material found in NFPA 99, as well as other NFPA publications such as the Life Safety Code (NFPA 101), the Standard for Bulk Oxygen Systems at Consumer Sites (NFPA 50), and Recommended Practice on Materials, Equipment and Systems Used in Oxygen-Enriched Environments (NFPA 53).

There are two other organizations that are important to the safe operation of hyperbaric facilities: the American Society for Testing and Materials (ASTM) and the Compressed Gas Association (CGA).

Established in 1898, ASTM is one of the world's largest developers of voluntary standards/

guidelines. The most relevant of these guidelines to hyperbaric facilities is developed through a special committee called the G-04 Committee. This committee, formally known as the Committee for Compatibility & Sensitivity of Materials in the Oxygen Enriched Environment, is most famous for its publication Safe Use of Oxygen and Oxygen Systems. This publication is highly recommended to all readers.

The Compressed Gas Association was formed in 1913. Its charter is to develop and promote guidelines for the safe use of gases. The guidelines most relevant to the hyperbaric community are:

- G-4 Oxygen
- G-4.1 Cleaning Equipment for Oxygen Service
- G-4.3 Commodity Specification for Oxygen
- M-1 Guide for Medical Gas Installations at Consumer Sites
- P-2 Characteristics and Safe Handling of Medical Gases
- P-2.7 Guide for the Safe Storage, Handling, and Use of Oxygen Systems in Healthcare Facilities
- P-39 Oxygen-rich Atmospheres

Current Regulatory Climate

As noted above, there are at least 18 organizations that have some level of interest for the practice of hyperbaric medicine. Unfortunately, there is little effective coordination or cooperation among the majority. For at least the last 12-15 years, there have been consolidated efforts to educate and coordinate but these have resulted in little or no success. While there has been limited action by the FDA exercising their authority through the release of warning letters, etc. and, federal and state agencies filing charges related to Medicare/Medicaid fraud, there has been a scarcity of oversight. Some readers may think this is a good thing. I disagree, because this lack of involvement facilitates the expanded use of hyperbaric chambers in situations and environments by untrained users that raise the risk of a major mishap, thus compromising patient safety and impacting the entire community.

The weaknesses in the regulatory community exist for many reasons. Even though we are growing rapidly, the hyperbaric medicine community is still relatively small. Being small frequently leads to being ignored. There are no mandatory staffing or training standards. There is no requirement that hyperbaric facilities be specifically licensed. There is little or no oversight over medical gas vendors who provide oxygen to users of personal hyperbaric chambers. The resources to educate the regulatory community are extremely meager and our safety record actually works against us.

Is there anything that you can do to improve the situation? Yes. Start by controlling what you can control. Know your community, know the types of facilities in your community and their scopes of service. Educate when you can. Develop a good working relationship with your local AHJ, etc. Most importantly, look for ways to differentiate your program from those with questionable operations. The hyperbaric community's credibility is at stake. One way to set yourself apart from others is to seek clinical hyperbaric facility accreditation.

Accreditation of Hyperbaric Medicine Facilities

When one thinks of accreditation programs for healthcare, visions of "running the gauntlet" may first come to mind. Unfortunately, there is basis for feeling that way. The road to defining and measuring quality of care and patient safety is frequently filled with speed bumps, stop signs, and check points making the journey a rigorous "road trip." Many organizations, however, have recognized that lessons learned along the route lead to improved outcomes and enhanced patient safety and are definitely worth the effort.

There are numerous hospital and specialty-specific accrediting organizations that provide high quality third-party assessment programs. The goals of accreditation in healthcare are generally universal, regardless of the specific focus of an individual accrediting body. Two primary goals are improved quality of patient care and enhanced patient safety by optimizing risk management processes. Perhaps the largest and most well-known is the Joint Commission (JC). Other hospital and specialty-specific accrediting programs are Det Norske Veritas (DNV), the American Osteopathic Association (AOA), the Accreditation Association for Ambulatory Healthcare (AAAHC) and the Commission on Accreditation of Rehabilitation Facilities (CARF), just to name a few. Of the above, the oldest program is that offered by the AOA being established in 1945, followed by the JC (1951). The newest to receive deemed status by Medicare is DNV. They were formally recognized by Medicare in 2008. None of the above accrediting bodies have program elements that are specific to the unique needs of the clinical hyperbaric medicine community.

What makes the hyperbaric medicine community different? The primary reason for the differentiation is the need to manage the risks associated with working with an oxygen-enriched environment. As a Class II medical device, a hyperbaric chamber (whether pressurized with air or oxygen) is the only medical device that has its own dedicated chapter in a nationally recognized fire safety standard (NFPA 99 as discussed above). In order to effectively manage the risks related to increased oxygen, hyperbaric chambers must be designed, installed, and operated with the highest respect to safety procedures and protocols. This is one element that makes hyperbaric facilities unique. Most accrediting bodies do not employ surveyors with the technical background and/or knowledge of hyperbaric systems. Therefore, should they assess processes in a hyperbaric facility, the veracity of that assessment is not as beneficial as it otherwise might be. Certainly, other accrediting bodies may be able to evaluate various clinical aspects, but they fall short in the assessment of installation, operational, and technical aspects of hyperbaric facility chambers.

Undersea & Hyperbaric Medical Society's Clinical Hyperbaric Facility Accreditation Program

It is primarily because of the uniqueness noted above that the Undersea & Hyperbaric Medical Society established a hyperbaric-specific sub-specialty accreditation program in 2001. There was also a secondary reason the Society took action. In October 2000, the Office of the Inspector General (OIG) of the Department of Health and Human Services published a report on the state of hyperbaric oxygen therapy in the United States. The report, "Hyperbaric Oxygen Therapy: Its Usefulness and Appropriateness,"[8] published findings that a lack of testing and treatment monitoring raised a variety of quality of care concerns and that Centers for Medicare and Medicaid Services (then known as the Health Care Financing Administration) guidance to the field of hyperbaric medicine was limited. Specific OIG recommendations were for CMS (HCFA) to initiate a national coverage decision policy for HBO; improve policy guidance (e.g. practice guidelines and physician attendance policy); and improve oversight by requiring contractors to initiate edits and consistent medical review procedures, and explore the creation of a national registry of facilities and/or physicians. Without a doubt, this report laid the foundation for a potential increase in government involvement and intervention. By creating a national clinical hyperbaric facility accreditation program, the UHMS responded proactively to the OIG findings and recommendations. This action was intended to be a sign to the various regulatory agencies that the organized hyperbaric medical community was concerned with the situation described in the report and promptly responded to the recognized need to assure that quality of care across the continuum of clinical hyperbaric facilities is achieved and maintained. More specifically, the Society believes that such a program is the most efficient method to ensure that:

- Clinical hyperbaric facilities are staffed with the proper specialists who are well-trained
- Clinical hyperbaric facilities are using quality equipment that has been properly installed and maintained, and being operated with the highest level of safety possible
- Clinical hyperbaric facilities are providing high quality of patient care
- Clinical hyperbaric facilities are maintaining the appropriate documentation of informed consent, patient treatment procedures, physician involvement, etc.

These objectives are achieved by undergoing a comprehensive two-day assessment by a team of three hyperbaric experts (physician, nurse and technician). The assessment concentrates on 24 individual areas:[9]

- Governance
- Administration
- Operations
- Maintenance
- Facility construction
- Chamber fabrication
- Chamber ventilation
- Chamber fire protection
- Chamber electrical systems and services
- Gas handling
- Patient rights
- Patient care
- Environment of care
- Patient education
- Quality improvement
- Professional improvement
- Leadership
- Human resources
- Information management
- Infection control
- Medical staff
- Teaching and publication
- Clinical research

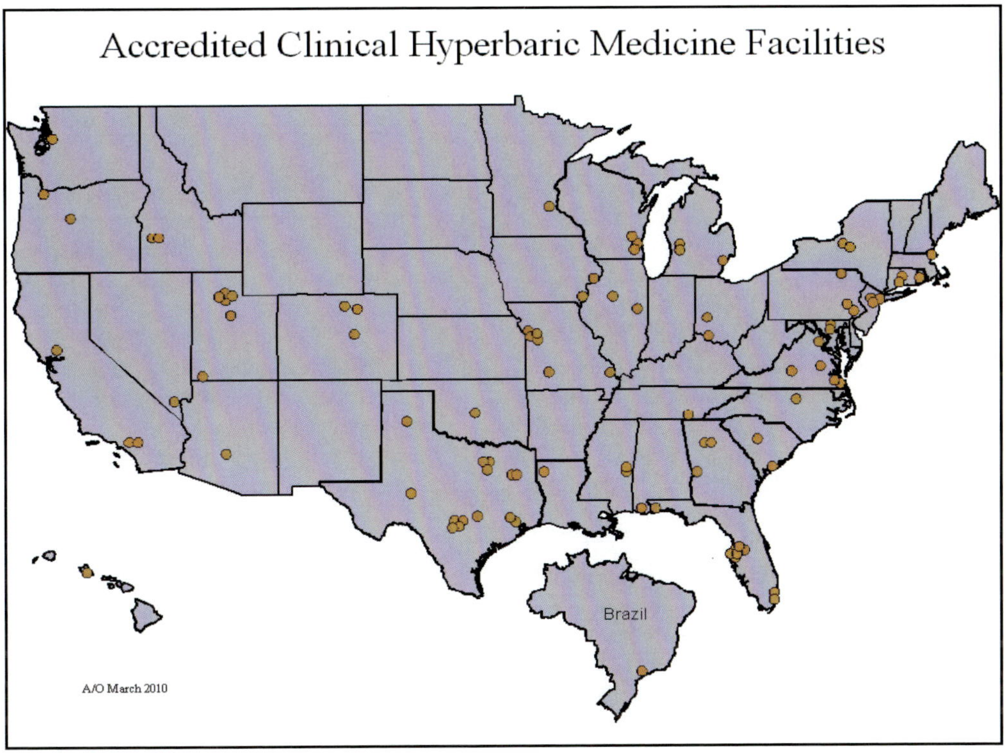

Figure 2: ***Accredited Clinical Hyperbaric Medicine Facilities.***

Even though the general benefits of accreditation have been mentioned above, one can anticipate specific benefits from the promotion of hyperbaric facility-specific accreditation. Although not all inclusive, some of the more obvious are:

- Improved quality of care
- Increased administrative efficiency
- More effective risk management programs (enhanced patient safety)
- Demonstration of compliance to industry standards of practice
- Possibly lower liability insurance pre-miums
- Staff motivation and esprit de corps
- Maximized public relations and mar-keting efforts
- Ability to recruit and retain quality staff
- Develop alliances with other provider groups
- Establish credibility of legitimate non-affiliated outpatient facilities among their professional referral base

It is beyond the scope of this chapter to describe the accreditation program in detail. The reader is encouraged to review the complete accreditation manual which can be downloaded free of charge from the UHMS website (www.uhms.org). It is important to know that it is the only hyperbaric-specific accreditation program of its kind in the world. The UHMS is an international professional medical society with members from over 50 countries. There is a growing interest among the international hyperbaric community to participate in this program. Actually, the program has already gone international, as there is a facility in Sao Paulo, Brazil, that has successfully achieved UHMS accreditation. Following this precedence, colleagues from Canada and Australia have formally taken steps to implement UHMS accreditation in their respective countries. Expressions of interest have been made by facilities in Mexico, Singapore, South Africa, and elsewhere. A special panel discussion on hyperbaric facility accreditation is planned for the 2011 meeting of the International Congress on Hyperbaric Medicine in Cape Town, South Africa.

What has been the impact of hyperbaric facility accreditation since this voluntary program was initially offered in 2001? From the more than 100 facilities that have been successfully accredited (see Figure 2), 32 changes have been approved for inclusion in the hyperbaric chapter of NFPA 99; new operational safety courses have been created; over 1,000 Safety Directors have been trained in their responsibilities as defined in NFPA 99; a significant increase in the number of hyperbaric technicians becoming certified by the National Board of Diving and Hyperbaric Technology and hyperbaric nurses becoming certified by the Baromedical Nurses Association has been noted; the level of safety awareness has been raised; and, accredited facilities that aggressively market the fact that they are accredited have enjoyed a significant increase in patient volumes which translates to increased revenue. While these are not the only improvements in the hyperbaric community, they represent tangible evidence that the level of care being provided to the hyperbaric patient is improving in all aspects, one accredited facility at a time. By improving the quality of care provided for hyperbaric patients in individual facilities, the quality of care is raised throughout the entire country. The UHMS's Clinical Hyperbaric Facility Accreditation Program is achieving its goals and will only improve over time.

As mentioned before, the program is currently voluntary. It is so in all cases with the exception of Utah. The Utah Medicaid program office mandates UHMS accreditation in order for a state-based hyperbaric facility to receive reimbursement for treatment of Medicaid eligible patients. New York's Medicaid program office has inquired about the Society's program. Is there a message there? Yes, there is. More agencies like Medicaid of Utah are evaluating whether to follow in their footsteps or not. There has also been a marked increase in requests for information on the UHMS accreditation program by Medical Directors of several MACS and a variety of third-party payers. Is there a message there? Again, yes. The message is that insurance companies, at all levels, are looking for ways to tighten their reimbursement criteria. It is clear to me that at some point in the not too distant future, organizations like Utah Medicaid will link reimbursement for hyperbaric therapy to accreditation.

In 1995, the JC established a program to help reduce costs and duplication of survey activities. In 2002, it was enhanced by creating the Cooperative Agreement Program to acknowledge other accrediting organizations. This program created two pathways to become formally recognized by the JC—Comparable and Complementary.

To become recognized as a Comparable Accrediting Body, the organization must demonstrate essential comparability with Commission's standards, process, methods, and policies. At the present time, there are only two organizations that are so designated: the College of American Pathologists and COLA (formerly known as the Commission on Office Laboratory Accreditation).

Organizations that are successfully recognized as Complementary are not required to maintain comparability as discussed above. Instead, the survey process of the Complementary body is more focused on the technical and clinical aspects of a specific department or service within a health care organization, and is not applicable to the entire organization. At present, there are only five accrediting organizations that are officially recognized by the JC as Complementary.[10] They are:

- American Society of Histocompatibil-ity and Immunogenetics
- American College of Surgeons- Bariatric Surgery Accreditation Program
- American College of Surgeons- Commission on Cancer
- American College of Radiology
- Undersea and Hyperbaric Medical Society (recognized in April 2010)

During JC surveys of the parent organization, the Commission could still visit the unit or service, even if the unit or service is accredited by one of the Complementary bodies. Due to the extremely unique technical requirements of a hyperbaric facility, the likelihood that the JC will visit the unit is remote (unless the pathway of their tracery methodology leads them to the hyperbaric department). It is of extreme benefit for the hyperbaric patient, knowing that a hyperbaric facility has voluntarily met quality and safety standards of both the JC and the UHMS. For hospital and hyperbaric facility management personnel, knowing that the JC has reviewed and validated the UHMS accreditation program is also extremely beneficial. This action should remove all doubt as to the veracity of the Society's program.

At the present time, DNV has no similar process to acknowledge specialty-specific accrediting programs. The UHMS is working with them to develop such a program.

Conclusion

You may be asking yourself what all of this has to do with hyperbaric nursing. The most obvious is that hyperbaric nurses frequently serve as the designated unit Safety Director. In the capacity as Safety Director, it is imperative that the nurse has a working knowledge of codes, standards, and regulatory requirements, especially those related to hyperbaric facility safety. The link to accreditation is that the survey process assesses, to a large degree, compliance to these codes and standards, and the incumbent should understand how they are intricately related to the survey process.

What is perhaps not as immediately obvious is that the nurse is just one member of a team of professionals, all working together toward the common goal of providing the highest quality of care possible. Even if the nurse is not the facility Safety Director, they are no less responsible for the safety of the hyperbaric patient. Each member of the team must be always diligent with regard to safety, with everyone doing their part to foster a healthy respect for hyperbaric safety.

While efforts at educating the regulatory community have met limited success, the hyperbaric community must continue to work together to take advantage of those few opportunities when they do present themselves. In the absence of significant external oversight, we have done a good job overall at "policing" ourselves- we must continue to do so.

Looking back over the last decade or so, I am amazed at the phenomenal success of hyperbaric facility accreditation. With the exception of Utah, no one is mandating hyperbaric accreditation. Even so, the community has begun to embrace the spirit of the effort and has recognized that it is a quality improvement program for the entire specialty of hyperbaric medicine. The list of facilities awaiting survey is getting longer and longer. Programs with any interest in seeking accreditation are strongly encouraged to submit applications as soon as possible. The program will continue to grow and exert a positive influence on our specialty. Years from now, when we look back and try to determine what has been the single most important thing that has made a real difference, I am convinced that it will be clinical hyperbaric facility accreditation. It is the right thing to do.

References

1. Foreman C, Weitershausen J. Regulation Of Hyperbaric Chambers As Medical Devices. In: Workman WT editor. Hyperbaric Facility Safety: A Practical Guide. Flagstaff: Best Publishing Company; 1999. p. 135.
2. ibid.
3. ibid. p. 143.
4. Swanson RP. Governing Directives. In: Workman WT editor. Hyperbaric Facility Safety: A Practical Guide. Flagstaff: Best Publishing Company; 1999. p. 29.
5. American National Standards Institute. Cited July 9, 2010. Available from: http://www.ansi.org/about_ansi/introduction/introduction.aspx?menuid=1
6. NFPA 99, Standard for Health Care Facilities, Chapter 20, Hyperbaric Facilities, 2005 edition. National Fire Protection Association, Quincy, MA. p. 18.
7. ibid. p. 127.
8. Office of Inspector General, Department of Health and Human Services. Hyperbaric Oxygen Therapy: Its Usefulness and Appropriateness. Report No. OEI 06-99-00090, October 2000.
9. Undersea and Hyperbaric Medical Society. Clinical Hyperbaric Facility Accreditation Manual, 2005 Edition, Rev 1. Undersea and Hyperbaric Medical Society, Durham, NC. p. 9.
10. The Joint Commission. Cited July 9, 2010. Available from: http://www.jointcommission.org/AboutUs/Fact_Sheets/coop_accreditation.htm

CHAPTER

7

Operational and Safety: *Common Elements Shared by Hyperbaric Facilities*

RICHARD BARRY

TO UNDERSTAND THE OPERATIONAL AND SAFETY elements of hyperbarics, one must first know what hyperbaric equipment is, where it comes from, where it can be placed, and how to properly use it. In the following chapter, we will attempt describe the common elements shared by all hyperbaric facilities, operational setups, center/facility safety, fire safety, and separate elements particular to the type of hyperbaric chamber one is utilizing. The intent of this chapter is to give the end user a base of operational and safety information that will allow one to design and implement operational and safety programs.

Hyperbaric chambers are currently built as either a multiplace or a monoplace unit, per the requirements of the current edition of American Society of Mechanical Engineers (ASME) PVHO-1, Safety Standard for Pressure Vessels for Human Occupancy. Multiplace chambers are termed Class A by the National Fire Protection Association (NFPA), and are pressurized with air. Patients breathe oxygen from devices such as a mask or hood. These types of chambers are designed to treat multiple patients simultaneously, hence the term multiplace. Monoplace chambers are termed Class B and are usually pressurized with oxygen. In some situations, monoplace chambers have been pressurized with air and have patients breathe oxygen from a mask or hood, as one would in a Class A chamber. Setups of this nature are the exception, not the standard. Class B chambers are designed for single person use, hence the term monoplace. Both style chambers are used for the same purpose- to deliver oxygen greater than sea level pressure to patients. The U.S. Food and Drug Administration (FDA) considers Class A and B chambers medical devices, and requires them to have a 510k Premarket Notification number. This number is applied for by the chamber manufacturer and must be issued prior to marketing the device to the public. All hyperbaric facilities should keep a copy of their chamber's 510k on hand. Copies can be requested from the chamber manufacturer or by visiting the FDA's website at www.fda.gov and searching "510k" and follow the links/instructions. This is a free service.

While the Class A and Class B chambers have different designs, they do share common elements regarding codes, standards, and guidelines. The two most common sources for the design and safety elements of hyperbaric facilities and chamber usage are: 1) The American Institute of Architects (AIA) "2006 Guidelines for Design and Construction of Health Care Facilities" (current edition at time of publication); and 2) The "NFPA 99: Health Care Facilities, 2005" (current edition at time of publication).

The AIA guidelines for hyperbaric suites outline the space required to house Class A and Class B chambers. The AIA guidelines of 5.10 Hyperbaric Suite should be consulted when designing a new hyperbaric facility or remodeling an existing facility. This is a tool for the facility's architect and design team. Additional information regarding AIA, or to purchase guidelines, can be found at www.aia.org.

The NFPA 99 scope for hyperbaric facilities is defined as:

> 1.1.20 Chapter 20, "Hyperbaric Facilities," covers the recognition of and protection against hazards of an electrical, explosive, or implosive nature, as well as fire hazards associated with hyperbaric chambers and associated facilities that are used, or intended to be used, or medical applications and experimental procedures at gauge pressure from 0 to 690 kPa (0 to 100 psi). Chapter 20 applies to both single and multiple occupancy hyperbaric chambers; to animal chambers, the size of which precludes human occupancy; and to those in which the chamber atmosphere contains an oxygen partial pressure greater than an absolute pressure of 21.3 kPa (3.09 psi) (0.21 atmospheres).

It is important to note that if you are utilizing a Class A chamber with hypobaric capability you will need NFPA 99B: Standard for Hypobaric Facilities, as well as NFPA 99. NFPA 99B is for "[...] hypobaric facilities in which humans will be occupants or are intended to be occupants of the hypobaric chamber." Additional information regarding NFPA 99 and 99B, or to purchase guidelines, can be found at www.nfpa.org.

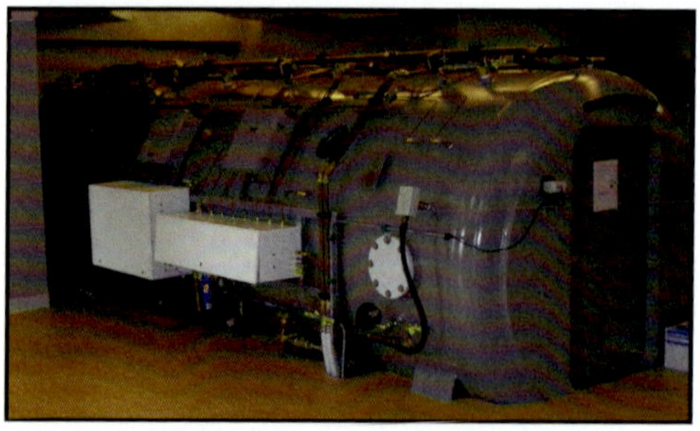

Figure 1: ***Class A.***

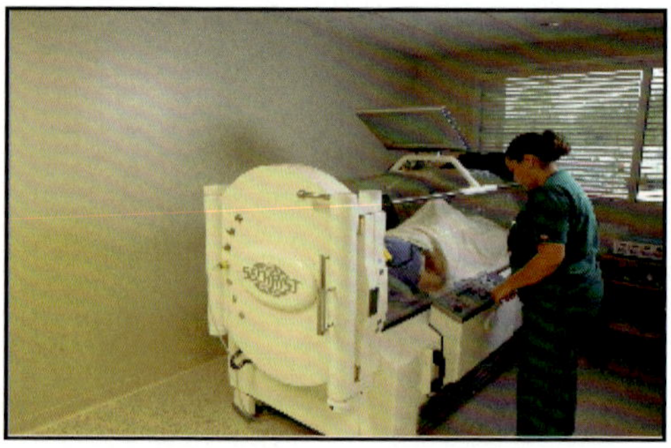

Figure 2: ***Class B (monoplace) hyperbaric chamber. Photo courtesy of Diversified Clinical Services, Inc.™***

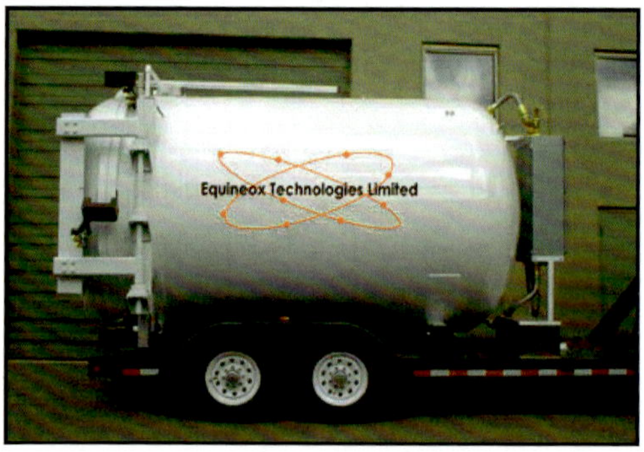

Figure 3: ***Class C (animal) chamber.***

Staffing and Initial Training

At the time of this publication, hyperbaric chamber operators (referred to as "techs") are those allied healthcare professionals that have received additional training in hyperbarics. Initial training in hyperbarics is gained by attending an introductory course in hyperbaric medicine as approved by The National Board of Diving and Hyperbaric Medical Technology (NBDHMT). The minimum requirement of those courses includes, but is not limited to:

1. Physics related to pressure exposures
2. Basic calculations for the conversion of common measurement units
3. Gas laws
4. Barotrauma
5. Decompression illness
6. Prevention and management of pressure related problems
7. Gas systems
8. Chamber operations and environment
9. Clinical skills
10. Transcutaneous oxygen monitoring.

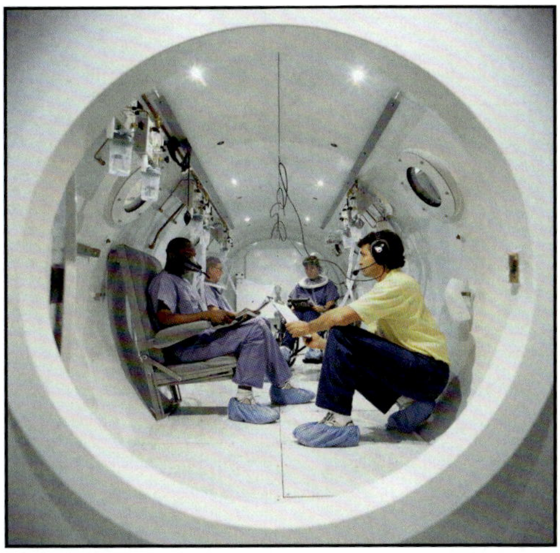

Figure 4: ***Inside Class A (multiplace) chamber.***

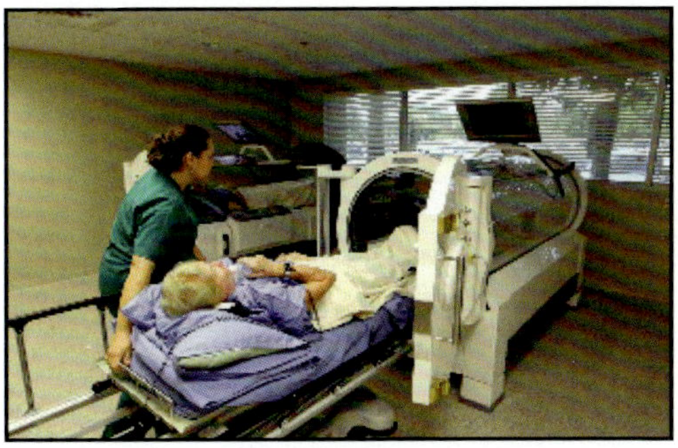

Figure 5: ***Class B (monoplace) hyperbaric chamber. Photo courtesy of Diversified Clinical Services, Inc.™***

The National Board of Diving and Hyperbaric Medical Technology has established guidelines for those medical professionals desiring to teach hyperbarics, and is the certifying body for individuals seeking to become certified as either Certified Hyperbaric Technologist (CHT) or Certified Hyperbaric Registered Nurse (CHRN). Additional information regarding the NBDHMT can be found at www.nbdhmt.org.

Hyperbarics, as a profession, is an added qualification to someone previously trained and competent in healthcare, i.e. an Emergency Medical Technician, Certified Medical Assistant, Respiratory Therapist, Registered, Licensed Practical Nurse, and Licensed Vocational Nurse. While certification in hyperbarics is not mandatory, it is becoming an industry standard and is highly recommended. Conversely, proper training in hyperbarics and an established method of showing competencies in the operation of the medical devices (Class A or B) is mandatory.

The Undersea and Hyperbaric Medical Society (UHMS) has published guidelines for staffing of the hyperbaric facilities which includes:

- Physician- Medical Director and panel physicians (physician supervision of hyperbaric treatments is necessary for the Class A and Class B chamber facility)
- Nursing- Clinical manager and center nurses
- Technical- Technical Directors (mostly seen in Class A chamber facilities), Safety Director (required per NFPA 99 at all hyperbaric facilities), and chamber operators
- Administrative- Program Manager as well as registration, coding, and billing support

These positions are general in nature and will take on different meaning from the facility located in a hospital with an accessible support structure versus the facility located in a medical office building some distance from a hospital, and even more so from the facility independent from a hospital. Each of these setups offers advantages and disadvantages, so the staffing guidelines are for the end user to implement the best practice according to their facility needs.

The Class B center utilizes a Safety Director as the lead hyperbaric tech, whereas the common practice for Class A centers is to utilize a Technical Director over the Safety Director; it is possible to have one person fill both roles. The primary reason for this is that Class B chambers do not have the intense amount of mechanical (technical) components as the Class A; therefore, a Technical Director is not needed for Class B operations.

Common practice for the Class B center is to have a staffing model of 1:2 ratio (1 tech per 2 chambers), but that does not mean a center should not have others trained in hyperbarics. A single tech (primary) can monitor 2 chambers that are next to each other, but there needs to be a designed backup to the primary tech. The backup tech is required for breaks, restroom visits, assisting during patient chamber turnover (i.e. completing one set of treatments and beginning another), and emergencies. For a center with an even number of chambers, this ratio is straightforward in application. One tech can monitor 2 patients and chambers, understanding that the tech's primary role during this time is to monitor the patients AND the equipment (chambers and auxiliary components). Once a third chamber is added, the primary tech loses the capability to effectively monitor 3 patients and equipment, unless those are the only things the tech is doing, but a 2nd tech is still needed to assist with patients on air breaks, removing patients from chambers, placing patients in chambers, and completing charting/documentation. The second tech can leave the room to gather patient charts, use the restroom, bring patients back for treatment, and other administrative duties as they pertain to hyperbaric operations. It is important to note that techs are monitoring patients during a medical treatment, and monitoring and adjusting the equipment delivering the treatment.

For the Class A chamber facility, the tech's role is still the same- to monitor patients and equipment during hyperbaric procedures. Staffing differs from Class B chambers in that a tech is required inside the chamber to assist patients and an additional tech is required outside the chamber to monitor the in-chamber activities, operate the chamber controls, and document the hyperbaric events.

Additionally, when the chambers are not in use, the role of the tech includes, but is not limited to, ensuring chamber equipment checks are completed and up-to-date, assisting with patient care (if wound care is being conducted), assisting with the identification of potential hyperbaric patients, conducting hyperbaric in-services, and assisting with insurance verification.

The examples above are just that- examples. Each facility will need to evaluate the center's operational flow and scope of practice to determine the preferred hyperbaric staffing mix.

Communications with facility associated and non-associated personnel

In any hyperbaric facility, it is important to understand who is responsible for interior and exterior building maintenance and upkeep. In a hospital setting, these responsibilities will generally fall under environmental services and facility/plant operations. Depending on the arrangement of the off-campus facility, like a medical office building, there could be hospital services within the building, and the building management or leasing company handling the exterior; or building management may be responsible for interior and exterior. For example, if the gas exhaust piping needed to be inspected or light needs to be fixed at the gas pad, you will know who to contact for this service based on your situation.

Safety Program

It is not enough to simply say, "We practice safety," or "We have a safety program." The center staff should define what safety means to them, and then implement a Safety Program. One approach to consider is forming a Safety Committee comprised of the Medical Director, Program Manager, Clinical Manager, and Technical or Safety Director to create and implement the Safety Program. In essence, the Safety Committee is an element of the Safety Program. Even though every facility is different in physical location, staffing, and scope of practice/care, there are a number of elements that can be considered common to a Safety Program.

The elements are:

1. **Support** from top management and mandated accountability- establish a charter statement
2. **Data analysis-** as part of continual improvement
3. **Safety training-** such as monthly in-services related to hyperbarics
4. **Motivation and communication-** newsletters, bulletins, awards for safety behavior
5. **Approved and prohibited items listing-** what the facility will or will not allow in the chamber
6. **Reporting-** such as incidents, accidents, safety meeting minutes, or other events
7. **Emergency procedures-** the establishment, training, and implementation of emergency procedures in and around the hyperbaric suite, as well as in the chamber

Safety Training

As mentioned earlier, NFPA 99 calls for an onsite hyperbaric safety director (HSD) at every hyperbaric facility. Those designated as the HSD should have a high level of maturity and be trained in hyperbaric operations at a minimum. This person should seek out advanced safety training, not only in hyperbarics, but in healthcare, facilities management, and oxygen as well. The more a HSD learns about safety as a whole concept, the better equipped they will be as a hyperbaric safety person.

Organizations such as the Undersea and Hyperbaric Medical Society and the National Board of Diving and Hyperbaric Medical Technology can provide information regarding hyperbaric safety courses that are available to the public. A commonly missed opportunity for general safety training is with the facility's risk or liability insurance carrier. When choosing safety training opportunities, one should contact their insurance agent and ask what their organization offers to its client base. It is not uncommon for insurance organizations to offer free training via classroom and/or online setting. Additionally, they may have a Safety Plan, Safety Committee, and in-service templates available for your use.

Fire Safety/Elements of a Fire

Fire safety is of the highest importance with hyperbaric operations as any time oxygen is used, the risk of harm is present. This is even more so in the hyperbaric environment where oxygen is used in a pressurized and enclosed area.

For a fire to occur and continue, there must be 3 elements present:

1. **Fuel**- burnable materials in hyperbarics could be, but are not limited to, pillows, linen, mattress, dressing, and hair.
2. **Heat**- anything that produces heat or static should be evaluated and deemed appropriate or not for the oxygen enriched atmosphere, and be thoroughly inspected prior to each operational use. Additionally, patients should be screened just before being placed in a chamber for any prohibited items, i.e. lighters, external items with batteries, or personnel warming device such as warming wraps or hand warmers.
3. **Oxygen**- this element is always present in chambers, both Class A and B. While oxygen is not flammable it does make fuel burn hotter, brighter, and faster.

Characteristics of Oxygen

Oxygen is approximately 10% heavier than air. It is for this reason that one needs to be cognizant of oxygen pooling, which can occur in areas of a Class A chamber due to hood or mask blow by or leaks. As the inside tech moves about the chamber, that person can stir the settled oxygen, thereby increasing the overall oxygen percentage. This is easily remedied by venting the chamber until acceptable oxygen levels are attained.

In the Class B chamber, pooling is not an issue as the chamber is filled and pressurized with oxygen; unless, of course, the chamber is filled with air and patients are administered oxygen via mask or hood. In this case, you will need to monitor the oxygen levels just as with a Class A chamber setup. Two areas to be aware of regarding pooling and the Class B chamber are the chamber exhaust location and the area around the chamber door. Oxygen dissipates quickly when exposed to atmospheric pressure and air, but you should know and understand your surroundings in order to prevent an incident related to high levels of oxygen.

No smoking signage should be visible around oxygen exhaust, regardless of the Class chamber or the exhaust location. This is to inform bystanders, staff, and workers of the presence of oxygen. Caution is needed to ensure machinery is not operated in the vicinity of exhaust, nor are open flames present.

When opening the door to a Class B chamber, upon depressurization one will notice the coolness of gas around the feet. This is due to the oxygen cooling during depressurization, and given that cool gas is heavier, coupled with oxygen's weight over normobaric air.

Regulatory

The following is a list of regulatory entities the hyperbaric facility should be aware of, as well as the impact each has to the facility.

- American Society of Mechanical Engineers (ASME)- chamber fabrication as seen in Pressure Vessels for Human Occupancy: PVHO-1
- American Society for Testing and Materials (ASTM)- particularly the Committee G4 for the compatibility and sensitivity of materials in oxygen-enriched atmospheres
- Compressed Gas Association (CGA)- for gas handling, transporting, and training
- National Fire Protection Association (NFPA)- for hyperbaric safety requirements
- State and local authorities
- One should seek out and determine who the local authorities are and where their responsibility and jurisdiction lies with hyperbaric facilities. Some states require a pressure vessel inspection of the chamber prior to use. There is not a right or wrong way to find this information, but it will take time and effort. If you are in a hospital setting, you can start by asking the Director of Plan Operations. If you are in a freestanding building, you can start by asking the local building inspector.
- U.S. Food and Drug Administration (FDA)- for premarket notification (510k)

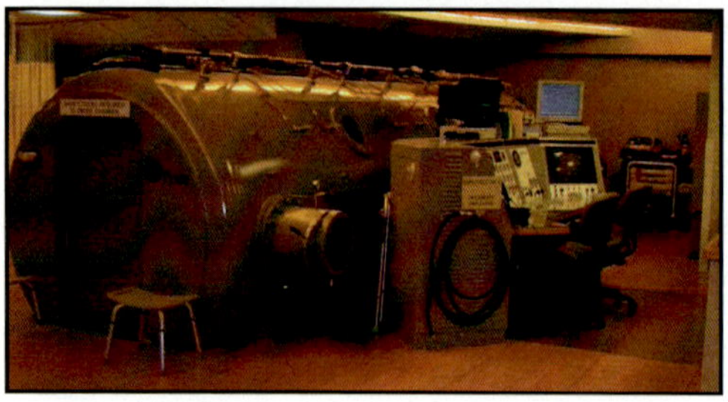

Figure 6: ***Class A.***

Approved and Prohibited Items for Inside the Chamber and Items Analysis

As part of the Safety Plan, each hyperbaric facility should have a list of items that will be allowed in the chambers and a list of prohibited items. At the time of this publication, there is no known listing of items approved or prohibited for use in hyperbarics, other than some generic term found in NFPA 99. It is up to the facility to determine what items will be listed for their given application of hyperbarics. Elements to consider are the facilities scope of practice/care and chamber type (Class A or B).

NFPA 99 allows for the physician in charge, with the concurrence of the hyperbaric safety director, to allow items not previously mentioned (items listed on your facilities approved or prohibited listing) or not previously known in the chamber. At the time of this writing, NFPA was vague on how to analyze or what method of analysis should be utilized in approving an item for use in hyperbarics. The chapter does state that if an item is to be allowed, then documentation is needed to support its use. This vagueness is due in part to there being no established standard for testing of a product for use in the hyperbaric application. That is not to say there are not oxygen-testing procedures that give the end user valuable information. Instead, this means you cannot send an item to a laboratory to be tested to Generic Hyperbaric Safety Analysis and receive a pass or fail grading for hyperbaric use.

The vagueness does allows flexibility for the end user to determine the best possible method for assessing the safety (oxygen compatibility) of a product. Below is a list of suggested information to review when researching a product for use in the hyperbaric chamber:

- Material safety data sheets
- Product specification sheets
- Chamber manufacturer
- Product supplier or manufacture. This is a suggested script when contact suppliers or manufacture:

Dear Tech Support,

I operate hyperbaric oxygen therapy chambers in (Hospital, City, and State). I am very cautious about the materials allowed in these chambers, as the chambers are pressurized with 100% oxygen to a depth of 2.0 ata or 2.5 ata (equal to 33 fsw or 50 fsw). We have a patient with a (implanted, prod product, device, wig-it) and (secondary item); that has been prescribed hyperbaric therapy. I am researching to see if (product) is compatible with the oxygen enriched atmosphere prior to starting this patient. Do you have any information describing what the (product) is made of?

Examples: Testing data, MSDS, make, manufacture, model, technical specification....

Has it been tested for use in:

Hyperbarics?

SCUBA diving?

Flying?

Driving through the mountains?

Operating room?

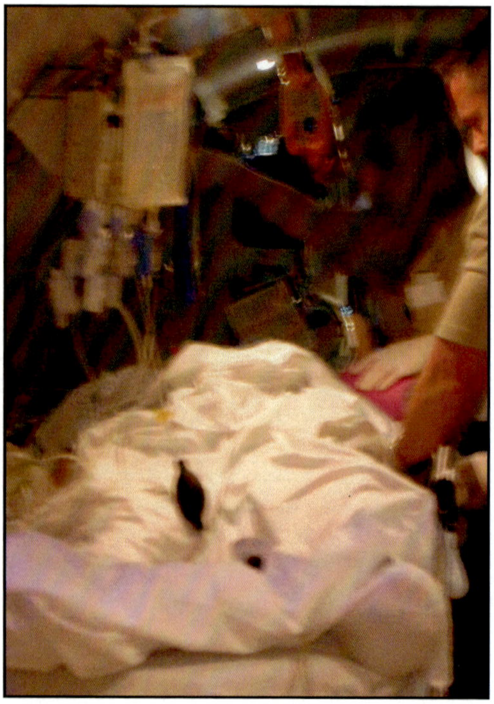

Figure 7: ***Inside Class A.***

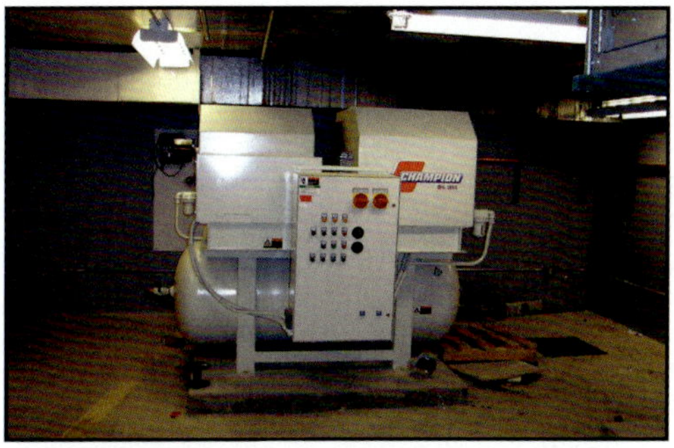

Figure 8: ***Class A.***

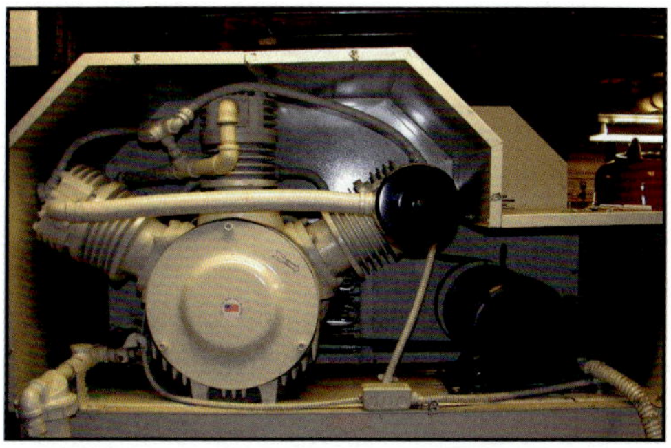

Figure 9: ***Champion comp. #1.***

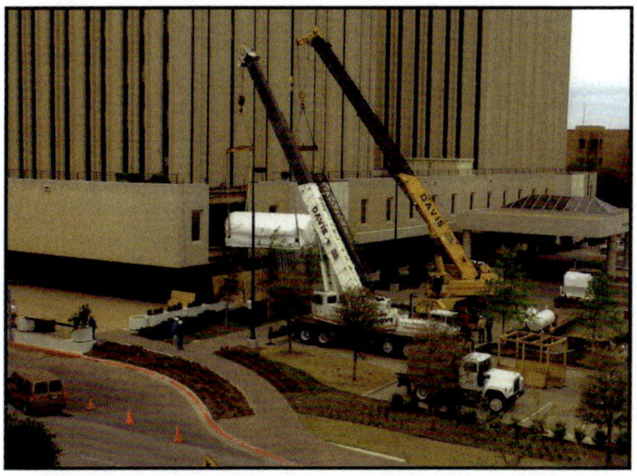

Figure 10: ***Class A.***

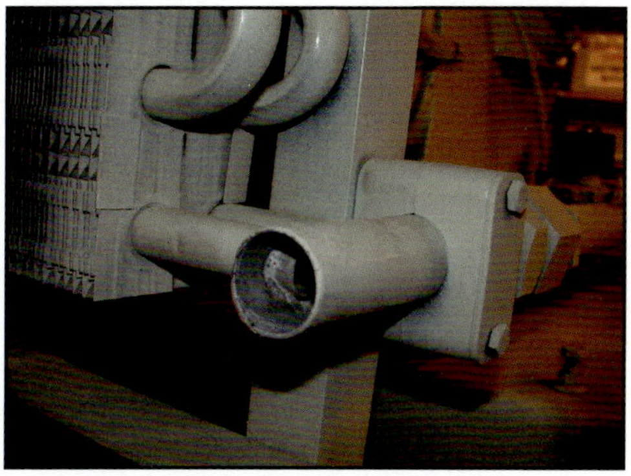

Figure 11: ***Comp. #2 damage at after cooler.***

Conclusion

When it comes to the operational and safety elements of a hyperbaric facility, the more information you have, the better equipped you will be. It is important to understand that we never stop learning about safety, its application, and its implementation as a practice, but if you approach safety as part of the daily routine and incorporate it in all of the facility processes, then it will be a continual process versus something to be re-taught.

References

1. NFPA 99 Health Care Facilities. 2005 Edition: National Fire Protection Association, 2005.
2. NFPA 99B Standard for Hypobaric Facilities. 2010 Edition: National Fire Protection Association, 2010.
3. Facility Guidelines Institute. Guidelines for Design and Construction of Healthcare Facilities. The American Institute of Architects.
4. The American Society of Mechanical Engineers. Safety Standard for Pressure Vessels for Human Occupancy. The American Society of Mechanical Engineers. 2007.
5. UHMS Guidelines for Hyperbaric Facility Operations. 2004 Edition: Undersea and Hyperbaric Medical Society, 2004.
6. National Board of Diving and Hyperbaric Medical Technology. http://www.nbdhmt.com/
7. ASTM International. http://astm.org/
8. U.S. Food and Drug Administration. http://www.fda.gov/
9. Compressed Gas Association. http://www.cganet.com/

CHAPTER

8

Management of the Critically Ill Patient in a Hyperbaric Setting: *Nursing Considerations and Preventions*

Julio R. Garcia, RN

As hyperbaric medicine has evolved as an accepted treatment modality and as an important adjunct in emergency indications, so has the knowledge base evolved for the hyperbaric registered nurse and the hyperbaric technician. The goal for this chapter is to provide an overview of the nursing management of the critically ill patient, assessment, and considerations as related to the hyperbaric setting. We will review critical care indications, general assessment, assessment tools, and associated nursing diagnoses in accordance with standards of the Baromedical Nursing Association (BNA).

The management of the critically ill patient can be a tremendous challenge in optimal intensive care settings such as our modern ICUs and emergency room. Now let us take that same patient and place them in an environment where we are going to have changes in their cardiac workload and respiratory effort. Let us also include the increased risk for seizure activity, hypoglycemia, and increased potential risk for fire. To top it all off, at least for most of us, in the monoplace setting you cannot place your hands on the patient when treatment is initiated. It seems like quite the daunting task that most of us would not readily volunteer for or place our patients in what appears to be such an uncontrolled setting. It is our responsibility to be proactive, to think ahead, and control as many variables as we can. Attention to detail is paramount. The challenge is great, but it is extremely fulfilling in helping deliver an adjunctive therapy we know will help provide a greater chance for a positive outcome for the patient.

Lastly, the art and science of treating the critically ill patient in the hyperbaric setting is becoming less and less available across the U.S. The perception by some contract services is that it is too costly, and there is not enough return on investment as related to the cost of skilled personnel, the training of personnel, and related medical equipment. Just as in any emergency, the value is never perceived until it becomes personal. In 2005, my hospital and contract service company were in negotiations to terminate emergency services. This would have left a void of emergency hyperbaric service along the central Gulf Coast from New Orleans, Louisiana, to Tallahassee, Florida.

In August of 2005, Hurricane Katrina devastated the Gulf Coast. In a matter of 3 days we treated over 30 patients for carbon monoxide poisoning related to gas generator usage. The youngest patient we treated was only 28 days old. In addition, two of the family groups we treated were staff physicians. This effectively ended any discussions of the need for the hospital to provide emergency coverage for our community. Emergency services can be managed in almost any center as long as you can effectively provide air breaks in order to deliver established treatment tables. Also, clearly define your scope of service. Determine which indications you are capable treating and which you cannot. Most hyperbaric patients can be broken down into two categories: those who are ventilator dependent and/or hemo-dynamically unstable, and those who have an emergent indication and are not ventilator dependent and/or hemo-dynamically unstable. It is ill conceived to place a blanket determination stating, "We do not treat any emergent indication," when the variables are so great. The 66-year-old female with central retinal artery occlusion (CRAO) who requires treatment within the first 24 hours of onset or a 6- year-old with a severe headache post-carbon monoxide exposure from a house fire, does not require the same level of intensity of supportive equipment as a necrotizing fasciitis patient who is ventilator dependent and hemo-dynamically unstable. It does require a facility and staff who are capable and willing to treat after "normal" hours of operation, call schedule, and willing physician coverage.

Since I became involved in the field in 1996, I fell in love with discipline. As a former U.S. Army combat medical specialist, SICU open heart recovery nurse, and emergency room nurse, I remember the first time I saw a lecture presentation on the management of the critically ill patient in a monoplace setting. The lecture was part of my Primary Hyperbaric Team Training with International ATMO in San Antonio. The lecturer was my friend and colleague, Ms. Valerie Larson-Lohr. I sat in the audience in awe of what was being presented. The implications to nursing were tremendous, as specialized as possible, exactly what I love in a challenge of specialty nursing. I would like for this chapter to provide a structure for assessment and the nursing considerations for the hyperbaric patient. Though it is not meant to be the be end-all in reference material, I do hope it provides food for thought and an insight into the incredible field of hyperbaric nursing.

General Nursing Considerations and Associated Nursing Diagnosis

Preparation is everything when dealing with the critically ill patient in a hyperbaric environment. You need to ensure you have suitable equipment for hemodynamic monitoring during transport and treatment, dependent on patient presentation. Due to the great variety of hyperbaric chambers, manufacturers, and monitoring equipment, you need communicate with the manufacturer of the both the chamber and the equipment you wish to utilize. Use the resources available to you in the field. Contact the Undersea Hyperbaric Medical Society (UHMS), the National Board of Diving and Hyperbaric Medical Technology (NBDHMT), and the Baromedical Nursing Association (BNA). The odds are someone in the field has experience with questions that may present as you are evaluating equipment for your center's needs.

Staffing

If your unit has decided to treat emergent indications, hire your staff accordingly. You will require a physician staff that is competent and comfortable in the management of the critically ill patient. RN staff is strongly recommended to have critical care experience. I like to say, "You can teach hyperbarics in a hyperbaric environment, but you will never have the opportunity to teach critical care nursing in a hyperbaric environment." That being said, ACLS is highly recommended for the nursing and physician staff. CHT or DMTs are preferred to have an EMT background or similar training. They are an extremely valuable part of the team and should be treated as such.

Equipment

Be sure your equipment is hyperbaric environment and operations compatible. This includes but is not limited to:

- Ventilator
- HBO compatible infusion pumps
- Non-invasive blood pressure monitoring
- ECG monitoring equipment

The treatment room should be equipped with, but not limited to, the following equipment:

- Bag Valve Mask (BVM) resuscitator bag
- Oxygen (either wall oxygen or an oxygen cylinder, i.e. an E cell or D Cell)

- Suction machine
- Oral pharyngeal airway devices
- Chest tube insertion trays
- Needle decompression kits for a pneumothorax
- Heimlich valve
- Availability of a crash cart or ability to get response from a code team/rapid response team

Monoplace Chamber Ventilator

Currently the only FDA approved ventilator for use in the monoplace hyperbaric environment in the Sechrist 500A (see Figure 1). This is a pneumatic time-cycled ventilator with the controls located outside the hull, and the ventilator circuit and block located inside the hull. The ventilator operates only in control mode with adjustments for flow, inspiratory time, and expiratory time. An oxygen driving pressure of 65 to 85 psig is required for adequate flow through the ventilator.[1] Oxygen flows through a single hose from the controller, passing through the ventilator pass-through in the hull of the chamber, and connecting to the inlet hose of the ventilator block. Tidal volume is measured inside the chamber with a spirometer connected to the limb of the ventilator circuit. Airway pressure is measured in the ventilator block with manometer, not at the proximal airway. Positive End Expiratory Pressure (PEEP) can be added by placing a PEEP valve or Emerson Water Column in the expiratory circuit. The ventilator will deliver 100% oxygen, or with modifications, 21% oxygen.[2] You cannot blend to obtain other oxygen concentrations. Whenever a patient is mechanically ventilated, the greatest risk of harm is from pulmonary barotrauma. The patient should be well sedated. If it is indicated, use a neuromuscular blocking agent to prevent this complication. If the patient is not sedated, asynchronous respirations with this control ventilator could occur, resulting in air-trapping or increasing auto-PEEP that could lead to a gas expansion injury.

Close monitoring and adjustment of ventilator settings to maintain the required tidal volume is required during compression and decompression. In testing of the 500A ventilator done by Weaver[3] it was found to have significant variability of tidal volume greater than was reported by the manufacturer.

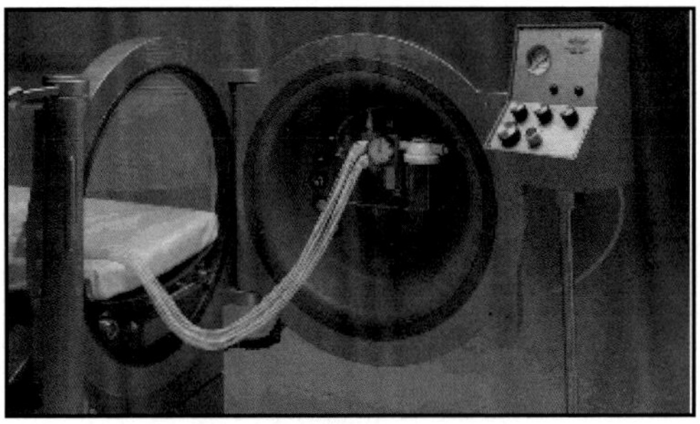

Figure 1: ***500a ventilator.***

Workup

Receive report from transporting unit. Take the time to assess the patient prior to transport to the hyperbaric medicine facility. Preparation time for a critical care treatment, depending on the unit and indication, is approximately 1 hour. Attention to detail is a requisite in the management of these patients. You need to be able to "see" possible complications before they happen. Communication among the ICU, ER and/or respiratory staff is crucial to eliminating mistakes or oversights. Perform your routine hyperbaric workup. This helps eliminate mistakes by following an established routine. Rule out contraindications to HBOT. Document and notify attending physician of absolute or relative contraindications. Obtain CXR and EKG if not already on the chart. Remember HBOT has profound effects on the cardiovascular system. Patients with a history of congestive heart failure or significant cardiac history may require an echocardiogram. Generally, an ejection fraction of 30% or greater is desired. This value is not written in stone. The staff should take into account the entire patient presentation, not simply making a decision based on a single value. Take note of and verify any implanted devices. Ensure the device is hyperbaric compatible.

Virginia Mason's Hyperbaric Medicine Team did an outstanding poster presentation detailing common implanted devices. This is not intended to be an all inclusive listing, but it does provide information on implantable devices. You should always contact the manufacturer of the device for definitive recommendations. Patients usually carry ID cards with device information with them. The following information is derived directly from the Virginia Mason presentation.

Implanted Devices

Device manufacturers were contacted for testing data. Data was pulled from manufacturers through phone calls, online posted data, and email.

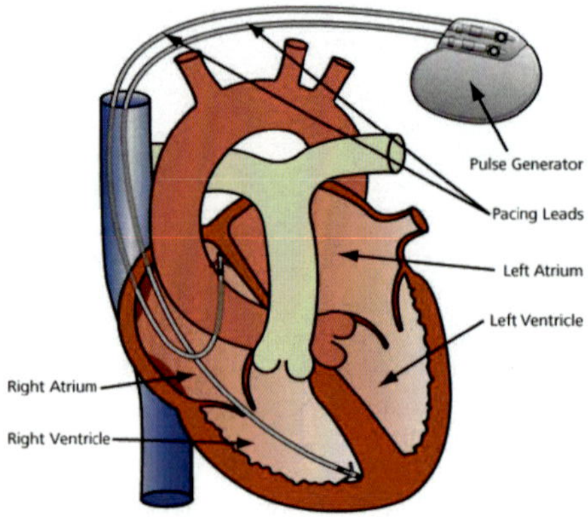

Figure 2: ***Automatic implanted cardiac defibrillators and pacemakers***

- Boston Scientific pacemaker to 2.35 ATA
- ELA Medical pacemaker to 4 ATA
- St. Jude/Ventritex pacemaker to 7 ATA
- St. Jude/Ventritex ICD to 3 ATA
- Medtronic pacemaker and ICD to 2.5 ATA
- Biotronic pacemaker and ICD to 3 ATA

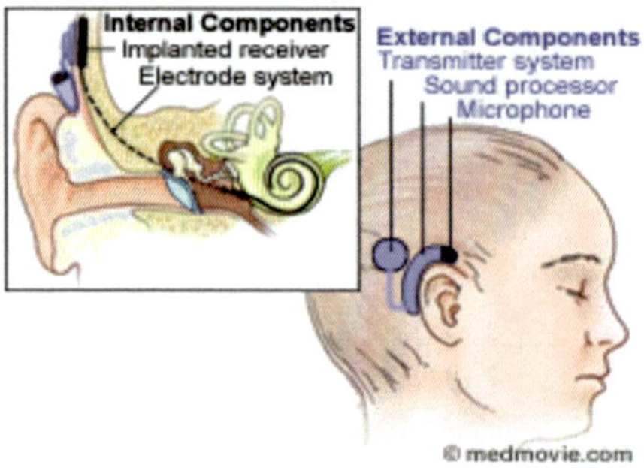

Figure 3: ***Cochlear implants.***

- Nucleus C124R and CI124M to 2.5 ATA
- Freedom to 4 ATA

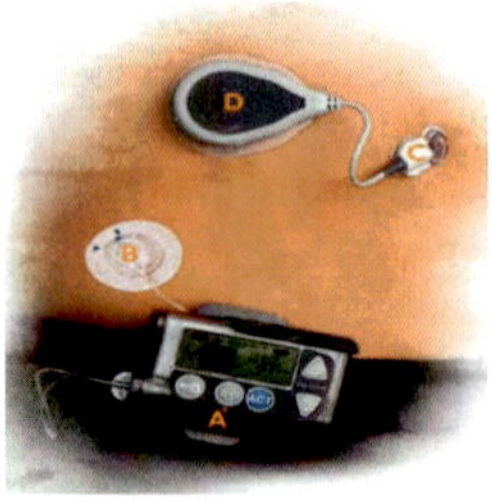

Figure 4: ***Implanted insulin infusion pumps.***

- PX 8 and Animus pumps are rated for swimming only, with 12 ft maximum depth
- Mini med pumps are not water proof or pressure tested for hyperbaric therapy

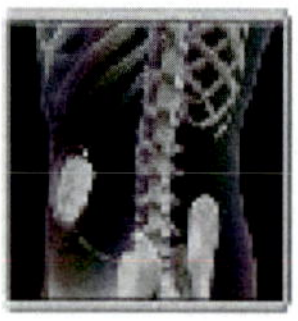

Special thanks to: Wreford-Brown CE and Bodwin DM, Virgina Mason Center for Hyperbaric Medicine

TEAM VIRGINIA MASON MEDICINE

Figure 5: ***ITB TherapySM (intrathecal baclofen therapy.***

- Medtronic Synchro Med II to 2 ATA

Continuing with your assessment, you need to note and document your Intra-Venous (IV) access. Note the location and type of ALL IV access available on the patient. Note if they are patent and flush per your hospital's protocols prior to initiation of pressurization. Central lines are preferred, if available. Note all IV solutions. Hold as many as possible without compromising patient care. Prioritize the fluids to be delivered in accordance with the number of pass-throughs available.

- Vasopressors
- Sedatives/Analgesics
- TPN/Insulin drips
- Antibiotics
- Maintenance fluids

Remember that IV pumps that are made for hyperbaric chamber operations are not extremely accurate at low or high rates of infusion. If the patient is on TPN and you are holding the infusion, convert the drip to a D10 solution. This will help prevent hypoglycemia and possible seizure activity. Check your blood glucose pre and post-treatment. Confer with your physician and pharmacists for the most suitable drip rate. Also, due to peripheral vasoconstriction, intra-muscular injections are not recommended within 1 hour prior to hyperbaric treatment.

Pulmonary

A complete and accurate pulmonary assessment is essential to avoid or prevent gas expansion problems. Many of the critically ill patients treated with HBO will have some degree of pulmonary dysfunction that requires supplemental oxygen. A number will also be intubated, requiring mechanical ventilator support.

Assessing the patient for a significant pulmonary history is a key starting point. Is there a history of asthma, chronic obstructive pulmonary dysfunction (COPD), fibrosis, spontaneous pneumothorax, or chest trauma? Has this patient developed adult respiratory distress syndrome (ARDS) due to their illness? Each of these conditions will impact patient preparation, the method of compression, and particularly decompression of the patient. In patients with reactive airways, COPD, or decreased pulmonary compliance, extra time for the exhalation period needs to be allowed. If a patient is not intubated, a slow decompression (1 psig/minute) is used. The same rate of ascent is used with a patient on mechanical ventilation and in addition to an adjustment of the ventilator to allow the exhalation time to be twice the inhalation time.

If there is chest trauma, has any pneumothorax been treated? A patient with a small, untreated pneumothorax can become a tension pneumothorax on ascent from HBO treatment.[4] Chest tubes can safely be placed in both monoplace and multiplace chambers. Adjustments will have to be made if the chest tube will be placed in a monoplace chamber. The use of a Heimlich valve (Figure 6) attached to the chest tube will allow the escape of air or fluid from the chest cavity and prevent air from entering the chest cavity. If there is drainage, a foley catheter bag or other small container may be attached to collect the drainage.

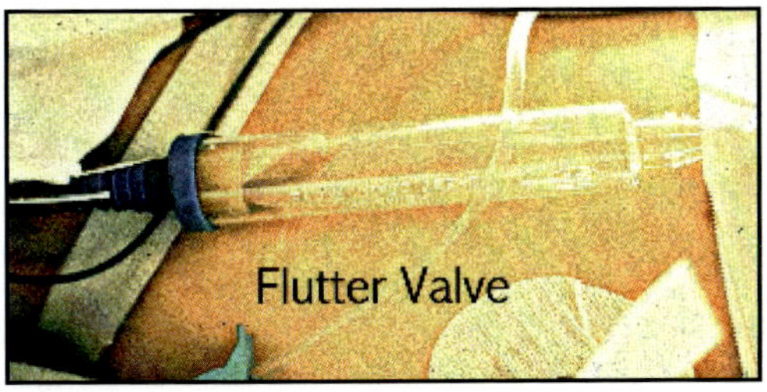

Figure 6: ***Heimlich valve.***

Physical assessment of the patient is the next step. Prior to each treatment, the lungs should be auscultated. If wheezing is present, an inhaled bronchodilator is recommended prior to treatment. Response of the patient to the bronchodilator needs to be assessed prior to placing the patient in the chamber. If there is not relief of bronchospasm, the risk/benefit to the patient needs to be weighed prior to placing the patient in the chamber. Patients with rales present prior to treatment should not be placed flat on the stretcher. Stretcher head will need to be elevated 30-45 degrees, depending on patient tolerance. Patients that are experiencing congestive heart failure (CHF) or dialysis patients with fluid overload should be carefully watched during the hyperbaric treatment. The effect of vasoconstriction from HBO may further exacerbate CHF or fluid overload.

If the patient is intubated and requires ventilator support, special attention to several key areas is required. The size of the endotracheal tube (ET) is important due to the change in gas density at pressure.[5] Adult ET tubes will have cuffs that are inflated with air. Prior to being placed in a hyperbaric chamber, the air needs to be removed and replaced with saline. This is done to prevent the compression of the air (Boyle's law) during HBO treatment. If the air is left in the cuff during HBO, the air will compress and the patient will develop an air leak, making ventilation difficult, if not impossible. At completion of the HBO, the saline will need to be removed and replaced with air. If the saline is left in, there will be a risk of tracheal erosion from increase in pressure at the cuff contact points.

ET tube position should be confirmed with a chest radiograph. The ET tube is well secured and distance noted at the teeth position. Observe the tube for any possible areas of pressure or erosion and make adjustments. Observe chest movement and position of trachea.

The degree of ventilator support is important as to whether or not that can be managed in a hyperbaric environment. Key factors are minute ventilation (Ve), fraction of inspired oxygen (FiO_2), and positive end expiratory pressure (PEEP). The ventilators used in the monoplace hyperbaric chamber are limited in the ability to deliver high Ve.[6] Ways to maximize the HBO ventilator will be discussed in the section on equipment.

In patients with pulmonary dysfunction that require supplemental oxygen, it may be difficult to elevate their PaO2 to what may be considered hyperbarically oxygenated. While a PaO2 level has not been defined, it would be possible to consider the effects of hyperbaric oxygen and at what PaO2 level these effects are activated.[7] Generally speaking, if a patient requires >50% oxygen, it may be difficult to elevate their PaO2 to the point of receiving benefit from HBO. This must be part of the risk/benefit equation in determining whether the patient should receive HBO.

PEEP can be added to the ventilator by placing PEEP valves in the expiratory circuit. Whenever PEEP is added, the patient should be carefully monitored. Auto PEEP can occur and cause cardiovascular compromise. If this should happen, expiratory time can be lengthened with a shortening of inspiratory time. While auto PEEP can be reversed with this maneuver, it can also result in hypoventilation of the patient.

One of the challenges of treating the critically ill patient with HBO is how to monitor their level of oxygenation. While techniques have been developed for use with a monoplace chamber[8] to sample arterial blood and accurately perform the test, this is not without risk and can be labor intensive. A simpler method is the use of a dual Clark electrode connected to a TINA 3, 30 or 400 (Radiometer, USA) transcutaneous monitor.

Cardiovascular

The cardiovascular assessment of a critical care patient receiving hyperbaric oxygen therapy is similar to any cardiovascular assessment of a critical care patient. Cardiac rhythm should be assessed and monitored during the treatment. If the patient would experience a cardiac emergency during HBO treatment, the staff should be trained to handle such an emergency. It is important to remember that a patient at depth is well oxygenated and will remain so for 5 to 8 minutes.[9] The safest way to bring a patient that has had a cardiac arrest to the surface is to bring them up at 5 psig (fastest rate on a monoplace chamber), while the staff prepares to deliver emergency care. Performing a rapid ascent using the emergency ascent button on monoplace chambers places the person at grave risk for air embolism due to expansion injuries. Once the patient has surfaced, move them to the point farthest away from the open chamber, remove the hyperoxygenated clothing, and if appropriate, defibrillate. Cold oxygen will fall to the floor and dissipate in 30 seconds,[10] so do not place the area at an increased fire risk with the use of a defibrillator. The staff needs to be able to respond quickly and appropriately to such an emergency, so it is our recommendation that the staff be Advanced Cardiac Life Support (ACLS) certified.

A wide range of intravenous therapy can be managed during HBO treatments. Blood products, vasoactive drugs, parental feedings, antibiotics, and simple crystalloids can be administered. Enteral feedings may also be administered if the feeding tube, such as the Miller-Frederick Feeding Tube, is placed in the small bowel. Gastric feeding during HBO therapy should be avoided. Vasoactive drugs can be safely managed and delivered to the patient through specially design infusion pumps. There are currently two pumps that are designed to be used with a monoplace chamber and are capable of pumping against increased atmospheric pressure. The two pumps are the IVAC 530 (IVAC Corp., San Diego, CA) and the Abbott Hyperbaric Pump (Abbott Laboratories, North Chicago, IL). Both pumps will have inaccuracies at very low and high infusion rates, particularly if they are pumping against greater than 2.0 atmospheres absolute[11,12]. Adjustments will need to be made to the drug infusion rate by the nurse to hold the blood pressure or cardiac function stable during the HBO treatment. If a vasoactive drug is being administered, cardiac rhythm as well as blood pressure should be monitored throughout the treatment. Overall, the blood pressure should be stable if supported by vasoactive medications before the patient is placed in the chamber. The blood pressure may fluctuate if on a support medication during compression and decompression. Before an adjustment is made in the medication during compression and decompression, it is recommended to observe the blood pressure for a brief period to determine if it will go back to an acceptable range once movement through pressure is complete.

Monitoring Arterial Oxygenation

In specific patients undergoing hyperbaric oxygen therapy, there can be a need to monitor arterial oxygenation and carbon dioxide levels. In patients on mechanical ventilation, it is necessary to evaluate the effectiveness of the minute ventilation being delivered. If the CO_2 is allowed to become elevated, the patient is potentially at greater risk for an oxygen toxic seizure to occur. In patients with pulmonary dysfunction and who require supplemental oxygen or other methods of ventilator support, hyperbaric oxygen can be dosed in order to achieve the desired PaO_2 level. In work done by Weaver,[13] it was found that in patients with abnormal pulmonary function it might be reasonable to treat this group of patients with higher chamber pressures than those patients with normal pulmonary function. It was also noted in their abstract that no decrement in pulmonary function occurred due to hyperbaric oxygen therapy.

There are two methods by which to monitor arterial oxygenation during monoplace hyperbaric oxygen therapy- arterial blood gas sampling and transcutaneous oxygen monitoring. In order to sample arterial blood gases during HBO treatments, a special setup is required and immediate access to a blood gas analyzer is necessary. Any blood sample obtained by this method must be held under pressure and analyzed in less than 2 minutes. The only blood gas analyzer that has demonstrated the ability to measure hyperbaric oxygen tensions is the ABL 330 (Radiometer, Copenhagen, Denmark). This method of determining hyperbaric oxygen and carbon dioxide levels is only recommended for staff with experience in this area and with support equipment readily available.

Determining oxygenation and carbon dioxide levels with the use of a transcutaneous monitor (TCOM) is much simpler and has demonstrated good correlation with arterial PaO2 and PcO2.14 In order to monitor both carbon dioxide and oxygen levels, a dual Clark electrode in required. In a monoplace environment, a TINA3, 30 or 400 (Radiometer) or a Periflux 5000 (Perimed) monitor may used. The electrode should be placed in a central area that does not have scar tissue present or had not previously been irradiated. Traditionally, the mid clavular, third intercostal space has been used for monitoring core oxygenation. There is no correlation found between PaO_2/PcO_2 and TCOM readings from a lower extremity.

Neurological and Assessment Tools

Neurological

Neurological assessment: The assessment of neurological status is dependent on the presentation of the symptomology and diagnosis. You can integrate your neurological examination with other parts of your physical examination. Assess some of the cranial nerves as you examine the head and neck, and inspect the arms and legs for neurological abnormalities as you are inspecting the musculoskeletal system.[15] Organize your thinking into five categories: (1) mental status and speech, (2) cranial nerves, (3) the motor system, (4) the sensory system, and (5) reflexes.

Mental status: The assessment of the mental status of patient in the hyperbaric setting can be crucial in the overall plan of care for that patient. Will the patient be able to follow instructions for Valsalva techniques? Will the patient be able understand directions as far as safety issues are concerned? What risk is the suicidal patient to self and your staff? These are some of the questions that the hyperbaric nurse must assess in a quick, thorough, and timely manner to ensure the proper management of the patient.

The assessment by the nurse begins immediately upon contact with the patient. Begin with the most notable feature, the level of consciousness (LOC). Is the patient alert and aware of his surroundings? Is the patient oriented to person, place, time, and self? These determinations come into play when assessing every patient, but particularly the carbon monoxide (CO) poisoned patient and the injured SCUBA diver with decompression sickness (DCS). The nurse should utilize a standard recognized qualitative format for the documentation of the patient LOC and cognitive function. The Glascow coma scale and the Mini-Mind set exam are examples of these measures (Figure 1). The form provided has combined both measures for a quick assessment tool by the nurse when indicated. A deficit in either of these measures should immediately be brought to the attention of the attending physician for appropriate intervention and documentation. The Mini-Mind set can be used to document cognitive impairment for such disorders as CO poisoning and DCS type II. Also, it can be related to the ability to understand teaching and the need for Pressure Equalization tubes (PE) in the impaired patient. This will eliminate the patient from having to experience any unnecessary middle ear barotraumas.

Speech needs to be assessed for hoarseness or nasal quality of tone. The hoarseness can be due to paralysis of the vocal cords, while a nasal voice can indicate a paralysis of the palate.[16]

Cranial Nerves: The assessment of the 12 cranial nerves can be very extensive. One should try to limit these to a quick screen when possible, unless there is a serious indication of possible impairment. Table 1 describes the function and evaluation of the 12 cranial nerves.[17]

Motor System: Although the examination of the nervous and motor system does not come into play for most hyperbaric patients, it is extremely important in the diagnosis of DCS. Assessment of the motor system can reveal deficits that can aid in the diagnosis of DCS. The following are examples of a few of the more common screening tests that are used.[18]

Gait and Legs

The heel-to-toe: A gait that lacks coordination, with reeling and instability, is called ataxic. Ataxia may be due to cerebellar disease, loss of position

Table 1: *Function and Evaluation of Cranial Nerves*

Name	Function	Evaluation
Olfactory (N1)	Sensory: smell	Volatile oils, coffee (each nostril should be tested separately
Optic (N2)	Sensory: vision	Visual acuity, visual fields (examine fundus to rule out papilledema, vessel integrity, consensual reaction)
Oculomotor (N3)	Motor: movement of eye upward and inward, elevation of eyelid, constriction of pupil (primary responsibility for consensual reactions)	Consensual reaction, pupil size, doll's eye maneuver, accommodation
Trochlear (N 4)	Motor: movement of eye down and out	Observation
Trigeminal (N5)	Motor and sensory: motor to masticatory muscles; sensory to face	Clenching of the jaw, corneal reflex, sensitivity to pinprick and temperature
Abducens (N6)	Motor: movement to lateral rectus of eye	Observation
Facial (N7)	Motor and sensory: motor to muscles of facial expression and stapedius muscle; sensory to anterior two-thirds of tongue (taste); salivary and lacrimal secretions	Uniformity of facial expression; taste (anterior tongue); normal tearing
Acoustic (N8)	Sensory: hearing and equilibrium	Hearing acuity, nystagmus, tuning fork on mastoid
Glossopharyngeal (N9)	Motor and sensory: motor to pharynx, salivary and parotid glands; sensory to pharynx, posterior one-third of tongue (taste); carotid sinus	Gag reflex, taste (posterior tongue), carotid sinus reflex
Vagus (N10)	Sensory and motor: lung, bronchi, heart, gastrointestinal tract, great vessels, esophagus, palate, pharynx, larynx	Gag reflex, symmetrical uvula movement when patient says "ah"
Spinal accessory (N11)	Motor: trapezius and sternocleidomastoid muscle movement	Shrugging of shoulders
Hypoglossal (N12)	Motor: tongue	Observation of tongue for deviation, tremor, atrophy

sense, or intoxication. Tandem walking may reveal an ataxia not previously noted.

Walk on the toes, then on the heels: These are sensitive tests respectively for plantar flexion and dorsiflexion of the ankles, as well as balance. Walking on the toes, then on the heels, may reveal distal muscular weakness in the legs. Further, weak dorsiflexion is a sensitive test for upper motor neuron weakness.

This particular series of screens can be somewhat strenuous on the patient. Utilize your judgment on the selection of screens as related to the patient's physical ability to perform the required actions.

Hop in place on each foot: The test requires a good sense of positioning and normal cerebellar function. Difficulty in hopping may be due to weakness, lack of position sense, or cerebellar dysfunction.

Shallow knee bend: Difficulty here suggests proximal weakness (extensors of the hip), weakness of the quadriceps (the extensor of the knee), or both. Supporting the patient's elbow lightly may be helpful. Alternately, you can have the patient rise from a chair or stool without the use of arm support. This can be useful for patients who are older or less robust.

Romberg Test: This is a functional test of position sense. The patient should first stand with feet together and eyes open, and then close both eyes for 20 to 30 seconds without support. Note the patient's ability to maintain an upright posture, and be sure not to allow a fall. Normally, only minimal swaying occurs.

Arms, Shoulders, and Hands: Check for pronator drift. Usually this test can be combined with the Romberg test. Ask the patient to hold both arms straightforward, palms up, and then close eyes and maintain this position for 20 to 30 seconds. The tendency of one forearm to pronate suggests a mild hemiparesis. A sideward or upward drift, sometimes with searching, writhing movements of the hands, suggests loss of position sense. At this point, you want to tap the arms briskly downward. The arms normally return smoothly to the horizontal position. This response requires muscular strength, coordination, and a good sense of position. When the position sense is lacking, the patient may not recognize the displacement, and if told to correct it, does so poorly.

Check grip strength: Ask the patient to squeeze two of your fingers as hard as possible and not to let them go. (Cross your fingers, middle finger over the index finger to prevent getting hurt by hard squeezes.) You normally should have difficulty removing your fingers from the patient's grip. A weak grip may be due to either upper or lower motor neuron disease.

Lower extremities: Grading for muscle strength should be evaluated on a uniform basis. The following is a grading scale for the muscle strength.

Muscle strength is graded on a 0 to 5 scale:

0 – No muscular contraction
1 – A barely detectable flicker or trace of contraction
2 – Active movement of the body part with gravity eliminated
3 – Active movement against gravity
4 – Active movement against gravity and some resistance
5 - Active movement against full resistance without evidence of fatigue.

This is normal muscle strength.

Additional muscle tone and strength can also be checked for deficits in the following areas:

1. Test flexion and extension at elbows
2. Test finger abduction
3. Test opposition of the thumb
4. Test flexion at the hip
5. Test abduction and adduction of the hip6.
   Test flexion and extension of the knee
6. Test dorsiflexion and plantar flexion of the foot

To complete a neurological examination, the only remaining recommended requirements are deep tendon reflex testing. Note the speed, force, and amplitude of the reflex response. Comparative testing should always be done.

Reflexes are usually graded on a 0 to 4+ scale:

4+ Very brisk, hyperactive; often indicative of disease; often associated with clonus (rhythmic oscillations between flexion and extension)
3+ Brisker than average; possibly, but not necessarily, indicative of disease
2+ Average; normal
1+ Somewhat diminished; low normal
0 No response

Reflex response depends partly on the force of the stimulus provided. Normally use only the amount of force required to illicit a response. It is easier to note deficits with contra-lateral testing than with symmetrical. Symmetrically diminished or even absent reflexes may be found in normal people.[19]

Some of the sites for deep tendon reflexes are

as follows:

1. Biceps reflex (C5, C6)
2. Triceps reflex (C6, C7)
3. Brachioradialis reflex (C5, C6)
4. Abdominal reflexes (T8, T9, T10)
5. Knee reflex (L2, L3, L4)
6. Ankle reflex (S1)
7. Plantar response (Babinski response) (L5, S1)

Special Considerations: The suicidal patient presents with unique considerations. The opportunity for injury within the hyperbaric environment still exists. The patient must be thoroughly examined for any ignition sources before entering the chamber. Also, note respiration patterns during any change of pressures to ensure no possibility of pulmonary barotraumas. Patient safety must always be in the forefront of our minds, even if it is not in theirs.

Restraints: If there is a need for the use of restraints with the hyperbaric patient, some issues need to be considered. In our facility, we employ the use of the Sigma II Perry Baromedical Dualplace chamber. In actuality, this is a large monoplace chamber that has the capability of a separate entry lock for tenders and is air compressed. The patients are delivered oxygen through a "built-in-breathing system" (BIBS). When we are treating a critical care patient that is ventilator dependent, the use of chemical intervention is usually required. Also, during this same scenario, soft wrist restraints are utilized to prevent the potential for patient injury to self. As always, in any setting in healthcare, ensure that the proper documentation is in place. JCAOH standards require a physician's order for the restraints, the purpose, and duration of application. Capillary refill times should be noted distal to the application sites, and should be less than 3 seconds. In addition, with the use of chemical restraints, special attention must be paid to the eyes. Provide a lubricant to both eyes and secure them with a small eye dressing or tape them shut. This will prevent the cornea from being injured during the absence of a blink reflex.

Assessment Tools: Objective, reproducible assessment is critical in medical management. Currently there are 2 indications that warrant utilization of validated neurological screening tools. These are decompression illness (DCI) and carbon monoxide poisoning. Both of these conditions can significantly impair cognitive function. Unfortunately, sometimes with these indications, cognitive impairment may be subtle. Utilization of the described screening tools for an objective measure can be extremely useful in detecting such impairment. In addition, there is significant research being performed on the use of HBOT for traumatic and anoxic brain injuries. If new indications are warranted, validated screening tools will be part of a routine work-up for treatment.

Below is an excerpt from Alert Diver Magazine, Fall 2009 issue that gives an excellent overview for neurological assessment of the injured diver. "Field Neurology for Divers" was written by Herbert B. Newton, M.D., and Eric Douglas, Director of DAN Training. The form detailed in the article is an excellent example on how to set up a neurological assessment form (Figure 7). The next form is a classic example of a simple cognitive function assessment frequently utilized in the geriatric setting, screening for dementia. The test is the Folstein Mini-Mind State Exam (MMSE). It can be used in our setting as a reliable quick screen for cognitive impairment (Table 2).

Gastrointestinal

Gastrointestinal Assessment: The management of the critical care patient in the hyperbaric setting always provides unique challenges. One must take into consideration any gastrointestinal involvement during the treatment regimen. Does the patient have a P.E.G. tube that may leak gastric content onto the skin and cause excoriation? Does the patient have a nasogastric tube that requires suction, or can it be clamped during treatment?

Inspection of the Abdomen: Note the four quadrants for any obvious abnormalities, such as pulsating masses or bulging organs. Auscultation of the right lower quadrant is usually sufficient in that peristalic bowel sounds transmit easily within the abdominal cavity. In the patient with suspected lower peripheral vascular disease, bruits can be heard above the iliac and femoral arteries.[20] Take note of hyperactive bowel sounds, and ask the patient about recent bowel habits. Nothing would be more embarrassing than an "accident" while in the chamber. A distended bowel from gas formation will actually be eased of pain at 2 ATA while breathing oxygen.[21]

Tubes: The attending nurse should take note of any presence of tubes, i.e., nasogastric (NG). If the patient does have a nasal gastric tube, one should note the amount of drainage from the nursing report prior to transport. Determine if can be clamped during treatment and obtain a physician order, or if intermittent low pressure suction will be required, if the chamber is so equipped. Tube patency and placement should be assessed prior to

NEUROLOGICAL ASSESSMENT

Vital Signs: Pulse rate____/Min Respirations_____/Min Blood pressure_____/_____

MENTAL FUNCTION

Consciousness:
❑ Alert
❑ Verbal
❑ Painful
❑ Unresponsive

Orientation:
❑ Person (what is your name?)
❑ Place (where are you?)
❑ Time (estimate what time it is?)

Ability to follow commands: Ask the diver to "Stick out your tongue and close your eyes." ❑ Yes ❑ No
Expression: Say "red, white and blue" or "no ifs, ands or buts." ❑ Yes ❑ No
Name 3 objects (e.g. comb, mask, scuba cylinder): ❑ Yes ❑ No
Read and interpret a sentence: ❑ Yes ❑ No
Example: "The small boy walked to the lake with a large dog."

Judgment:
Why are you here?
❑ Yes ❑ No

Memory: 3 items/3 minutes
Repeat 3 objects identified earlier
❑ Yes ❑ No

Calculations: (circle misses) 93, 86, 79, 72, 65, 58, 51, 44, 37, 30, 23, 16, 9, 2
Able to complete? ❑ Yes ❑ No

Abstract reasoning/proverbs: Interpret a proverb such as "A birc in the hand is worth two in the bush." Or "A stitch in time, saves nine."
Could the diver explain the proverb? ❑ Yes ❑ No

CRANIAL NERVES

EYES: Forward Left Right Up Down   Nystagmus (eye twitching): ❑ Yes ❑ No
Circle any direction the diver cannot look.
FACE: Close eyes and smile.   HEARING: Symmetrical ; >1 foot ❑ Yes ❑ No
Is the face symmetrical? ❑ Yes ❑ No
LIGHT TOUCH: Forehead L ❑ R ❑ Cheek L ❑ R ❑ Jaw L ❑ R ❑ Chin L ❑ R ❑
Identify any area where the diver identifies altered sensation.

MOTOR FUNCTION

Grading scale: No movement (0), Movement but weak (3), Normal (5)

Arms:			Legs:		
Shoulders	L___	R___	Hip flexors	L___	R___
Biceps	L___	R___	Quadriceps	L___	R___
Triceps	L___	R___	Hamstrings	L___	R___
Finger spread	L___	R___	Foot (up)	L___	R___
Grip strength	L___	R___	Foot (down)	L___	R___

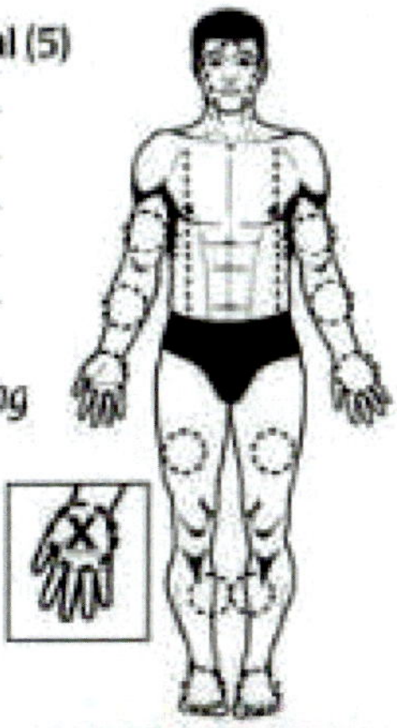

SENSORY FUNCTION

Shade in any areas on the figure at right with decreased sensation using the symbols below.
LIGHT TOUCH: X PIN: P BOTH: B

COORDINATION AND BALANCE

WALK: ❑ Normal ❑ Wobbly ❑ Unable to complete
FINGER-NOSE-FINGER: Able to complete? ❑ Yes ❑ No

COMMENTS:____
____
____

DAN
DIVERS ALERT NETWORK
1-919-684-4DAN

Figure 7: *DAN Neurological Assessment.*

TABLE 2: *Folstein Mini-Mental State Exam*

Folstein Mini-Mental State Exam	SCORE
I. ORIENTATION Ask the following questions: correct = ☑ **Record Each Answer:** (Maximum Score = 10) What is today's date? Date (e.g., May 21) 1 ☐ What is today's year? Year 1 ☐ What is the month? Month 1 ☐ What day is today? Day (e.g., Monday) 1 ☐ Can you also tell me what season it is? Season 1 ☐ Can you also tell me the name of this hospital/clinic? Hospital/Clinic 1 ☐ What floor are we on? Floor 1 ☐ What city are we in? City 1 ☐ What county are we in? County 1 ☐ What state are we in? State 1 ☐	
II. IMMEDIATE RECALL correct = ☑ (Maximum Score = 3) Ball 1 ☐ Flag 1 ☐ Tree 1 ☐ Ask the subject if you may test his/her memory. Say "ball, "flag," "tree" clearly and slowly, about one second for each. Then ask the subject to repeat them. Check the box at right for each correct response. The first repetition determines the score. If he/she does not repeat all three correctly, keep saying them up to six tries until he/she can repeat them NUMBER OF TRIALS: __________	
III. **ATTENTION AND CALCULATION** **A. Counting Backwards Test** (Record each response, correct = ☑) (Maximum Score = 5) 93 1 ☐ 86 1 ☐ 79 1 ☐ 72 1 ☐ 65 1 ☐ Ask the subject to begin with 100 and count backwards by 7. Record each response. Check one box at right for each correct response. Any response 7 or less than the previous response is a correct response. The score is the number of correct subtractions. For example, 93, 86, 80, 72, 65 is a score = 4; 93, 86,78 70, 62 = 2; 92, 87, 78, 70, 65 = 0. **B. Spelling Backwards Test** Ask the subject to spell the word "WORLD" backwards. Record each response. Use the instructions to determine which are correct responses, and check one box at right fore each correct response. D 1 ☐ L 1 ☐ R 1 ☐ O 1 ☐ W 1 ☐ **C. Final Score** Compare the scores of the Counting Backwards and Spelling Backwards tests. Write the greater of the two scores in the box labeled FINAL SCORE at right, and use it in deriving the **TOTAL SCORE.** **FINAL SCORE**______ (Max of 5 or Greater of the two Scores)	
IV. RECALL (correct = ☑) (Maximum Score = 3) Ball 1 ☐ Flag 1 ☐ Tree 1 ☐	
Ask the subject to recall the three words you previously asked him/her to remember. Check the Box at right for each correct response. **V. Language** (correct = ☑) (Maximum Score = 9) **Naming** Show the subject a wrist watch and ask him/her what it is. Repeat for a pencil. Watch 1 ☐ Pencil 1 ☐ **Repetition**	

Ask the subject to repeat "No, ifs, ands, or buts." Repetition 1 ☐	
Three -Stage Command Establish the subject's dominant hand. Give the subject a sheet of blank paper and say, "Take the paper in your right/left hand, fold it in half and put it on the floor." Takes paper in hand 1 ☐ Folds paper in half 1 ☐ Puts paper on floor 1 ☐	
Writing Give the subject a sheet of blank paper and ask him/her to write a sentence. It is to be written spontaneously. If the sentence contains a subject and a verb, and is sensible, check the box at right. Correct grammar and punctuation are not necessary. Writes sentence 1 ☐	
Copying Show the subject the drawing of the intersecting pentagons. Ask him/her to draw the pentagons (about one inch each side) on the paper provided. If ten angles are present and two intersect, check the box at right. Ignore tremor and rotation. Copies pentagons 1 ☐	
Reading Hold up the card that reads, "Close your eyes." So the subject can see it clearly. Ask him/her to read it and do what it says. Check the box at right only if he/she actually closes his/her eyes. 1 ☐	
Add the number of correct responses. The maximum is 30. **Folstein MF, Folstein SE, and McHugh PR, 1975**	TOTAL SCORE __________ 23-30 = Normal 19-23 = Borderline <19 = Impaired Up to Grade 8 Level

entry into the chamber.[22] PEG tubes need to be secured to the skin to prevent pulling. Reinforce the dressing to prevent leakage onto the underlying tissue.

Genitourinary

Assessment of Genitourinary system: There really is no required examination of genitourinary system, but there may be situations that must be accounted for. The most common is the need for some type of urinal device for the elderly patient who is taking a diuretic. It would be greatly preferred if the patient can time their dosage so that the medication does not peak while the patient is treatment. Another consideration is the congestive heart failure patient. If this patient and physician decide to withhold the diuretic until after treatment, the patient will be at increased risk for pulmonary edema during the course of the treatment. Monitor breath sounds and saturation levels closely on these patients pre- and post-treatment.

One of the goals in the treatment of DCI is re-hydration of the patient. Most divers are commonly dehydrated to some degree. During the course, a USN treatment Table 6, while pushing fluids either orally or intravenously, the need for a urinal is bound to arise. Be sure and have the forethought to have one in the chamber prior to initiating treatment.

Foley Catheters: Empty the reservoir bag prior to treatment. Ensure that the retention balloon is filled and secure. Place the reservoir bag between the patient's legs in a dependent position. Inspect the catheter for any kinks or leakage. No other special attention is required with a foley catheter except that it does not get pulled or dislodged upon entry into the chamber.[23]

Nursing Standards of Care

Established in 1985, the Baromedical Nursing Association (BNA) has provided a professional organization for hyperbaric nurses to flourish in the field. Leadership and collaboration of colleagues have advanced the professional society to provide certification exam via National Board of Diving and Hyperbaric Medical Technology. It has provided scholarships and funding for research within the field. Arguably, one of the biggest contributions from the BNA in recent years has been the publication of Nursing Standards of Care for Patients Receiving Hyperbaric Oxygen Therapy, revised 2007. As a surveyor for the Undersea Hyperbaric Medical Society (UHMS) accreditation teams, I can attest that it is utilized to assess nursing plans of care. You should be versed

Table 3: ***Nursing Standards of Care***

PROBLEM	GOAL/RATIONALE	ACTONS
1. Anxiety related to knowledge deficit of hyperbaric oxygen therapy and treatment procedures. Definition: Anxiety is a practical risk with hyperbaric oxygen treatments. It can occur before, during or after the treatment. Identify signs and symptoms of anxiety • Patient verbal admission of anxiety Clenching of fists Flushed face Complaint of nausea or diarrhea Sudden complaint of pain or discomfort Feelings of being smothered or suffocated Urgency to empty bladder Defensive attitude Profuse diaphoresis Flat affect Tachycardia Restlessness	Patient and/or family will state: 1. Rationale for hyperbaric oxygen therapy. 2. Goals of therapy. 3. Procedures involved with hyperbaric oxygen therapy. 4. Potential hazards of hyperbaric oxygen therapy. Purpose: Familiarize the patient with the procedure, potential beneficial effects and safety precautions relating to his/her treatments to ensure patient's emotional comfort.	1. Assess and document patient and/or family's understanding of rationale for and goals of hyperbaric oxygen therapy, procedures involved with, and potential hazards of hyperbaric oxygen therapy. 2. Identify barriers of learning. • Involve interpreter if indicated • Apply age-specific teaching • Consider cultural/religious factors • Assess readiness to learn 3. Include information on the following when identified as a learning need: • Purpose and expected outcomes of hyperbaric oxygen therapy • Sequence of treatment procedures and what to expect, e.g., pressure, temperature, noises, wound care • Gas delivery systems; hands-on practice of applying mask or hood • Ear clearing techniques • Pulmonary barotrauma • Prevention of oxygen toxicity 4. Provide continued opportunities for discussion and instruction. 5. Provide patient and/or family with information brochure on hyperbaric oxygen therapy. 6. Keep patient and/or family informed of all procedures. 7. Document patient/family instruction, using the confirmation of instruction form and the general patient instruction form.
2. Potential for injury related to transferring patient in/out of chamber and within hyperbaric facility Identification: Equipment located in the hyperbaric facility should only be items necessary to provide patient care. Excess items like personal belongings or other medical equipment unrelated to the function of HBO treatment contribute to potential injury hazards and therefore should be removed. All necessary equipment in the facility should be in good working order at all times. Only those personnel trained to operate the equipment should do so.	Patient will not experience any injury. Purpose: The patient has the right to expect safe care delivery throughout the admission.	1. It is the responsibility of all staff, led by the Safely Director to inspect the facility and identify equipment with the potential of causing harm to a patient in any state. 2. Comply with the local Fall Risk Policy; assess patient's potential risk for fall and apply precautions as appropriate. 3. All equipment with the potential for injury will be secured to prevent harm. 4. Assist patient in and out of the chamber appropriately. • 1-2 person assist, as necessary • Use of gait belt, as necessary • Use of foot stool and/or lower gurney to load patient • Use of slide board, as necessary • Use side rails on stretcher, as appropriate 5. Communicate transfer plan with patient and staff involved prior to taking action.

3. Potential for barotraumas to ears, sinuses, teeth, and lungs or cerebral gas embolism related to changes in atmospheric pressure inside hyperbaric oxygen chamber.	Prevention of barotraumas during HBO2	Ear Barotrauma • Administers decongestants, per physician orders, prior to HBO2 • Patient education prior to HBO therapy should include: methods to equalize pressure in middle ear during therapy; patient demonstration of equalization techniques and importance of notifying chamber operator immediately when pressure or fullness is felt in middle ear Nursing interventions include: • Assess tympanic membrane pre and post HBO treatment, recording level of barotrauma using TEED scoring system • Assess patient's ability to equalize pressure • Have HOB elevated during HBO therapy to assist in equalization of middle ear • Ensure operator of chamber understands chamber descent should stop when patient is unable equalize pressure and should return to the point of no pain/pressure prior to asking patient to equalize ears. Pneumothorax • Identify those patients at greater risk for development of a pneumothorax • Implement protocols to decrease risk of pneumothorax in high risk patients • Observe for: - sudden, sharp chest pain - difficult, rapid breathing - abnormal chest movements on the affected side Nursing interventions include: • Notify physician, follow physician's orders for patient management • Chamber should not be decompressed until preparations are made for emergency decompression of pneumothorax Document assessments.

4. Potential for oxygen toxicity seizures related to delivery of 100% oxygen at an increased atmospheric pressure	Signs and symptoms will be recognized and promptly addressed. Seizing patients will suffer no harm.	1. Report patient assessment outcome to hyperbaric physician of: • elevated body temperature • history of steroid use • history of oxygen seizures • other high risk factors as appropriate 2. Monitor patient during HBO_2 and document signs and symptoms of central nervous system oxygen toxicity including: • Numbness and twitching • Ringing in the ears or other auditory hallucinations • Vertigo • Blurred vision • Restlessness and irritability • Nausea (Note: CNS oxygen toxicity can ultimately result in a seizure.) 3. Change 100% oxygen source to air for patient if signs and symptoms appear and notify the hyperbaric physician. 4. Protect patient during seizure.

5. Potential for inadequate therapeutic gas delivery related to delivery systems and patient's needs/limitations.	Signs and symptoms of inadequate oxygen delivery will be recognized and reported promptly.	1. Assess the patient's condition, needs, and limitations for the best suited gas delivery systems: • head hood for children with facial deformities, or per patient preference (customize neck dam when possible for best fit). • face mask • "T" piece (Briggs adapter) for patients who are intubated or with tracheostomy or laryngectomy. • Ventilator for intubated patients who require ventilation assistance. 2. Monitor the patient's response to the oxygen delivery system, including their ability to tolerate chosen system. 3. Assist the hyperbaric technician with the delivery system, as appropriate. Head Hood a. Assist patient with application and removal of hood. b. After assembly, check for leaks c. Observe patient for signs and symptoms of CO_2 build- up, including restlessness. Face mask/Mouth Piece a. assist patient with mask, application and removal, and reposition mask/ mouth piece as needed. (i.e. monoplace) b. Check form leaks, continuity of seal against the patient's face, keep tight fit around mouth piece. T-Piece (Briggs adapter) a. set-up process b. monitor patient's rate and depth of respirations, listen to breath sounds. c. notify the hyperbaric physician if patient is experiencing difficulty breathing. Have IV access for medication administration if needed. d. suction as needed. Ventilator a. document management of ET cuff with NS prior to descent. b. Keep suction equipment nearby and ready to use. Suction PRN. c. Monitor and document patient's tidal volume, respiratory rate and breath sounds prior to chamber pressurization, after chamber pressurization, then every 10-15 minutes, or as ordered. d. Monitor patient for respiratory distress. Notify hyperbaric physician if apparent. e. Manually oxygenate the patient if necessary (resuscitator bag). f. Monitor PtcO2 levels, pulse oximetry, or ABG levels, if possible, and as ordered. Notify hyperbaric physician of abnormal readings.

6. Anxiety related to feelings of confinement associated with the hyperbaric oxygen chamber. Definition: Confinement anxiety is a practical risk with hyperbaric oxygen treatments. It can occur before, during or after the treatment. Identify signs and symptoms of anxiety • Patient verbal admission of anxiety • Clenching of fists • Flushed face • Complaint of nausea or diarrhea • Sudden complaint of pain or discomfort • Feelings of being smothered or suffocated • Urgency to empty bladder • Defensive attitude • Hyperventilation • Profuse diaphoresis • Flat affect • Tachycardia • Restlessness	Patient will tolerate the hyperbaric oxygen therapy treatment. Purpose: • To prevent confinement anxiety during treatment. • To assess the degree of confinement anxiety when it may occur and manage it effectively. • By relieving or decreasing contributing or precipitating factors, its incidence may be reduced.	1. Patient interaction: • Address patient calmly. • Establish eye contact with the patient. • Reassure patient that he/she is safe. 2. Assess patient for any history of confinement anxiety. 3. Engage patient in problem-solving his/her feelings of confinement anxiety. 4. Identify barriers of learning. • Involve interpreter if indicated • Apply age-specific teaching • Consider cultural/religious factors • Assess readiness to learn 5. Implement preventative measures as appropriate: • Education • Chamber tour • Anti-anxiety medication • Eliminate preconceived notions • Empower patient; he or she is in charge and may request to end treatment at any time. • Offer diversional activities: TV, music, books on tape, family member chamber side. • Assure patient of nurse presence throughout treatment. 6. Prior to, during, and after the hyperbaric oxygen therapy treatment, monitor and assess for signs and symptoms of confinement anxiety. 7. Notify hyperbaric physician of patient's response to the anti-anxiety measures and ability to tolerate confinement. 8. Document results of interventions.
7. Pain related to associated medical problems.	Patient will state satisfaction with pain management	1. Assess patient's experience of pain and whether pain is increased during HBO_2. 2. Medicate patient for pain before HBO_2 as needed. Document efficacy of analgesic. 3. Have analgesic available during HBO2 treatment. 4. Reposition patient for comfort. 5. Avoid IM medications immediately prior to treatment.

8. Discomfort related to temperature and humidity changes inside hyperbaric chamber. Definition: According to Charles' law, when gas volume is kept constant the temperature of the gas will vary with the absolute pressure. As pressure increases, so does temperature; the reverse is true during decompression.	Patient will tolerate the internal climate of the chamber. Purpose: Slowing the rate of gas flow through the chamber increases the relative humidity. This effect is the result of a greater accumulation of the patient's evaporative moisture loss within the chamber. The increased humidity in a monoplace chamber decreases the risk of static electricity.	1. Identify barriers of learning: • Involve Interpreter if indicated • Apply age-specific teaching • Assess readiness to learn 2. Discuss with patient prior to treatment how the pressure environment affects the temperature. 3. Discuss with the patient how their exhalation contributes to the relative humidity in the chamber. 4. Periodically assess patient's comfort with humidity and temperature. 5. Offer the patient comfort measures: • If the patient complains of being cold, first decrease the purge flow of the monoplace chamber; slowing the flow, increases the temperature. • If the patient continues to be cold, next offer a blanket keeping in mind that should a fire occur within the chamber, more fuel is available. • If the patient complains of being warm; slow compression rate and increase the chamber purge flow; offer a cool moist cotton cloth to take into the chamber. • Ensure the chamber facility temperature is maintained according to manufacturer recommendations; usually 68-72 Degrees F.
9. Potential for ineffective individual coping related to stresses of illness and/or poor psych-social support systems.	Patient will be able to comply with HBO2 treatment procedures	1. Provide support and encouragement without exceeding treatment outcome expectations. 2. Discuss with patient ability to cope with other caregivers. Stay informed of progress and helpful approaches. 3. Facilitate communication between patient and/or family and other HBO2 staff members. 4. Encourage patient, if able, to discuss concerns and feelings. 5. Document pertinent discussions and assessments.
10. Potential for dysrhythmia related to disease pathology	Signs and symptoms of dysrhythmia will be recognized and promptly addressed	1. As ordered, monitor EKG readings while patient is inside the chamber, (especially if IP on telemetry) . 2. Monitor and document blood pressure as indicated (by invasive or non-invasive methods). 3. Assess and document any signs of hypokalemia in patients with acute necrotizing infections. 4. Maintain IV infusions as ordered. 5. Maintain invasive pressure monitoring and record values, as indicated (make sure infusion pumps are plugged into D/C). 6. Obtain lab samples as ordered. 7. Notify hyperbaric physician as needed.

11. Potential for fluid deficit related to dehydration or fluid shifts.	Signs and symptoms of fluid volume deficit will be recognized and promptly reported	1. Assess fluid and electrolyte balance. Maintain hydration and/or pressure support as per physician order. 2. Monitor patient's I & O as indicated. 3. Monitor patient's vital signs as indicated.
12. Altered cerebral tissue perfusion to: a. carbon monoxide poisoning b. decompression sickness c. gas embolism d. other	Signs and symptoms of changing neurologic functioning will be recognized and promptly addressed.	1. Perform baseline neurological assessment prior to treatment. 2. Monitor neurological checks per established protocol. 3. Use a common language such as Glasgow Coma Score to facilitate communication and determination of altered level of consciousness. 4. Assess and document patient's motor and sensory functioning. 5. Provide reorientation and emotional support as needed. 6. Notify physician of changes as per facility protocol.
13. Potential for alteration in comfort, fluid, and electrolyte balance to nausea and vomiting.	Patient will experience decreased symptoms of nausea and vomiting	1. Assess and document patient's complaints of nausea. 2. Maintain airway integrity to prevent aspiration. 3. Notify hyperbaric physician of patient's nausea and administer medication as ordered. 4. Place NG tube if ordered. 5. Monitor and document amount of emesis on patient's I & O record.

14. Altered health management related to knowledge deficit.	Patient and/or family will be able to state/ discuss factors appropriate to the management of their disease process during treatment.	1. Assess for knowledge deficits related to underlying pathology. 2. Identify patient's expectations of treatment. 3. Begin discharge planning with patient during first visit. Supply information in format to match patient's preferred learning method. 4. Document patient/family teaching, their understanding of instructions, and any return demonstrations. 5. Provide orientation to the hyperbaric environment to include: chamber orientation; middle ear equalization, fire hazards; safety policies and procedures; and risk and benefits of hyperbaric oxygen therapy. 6. Appropriate information specific to the patient's disease process should be provided. 7. Upon discharge, written instructions should be provided to patient and /or family. Monitor the patient during HBO2 and document signs and symptoms of pulmonary oxygen toxicity including: • substernal irritation or burning • tightness in the chest • dry, hacking cough • difficulty inhaling a full breath • Dyspnea on exertion • Monitor Units of Pulmonary Toxicity Dose (UTPDs) to max of 1425/ day. • Notify the hyperbaric physician if signs and symptoms of pulmonary oxygen toxicity appear. • Add humidity to oxygen as needed to reduce chest discomfort.
15. Potential for pulmonary oxygen toxicity related to delivery of 100% oxygen at an increased atmospheric pressure	Signs and symptoms of pulmonary oxygen toxicity will be recognized and promptly addressed Problem: Hyperbaric oxygen involves placing a patient (fuel) in 100% oxygen (oxidizer) under pressure in a chamber. To complete the fire triad, an ignition source is necessary and this can occur from a spark in the chamber.	1. Follow fire prevention procedure per established policy and procedure. 2. Hyperbaric oxygen treatment teaching and consent of the patient will include the risks of fire in the hyperbaric environment. 3. Provide the patient and family an educational pamphlet that discusses the fire risks with HBO and the materials to be avoided during treatment. 4. Staff will conduct a safety inspection prior to each treatment to ensure fire safety precautions are met. Prohibited items will not enter the chamber. 5. The Safety Director will: • Screen patients with special circumstances (prohibited items). • Collaborate with the Medical Director to determine medical necessity. • Identify ways to reduce fire risk. • Sign a Prohibited Items release form, if indicated, to allow certain materials to enter the chamber. 6. The chamber and patient will be confirmed as grounded prior to treatment. 7. Staff will participate in quarterly unit fire drills to ensure preparedness.

16. Potential for injury related to fire within the hyperbaric chamber. Problem: Hyperbaric oxygen involves placing a patient (fuel) in 100% oxygen (oxidizer) under pressure in a chamber. To complete the fire triad, an ignition source is necessary and this can occur from a spark in the chamber.	Patient will not experience any injury related to fire. Purpose: The patient has the right to expect safe care delivery throughout the admission.	1. Follow fire prevention procedure per established policy and procedure. 2. Hyperbaric oxygen treatment teaching and consent of the patient will include the risks of fire in the hyperbaric environment. 3. Provide the patient and family an educational pamphlet that discusses the fire risks with HBO and the materials to be avoided during treatment. 4. Staff will conduct a safety inspection prior to each treatment to ensure fire safety precautions are met. Prohibited items will not enter the chamber. 5. The Safety Director will: • Screen patients with special circumstances (prohibited items). • Collaborate with the Medical Director to determine medical necessity. • Identify ways to reduce fire risk. • Sign a Prohibited Items release form, if indicated, to allow certain materials to enter the chamber. 6. The chamber and patient will be confirmed as grounded prior to treatment. 7. Staff will participate in quarterly unit fire drills to ensure preparedness.

in the document and incorporate it in your plans of care. Below is listed the Nursing Standards of Care as available on the website www.hyperbaricnurses.org. Note how the nursing diagnoses are relevant to the emergent indications.

Critical Care Indications

You have assessed your patient. You know your indication and the patient status. You have your equipment ready, everything is zeroed and calibrated. IV lines are labeled and ready to go. Now what? Your treatment table is determined by the diagnosis type. The following is intended to be an overview of the common emergent indications, not a comprehensive guide. Any good hyperbaric medical library will include copies of Hyperbaric Oxygen Therapy Indications, UHMS, L.B. Gesell, 12 Edition, a UHMS committee report, and Hyperbaric Medicine Practice, 3rd Edition, Kindwall and Whelan. These publications are revised periodically, so keep abreast of the changes. They also give details in the science, research, and physiology behind the treatment rationales. The tables listed are not the only treatment tables available in the field, but some of the more commonly utilized. Whatever treatment tables are utilized, ensure they are provided by a reputable professional organization and recognized within the industry as being effective.

- Arterial Gas Embolism– USN Treatment Table 6 or equivalent
    - Utilization review after 10 treatments, resolution usually after 1 treatment
- Carbon Monoxide– USAF Treatment CO
    - After initial treatment, patients with persistent cognitive sequela may require additional treatments until there is no further improvement
    - Baseline neurological exam
    - Utilization review after 5 treatments
- Clostridial Myonecrosis (Gas Gangrene)– (USAF Gas Gangrene Treatment Table)
    - This one takes coordination with the surgeon and the surgery schedule.
    - Provide 3 treatments within the first 24 hours. Provide at least a 2 hour surface interval; preferably 4 hours between treatments.
    - Then twice a day treatments for the next 2-5 days.
    - Utilization review is indicated after 10 treatments.
    - Collaborate with the surgeon for patient response of the abating necrosis.
- Crush injuries and Compartment Syndromes – (USAF Wound Care table/ USN treatment table 9)
    - Treatment protocol depends on the severity of the injury.
    - At minimum, twice a day treatments should be initiated utilizing the USAF Wound Care table or the USN treatment table 9 within the first 24 – 36 hours. The earlier, the better the chance for a positive outcome.
    - Utilization review is recommended after 7 days or 14 treatments. Supportive HBOT may be required under a wound care protocol.
- Decompression Sickness– (USN Treatment Table 6)

The formation of inert gas bubbles in the tissues and vascular system after rapid decompression from increased atmospheric pressures or rapid ascension in altitude.

If the patient has been in a compressed air environment (SCUBA diving, rapid altitude changes) prior to onset of symptoms and if the patient presents with signs and symptoms of DCS, whether it is:

- Type I – Musculoskeletal pain only, skin manifestations, "chokes" without neurological symptoms
- Type II – Numbness, tingling, motor weakness, ataxia, etc.

- One must assume a DCS injury. There is no definitive diagnostic testing for DCS.
- Considerations with DCS injuries
    - Baseline neurological exam
    - Elevated correlation with dehydration and DCS
    - Provide IV fluids
- On scene management should include 100% O_2 via non-re-breather mask.
- If patient is being air medevaced, keep cabin pressure to less than 7,000 feet or if on a helicopter, a ceiling of 1,000 feet, if possible

There are a wide variety of treatment tables available for DCS. You cannot go wrong by utilizing a USN Treatment Table 6. It can be administered in any monoplace with air-break capability. Extensions during the administration of the treatment are dependent on patient response and determined by physician/technical assessment. Resolution of symptoms usually occurs after a single treatment. Repetitive treatments may be required. Once there is no improvement of symptoms for two consecutive treatments, general consensuses is to hold HBOT.

- Utilization review is recommended after 10 treatments.

- Central Retinal Artery Occlusion (CRAO)-(USAF Wound Care table/USN Treatment Table 9)
  - The sudden painless onset of loss of visual fields and/or light perception due to a thrombus or emboli in the central artery.
  - Considered an emergent indication
  - Provide the highest level of surface level FIO_2 as soon as possible.
  - For the highest possibility of resolution, HBOT must be initiated within 24 hours of onset of symptoms.

Alabama Blue Cross Blue Shield has included CRAO in their local coverage determination since 2006. More and more local coverage determinations are providing coverage for the indication. Check with your local coverage determinations.

- If there is no response to surface level O2 within 5 minutes, refer to HBOT.
- Compress to 2.0 or USN TT9 - 2.4 ATA x 110 minutes.
- If vision improves, continue with twice a day treatments for a minimum of 3 days.
- If there is no improvement in vision after 20 minutes of O2 at 2.0/2.4 ATA, compress to 2.8 ATA. Consider continuing with a USN TT6.
- Clinical plateau should be reached within 1 week of treatment. Utilization review is indicated after 3 days of treatment or stabilization of vision has occurred.

Conclusion

There are 13 recognized indications for treatment with hyperbaric oxygen therapy. Of those, only two are treated with HBOT as the primary mode of therapy: arterial gas embolism and decompression illness. All other indications for HBOT are an adjunct to the primary treatment course. If HBOT is not available, as noted in the cases of CO poisoning and CRAO, normobaric oxygen therapy is indicated. In addition, I would also argue that the true definition of a compromised graft/flap could be categorized as an emergent indication due to twice a day treatment schedules. This means thhat of the 13 indications, 9 of those have an emergent component to the treatment protocols. Proper preparation, planning, and defining the scope of service can increase the delivery of hyperbaric services to your community. It enhances outcomes, provides a needed service, and can potentially save lives. Become familiar with your resources and equipment. Acquire a good medical library for reference material. Establish working relationships with other hyperbaric medicine centers within your area. And lastly, become involved in your professional organizations. With these tools in mind you can increase your scope of service and provide a truly wonderful service unlike any other in medicine.

References

1. Weaver LK, Greenway L, Elliott CG. Performance of the Sechrist 500A ventilator in a monoplace hyperbaric chamber. In: Kindwall EP, ed. Hyperbaric Medicine Practice, 1995; 235-245.
2. Weaver LK. Air breaks with the Sechrist 500A monoplace hyperbaric ventilator. J. Hyperbaric Medicine 1988;3(3):179-186.
3. Kindwall E. Gas Embolism. In: Kindwall EP, ed. Hyperbaric Medicine Practice, 1995; 328-341.
4. Kindwall E. Gas Embolism. In: Kindwall EP, ed. Hyperbaric Medicine Practice, 1995; 328-341.
5. Weaver LK. Management of critically ill patients in the monoplace hyperbaric chamber. In: Kindwall EP, ed. Hyperbaric Medicine Practice, 1995;174-235.
6. Weaver LK. Appendix V. Performance of the Sechrist 500A hyperbaric ventilator in a monoplace hyperbaric chamber. In: Kindwall EP, ed. Hyperbaric Medicine Practice, 1995;235-
7. Weaver LK, Howe S, Berlin SL. Normobaric measurement of O2 tension of blood and saline tonometered under hyperbaric oxygen conditions. J Hyperbaric Med. 190;5(1):29-38.235-245.
8. Weaver LK, Howe S, Berlin SL. Normobaric measurement of O2 tension of blood and saline tonometered under hyperbaric oxygen conditions. J Hyperbaric Med. 190;5(1):29-38.235-245.
9. Holcomb JR, Matos-Navarro AY, Goldmann RW. Critical care in the hyperbaric chamber. In: Problem Wounds. (Davis JC, Hunt TK, eds.) New York:Elsevier, 1988; 187-209.
10. Personal communication with Weaver LK 1993.
11. Evans P, Weaver LK. The use of IVAC 530 infusion pumps in the monoplace hyperbaric chamber. Undersea Biomed Res. 1991;18 (supplement):18-19.
12. Ziegler BA, Weaver LK. Intravenous infusion pumps: evaluation for use with the monoplace hyperbaric chamber. Undersea Biomed Res. 1991;18 (supplement):91.
13. Weaver LK, Howe S. Arterial oxygen tension of patients with abnormal pulmonary function during hyperbaric oxygen therapy. Undersea Biomed Res. 1991;18 (supplement):107-108.
14. Howe S, Hein S, Weaver LK, Larson-Lohr VL, Kristo D, Haberstock D. Response of arterial oxygen tension and transcutaneous oxygen to changes in alveolar PO_2. J. Undersea and Hyperbaric Medicine 1995:22 (supplement): 76.
15. Bates, Barbara. Techniques of Examination, THE NERVOUS SYSTEM, In: A guide to physical examination and history taking, 5th ed., pp 514-517
16. Bates, Barbara Techniques of Examination, THE NERVOUS SYSTEM, In: A guide to physical examination and history taking, 5th ed., pp 518
17. Means, B, Taplett, L. Quick Reference to Critical Care Nursing, Aspen Publishers 1986, p.161
18. Bates, Barbara. Techniques of Examination, THE NERVOUS SYSTEM, In: A guide to physical examination and history taking, 5th ed., pp 520-530
19. Bates, Barbara. Techniques of Examination, THE NERVOUS SYSTEM, In: A guide to physical examination and history taking, 5th ed., pp 531-537
20. Bates, Barbara Techniques of Examination, THE GASTROINTESTINALSYSTEM, In: A guide to physical examination and history taking, 5th ed., pp 344-345
21. Kindwall, Eric Hyperbaric Medicine Practice, Best Publishing Co., pp18
22. Kindwall and Goldman Hyperbaric Medicine Procedures, Aurora Health Care, pp 68
23. Hyperbaric Oxygen Therapy Indications, UHMS, L.B. Gesell, 12 Edition
24. Diving Medicine, Saunders Publishing 1990, Bove and Davis
25. Hyperbaric Medicine Practice, 2nd Edition Revised, Best Publishing Company 2002, Kindwall and Whelan
26. Hyperbaric Nursing, Best Publishing Company 2002, Larson-Lohr and Norvell_Folstein MF, Folstein SE, and McHugh PR, 1975
27. Field Neurology for Divers Alert Diver, Issue: Fall 2009, Newton, M.D., and Douglas

Notes

CHAPTER

9

Essentials of Wound Management

Patrick N. Kimbrell, MD and Heather A. Mckenzie, MD

Over the last 15 years, interest in developing strategies to effectively manage high risk, difficult, or non-healing wounds has blossomed. Pharmaceutical companies have perfected basic dressings and developed interactive and biological dressings that maintain a proper healing environment or stimulate the healing cascade. These advanced dressings have undoubtedly given the clinician a much wider array of options for managing or stimulating the wound bed. Which of these dressings will prove to be superior in helping "heal" the wound is still an area under investigation.

During this same period of time, interested and astute researchers and clinicians have worked to expand our understanding of wound healing, as well as conditions that inhibit or disorder the healing process. Through this improved understanding, we continue to develop and perfect management strategies, improving our ability to heal problem wounds and significantly improve patient outcomes.

Emerging from this explosion of wound activity appear the modern day clinical wound specialists: physicians, nurses, and technicians, all trying to assimilate and make sense of this plethora of information, dressings, and products, merging the new concepts with the old rules in hopes of finding a "best way" to manage problem wounds.

This chapter is not written to be all-inclusive. Its goal is to guide the wound specialist towards a logical sequence of evaluation and thought that will allow the clinician to consistently evaluate wounds and formulate effective treatment plans for all wound types.

The concepts that make up the "Essentials of Wound Management" were initially developed as a teaching tool to help physicians and nurses understand how to logically approach the evaluation of a wound patient. Its success in quickly bringing a working understanding to these topics, emphasizing the most important concepts of wound management, has helped numerous clinicians establish a solid foundation on which to expand and build on through clinical practice and experience.

This chapter will review each of the essentials, and explain the concept and its effect on wound healing and management strategies. The chapter is written to help the reader to focus on a logical sequence of evaluation and management with the goal of limb salvage, healing, and improved outcomes. The emphasis is on what you need to do upon initial evaluation of the wound, and in the subsequent hours and days. These same essentials should also serve to help you focus on the most important concepts of ongoing wound management.

The Essentials of Wound Management

1. Managing bioburden
2. Maximizing perfusion and oxygenation
3. Managing necrotic and non-viable tissue
4. Controlling edema
5. Stopping repetitive trauma and pressure
6. Reducing excessive inflammation
7. Maintaining the healing environment

Essentials as a Tool

There are many potential causes of chronic wounds, and it is likely that any single wound has multiple contributing factors, all of which must be addressed in order for sustained wound closure to occur. Successful management of chronic wounds depends not so much on topical products, but on the ability of the clinician to identify the underlying causes of the wound and then aggressively address them through proper wound management.

The steps that make up these essentials have been successful in guiding the wound specialist towards effective wound management strategies when utilized, in earnest, each time the patient's wound(s) are evaluated, from initial contact through final resolution. Once mastered, each step can be part of your evaluation thought process, easily fitting into the time frames typically allotted for an initial evaluation as well as follow up visits.

Just as the disease processes that disorder and inhibit the wound healing cascade are often complex and overlapping, you will notice that as you read through each essential of wound care that content and concepts also overlap. Such is the thought process of a successful wound specialist: to be able to identify the processes that are inhibiting a wound from healing, then resolving or temporizing as many as possible until the body is able to once again progress positively towards the biologically preferred process of healing.

Essential 1: Managing Bioburden

The term bioburden has been coined in recent years to refer to organic and inorganic material(s) generated in the wound bed such as necrotic tissue, colonizing bacteria, slough, chronic wound fluid, cell debris, foreign bodies, and enzymes. This bioburden stimulates an inflammatory response or activates a host immune response. Bioburden can add to the physical barrier in the wound base, creating a metabolic stress load and, in excess, can rob the wound of vital nutrients and oxygen needed to feed the normal healing process. Although bioburden is essential in kicking off the healing cascade, if it becomes excessive or prolonged these factors can collectively disorder healing and lead to a delay or inhibition of wound healing.

Bacterial Burden and Biofilms

All chronic wounds have a bacterial load, usually consisting of normal skin flora. If bacterial growth goes unchecked in a compromised host, bacterial colonies can increase to a "critically colonized state," which begins to impede wound healing by creating a pro-inflammatory environment with secreted proteases which decrease available wound growth factors, while at the same time robbing the wound bed of healing nutrients and oxygen. The wound will start to exhibit excess drainage, pain, odor, friable granulation tissue, or increasing non-viable or necrotic tissue. This is the stage of bacterial burden termed infection.

To complicate matters further, many of these wounds will have more than one bacterial or infecting organism contributing to the wound bacterial burden which can lead to the formation of wound biofilms. Biofilms appear when a community of bacterial organisms within the wound secretes a polysaccharide and protein slim coat that protects them from host defenses and antibiotics. The organisms, bacteria, yeast, or viruses in the protective biofilm secrete toxins into the wound bed which can promote a prolonged inflammatory state, tissue destruction, and contribute to a chronic non-healing wound condition. For wound

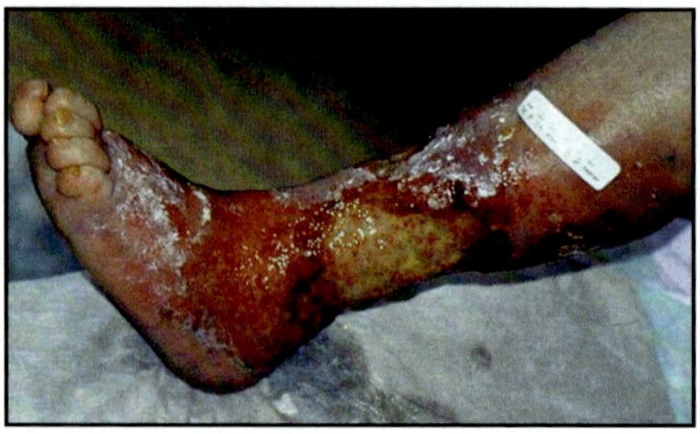

Figure 1: ***Arterial venous ulcer with high bioburden.***

healing to progress, wound balance must be reestablished by decreasing these invasive organisms, biofilms, and ultimately bioburden, to a level that can be managed by host defenses.

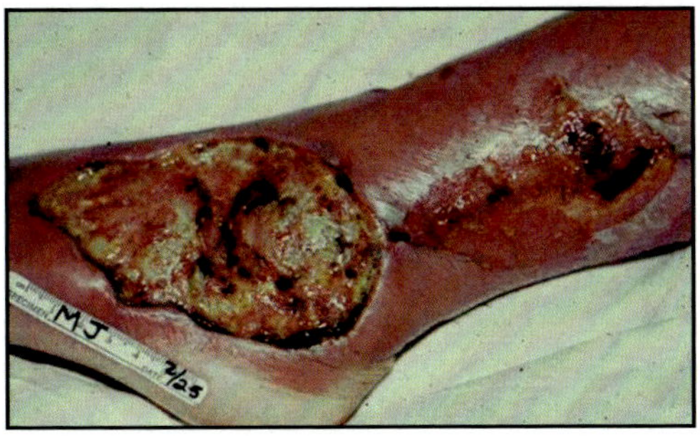

FIGURE 2: ***Infected wound.***

ESTABLISHING WOUND BALANCE

Tissue cultures should be obtained and sent from the leading edge of the tissue-bioburden interface to help guide possible antibiotic needs. If your clinical impression is consistent with critical colonization or infection, then appropriate systemic antibiotic coverage must be started and a decision on topical wound treatments made. Systemic and topical antibiotics have a place in managing bacterial burden therefore decreasing overall bioburden within a wound bed. Topical antibiotics (bactroban, bacitracin, silver, etc.) have been commonly and successfully used to manage local bioburden either alone or in combination with systemic antibiotics, depending on the severity of tissue invasion or infection.

Antiseptics are effective against gram positive and gram negative bacteria, viruses ,and fungus, all useful in the management of chronic wounds which are usually colonized by polymicrobes. Topical antiseptics such as boric acid (2%), acetic acid (2%), or sodium hypochloride (Dakins) can be used in both the early and late stages of bacterial bioburden control when immediate bacteriostatic or bactericidal activity is required to quickly suppress and control bacterial growth. Although very effective in decreasing bacterial bioburden, these clinically useful strengths of antiseptics can still interfere with cellular proliferation and, therefore, healing. Once the wound is brought back into balance, antiseptics should be discontinued and replaced with topical antibiotics or appropriate moisture balancing wound dressings.

Although many wound dressings have been developed with the goal of mediating bioburden, to date the most effective and immediate treatment that can be applied by the wound specialist remains sharp debridement. This action will remove non-viable, necrotic tissue and bioburden that serve as a nutritional source and safe haven for bacterial growth (see "Managing Necrotic and Non-Viable Tissue"). You will realize as you continue to read that the subsequent steps of the essentials all have feedback that helps decrease bioburden. All clinical treatments that bring the wound back into balance serve to ultimately decrease wound bioburden.

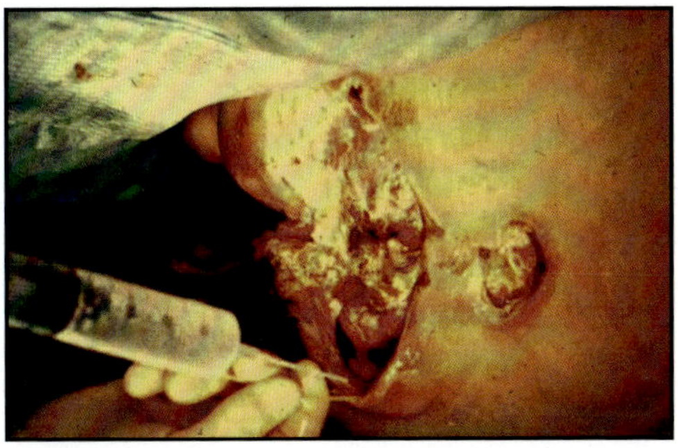

FIGURE 3: ***Lavaging wound with 2% boric acid.***

ESSENTIAL 2: MAXIMIZING PERFUSION AND OXYGENATION

Oxygenation from adequate arterial perfusion is essential for support of tissue metabolism, growth, integrity, and viability. We are born with a redundancy of tissue perfusion, enabling the healthy arterial bed to quickly increase oxygenation to meet increases in metabolic demand.

Tissue aging, chronic disease, and arthrosclerosis eventually results in a decrement of this perfusion reserve. Over time, this may progress to the point where arterial function fails to adequately respond to an increased need for tissue oxygenation (hypoxia). If this perfusion response worsens, a severe deficit in tissue oxygen can result in loss of tissue integrity or even tissue death (ischemia).

The concept of tissue perfusion-oxygenation and healing is not as straightforward as some clinicians think. For example, intact and undamaged skin and tissue can survive at relatively low levels of oxygen-perfusion (20 mmHg). Only after an insult results in skin or tissue damage does the oxygen and, therefore, perfusion need to increase ($\geq$40 mmHg) in order to support normal healing. Once healing is complete, a subsequent return to lower oxygen levels may be tolerated, as long as further wounding can be avoided. Critically ischemic limbs (<20mmHg or ABI < 0.6) should be quickly referred for a full vascular evaluation since this group of wound patients is at high risk of healing failure in spite of proper wound care.

Establishing Wound Balance

In patients with marginal tissue perfusion (>20mmHg or ABI > 0.6), the evaluating wound specialist should expeditiously evaluate the patient's wound(s) using the essentials and start aggressively managing, reversing, or ameliorating as many of the barriers to healing as possible. Often, this will improve the wound bed to the extent that it contributes to improved perfusion and oxygenation, placing the wound back onto a positive healing trajectory.

Wound bed perfusion and oxygenation must be reassessed during weekly follow-up visits. Sometimes the wound bed will fail to show improvement and oxygenation will remain marginal, even with good wound management. Instigation of a full vascular evaluation for these patients then becomes the prudent course of action.

In addition to revascularization, other adjuncts for increasing wound bed oxygenation include the appropriate application of hyperbaric oxygen therapy and negative pressure wound therapy (NPWT).

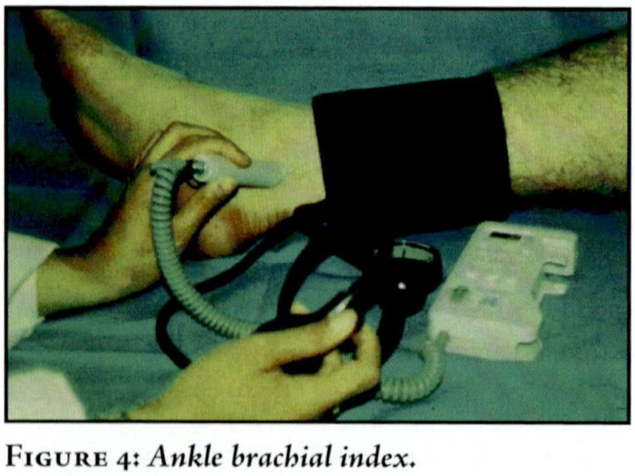

Figure 4: ***Ankle brachial index.***

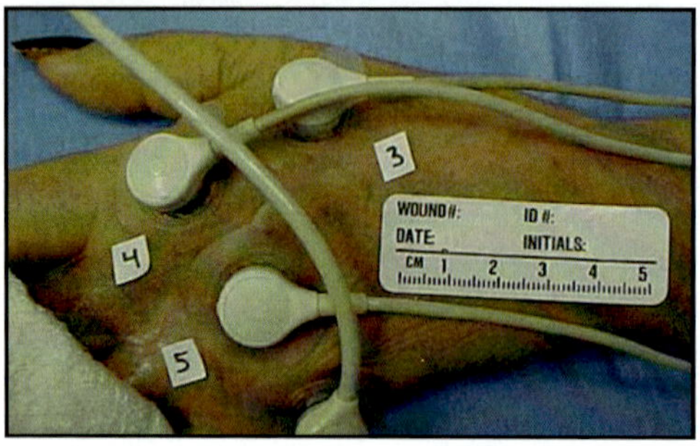

Figure 5: ***Evaluating tissue oxygenation with TCOM.***

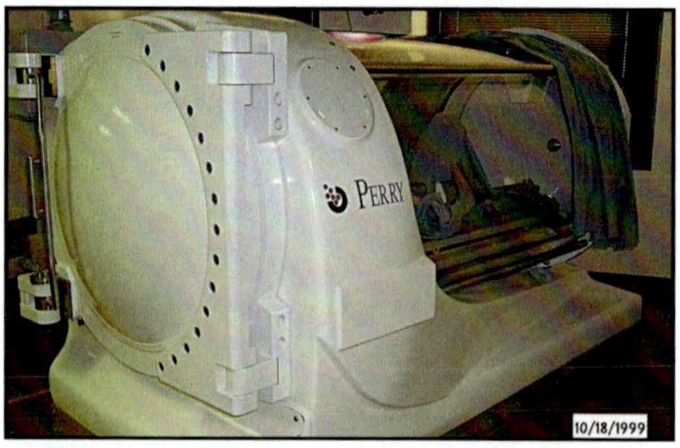

Figure 6: ***Monoplace hyperbaric oxygen chamber.***

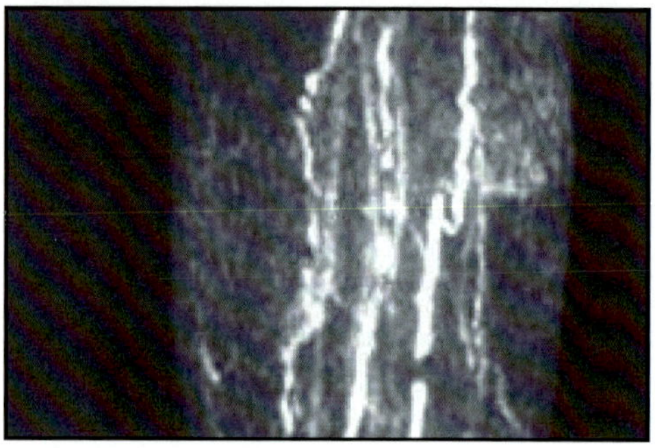

Figure 7: ***Arteriogram.***

Essential 3: Managing Necrotic and Non-Viable Tissue

Dead and nonviable tissue within any wound bed is a major impediment to healing, no matter whether the host is healthy or compromised. Necrotic tissue serves as a significant oxygen sink to the wound bed, enabling bacteria and bioburden to flourish while contributing to drainage, inflammation, and edema.

Once damaged tissue loses its blood supply and dies, it becomes a foreign body with all its associated complications. It has the potential to overstimulate the inflammatory cascade and serves as a nidus for infection by providing a non-perfused interface for bacteria to hide from the host immune response or escape from normally effective antibiotic regiments. While necrotic tissue is better tolerated by the well-perfused tissue envelope and wound bed, it becomes a significant contributor to wound chronicity or deterioration when present in a marginally perfused or hypoxic wound.

Establishing Wound Balance

Nonviable tissue can consist of skin, subcutaneous tissue, fat, muscle, fascia, tendon, bone, or any combination of these tissues. The fastest and usually most effective means to remove this healing impediment is through sharp debridement.

Stable but marginally perfused wounds benefit from an early debulking debridement to near viable tissues. As the initial wound assessment and management plan improves tissue perfusion, a more complete debridement to bleeding and viable tissue should be accomplished.

Adequately perfused wounds can be debrided to viable and bleeding tissues as early as the initial wound evaluation. In both wound types, as the tissue around the wound bed improves and begins to heal, the wound often expels non-viable and necrotic debris from deep in the tissue bed necessitating repeat interval wound debridements.

Critically ischemic wounds should be quickly referred for a full surgical-vascular evaluation since this group of wound patients is at high risk of healing failure in spite of proper wound care and debridement. These patients will benefit from returning to the care of a wound specialist after the surgical-vascular intervention has been accomplished.

While sharp debridement continues to be the most effective means to rid a wound of necrotic and non-viable tissue(s), pulse lavage, ultrasonic, and enzymatic techniques have shown to be effective debridement adjuncts when appropriately applied.

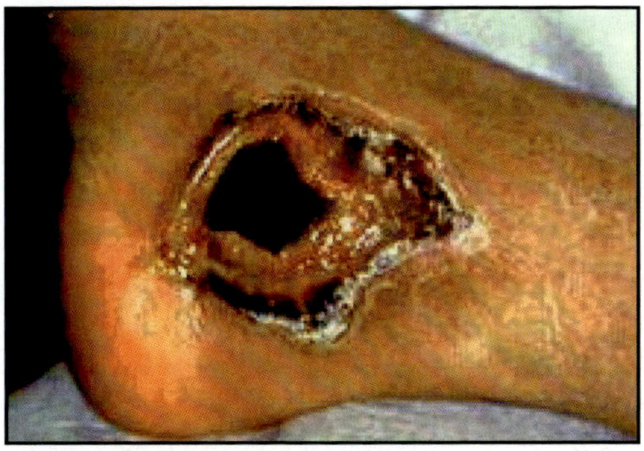

Figure 8: ***Necrotic wound bed.***

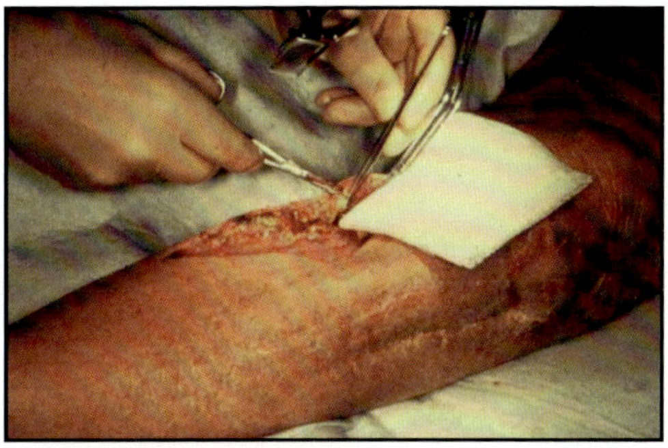

Figure 9: ***Sharp debridement of non-viable tissue.***

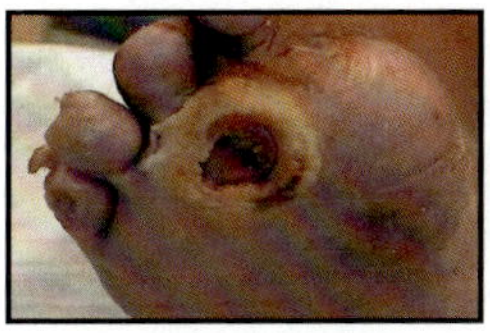

Figure 10: ***Chronic wound bed before debridement.***

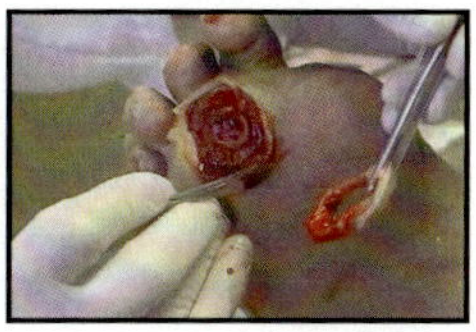

Figure 11: ***Debridement of callus and non-viable skin.***

Essential 4: Controlling Edema

Often ignored, overlooked, or underestimated, chronic tissue edema (swelling) has a powerful negative effect on the body's ability to heal all wound types. Healing involves fluid release into the wound and periwound tissues as part of the normal healing cascade. Excessive edema becomes destructive when present chronically. Causes of edema are multiple and can be simple or complex. Venous stasis, infection, trauma, necrotic tissue, hypoxia, and inflammatory diseases can all contribute to edema. Whatever the origin, edema originates from plasma leakage from the damaged vascular system into the surrounding wound and periwound tissues.

Under chronic conditions, this protein rich fluid becomes inflammatory and can initiate a series of enzymatic processes such as activation of matrix metalloproteinases (MMPs), which can ultimately be destructive to the healing process, degrading the extracellular matrix, interfering with collagen formation, and binding growth factors. The protein rich fluid leads to pericapillary cuffing and increases the diffusion distance from the arterial bed to the skin and tissues, starving them of oxygen and nutrients needed to repair or sustain tissue integrity. Fibrin plugs, due to coagulation of the protein rich fluid, can block and scar lymphatic channels, leading to a progressive worsening of the edema, dermatosclerosis, and inflammatory dermatitis. It becomes obvious that controlling edema should be a major focus in both the prevention and healing of wounds.

ESTABLISHING WOUND BALANCE

The wound specialist will positively influence and reduce wound edema with each wound essential that is managed, treating hypoxia, infection, necrotic tissue, trauma, and inflammation will all result in edema reduction. The lower extremity, where 75% of all problem wounds occur, often requires additional treatment to reduce edema. Presently, the most effective way to accomplish this is through the use of gradient compression bandages or wraps. 2 to 4 layer gradient wraps are very effective and are able to treat patients with ankle-brachial indexes between 0.5 and 1.2. Properly placed and managed, gradient leg wraps will augment venous and lymphatic flow, reversing the problems associated with destructive tissue edema, while simultaneously serving as a secondary wound dressing, and have been proven a powerful tool when applied to edema management. Once the wounds are healed, patients with chronic venous stasis or lymphedema will benefit by being placed in maintenance gradient stockings in order to reduce the risk of forming future non-healing wounds.

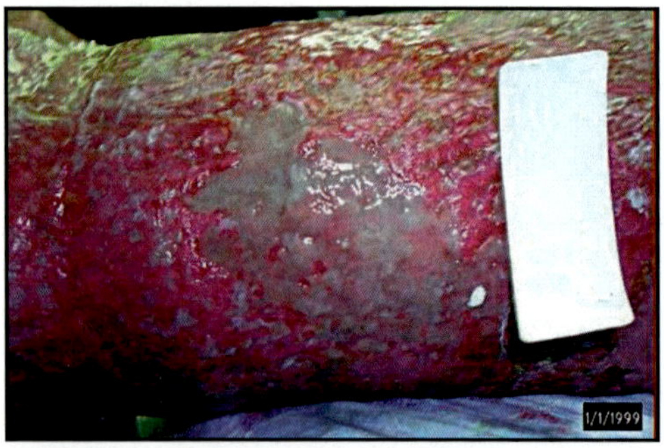

FIGURE 12: ***Edema with inflamed wound.***

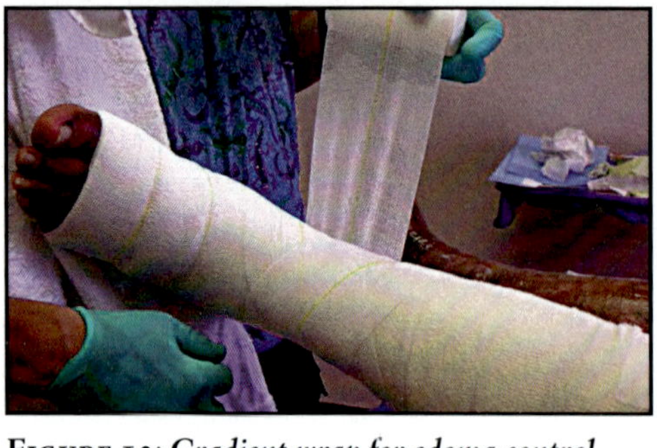

FIGURE 13: ***Gradient wrap for edema control.***

ESSENTIAL 5: STOPPING REPETITIVE TRAUMA AND PRESSURE

The most expensive or elaborate dressing available will not protect or overcome the damage of sustained repetitive pressure or trauma to tissue or a wound bed. While the concept behind avoiding pressure and trauma appear basic, it can be one of the most difficult to achieve because it involves strict patient compliance and often assistance from family or other healthcare providers.

The 3 main trauma types are: friction and shear, static pressure, and repetitive trauma. All have the ability to cause, as well as perpetuate, wounds.

Friction and shear are common forces seen with bed mobility and transfer from flat surface and describe when the skin surface rubs (friction) and then tears (shears). Friction and shear not only have the ability to cause tissue damage, but they are also sensitizers, making skin more susceptible to damage from both static and repetitive traumas.

Static pressure usually results from laying, sitting, or standing, and describes the forces and damage that occur at the interface of skin and a boney prominence. When sustained, the skin and underlying tissues become ischemic as the microcirculation becomes occluded and damaged leading to tissue necrosis and ulceration.

Repetitive trauma is most frequently seen in ambulatory patients with diabetic neuropathy and results in non-healing wounds of the forefoot and toes.

The wound specialist cares for patients that have a multitude of diseases that lead to susceptibility to trauma and pressure related injuries. Diabetes mellitus, peripheral neuropathy, peripheral vascular disease, and Charcot's arthropathy are definite risk factors, and it is not uncommon for wound patients to suffer from one or more these conditions. The loss of protective sensation that occurs with peripheral neuropathy and vascular disease is a common theme in the recurrence of trauma and pressure related injuries. Conditions that lead to patient immobility are a major risk factor for pressure injuries including stroke, multiple sclerosis, spinal cord injuries, and critical illness resulting in prolonged hospital stays. Finally, moisture, urine, and stool all act as sensitizers when chronically present on the skin, resulting in accelerated tissue breakdown when coupled with pressure or trauma.

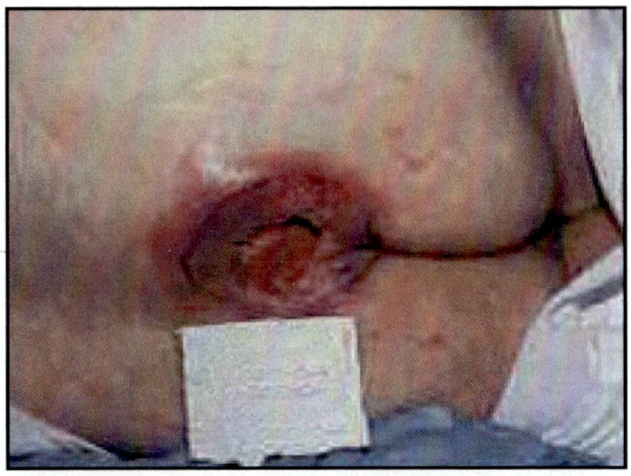

Figure 14: ***Sacral pressure ulcer.***

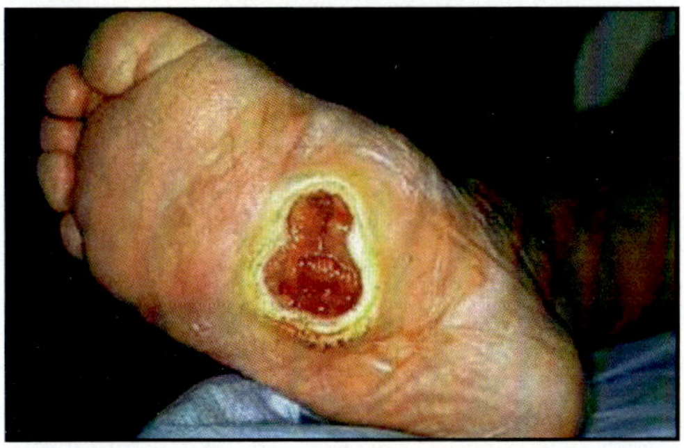

Figure 15: ***Charcot neuropathic foot ulcer due to repetitive trauma.***

Establishing Wound Balance

Early resolution of repetitive trauma and pressure is essential to wound healing and is best attacked using a multifaceted approach involving the wound specialist, patient, medical staff, family, friends, and a trusted orthotist. Wound off-loading can be broken down into acute and maintenance phase off-loading. Examples of acute phase off-loading include: total contact cast, removable cast walkers, Darco wedge shoes, and off-loading boots such as multi-podis or prevalon. Mobility off-loading aids include crutches, walkers, and wheelchairs. Bed off-loading cushions reduce static pressure and limit shear/friction and can even manage moisture. In severely debilitated or bed-bound patients an "every 2 hour" patient repositioning (off-loading) schedule is a must.

After wound healing, it is important to reduce the very real risk of wound recurrence. Aggressive maintenance phase off-loading must be instigated by the treating wound specialist. Proper orthotic shoes, inserts, and braces are critical as well as correct maintenance off-loading cushions. The patient, caregivers, and family must be educated in proper off-loading techniques and the importance of maintenance off-loading. Physical therapy aimed at strengthening the patient and returning a level of mobility should not be overlooked. It bears repeating that "the most expensive or elaborate dressing available will not protect or overcome the damage of sustained or repetitive pressure or trauma to tissue or a wound bed."

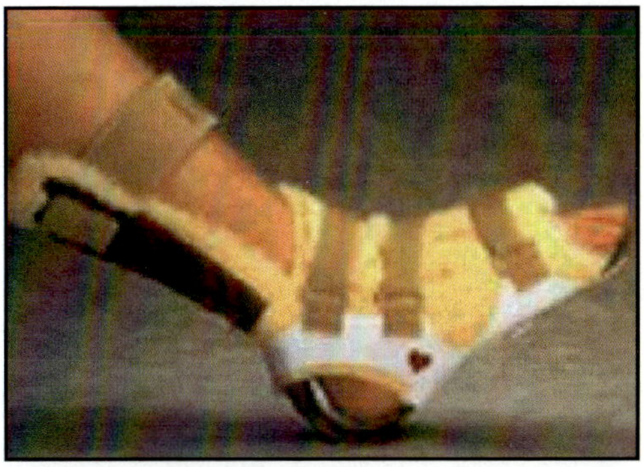

Figure 16: ***Off-loading boot.***

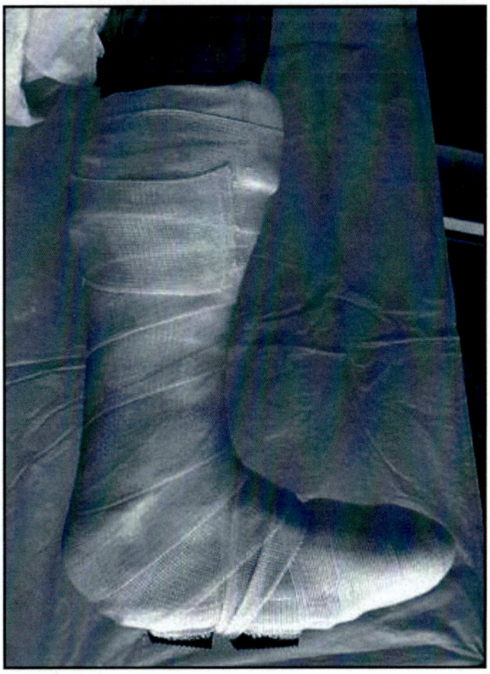

Figure 17: ***Total contact cast.***

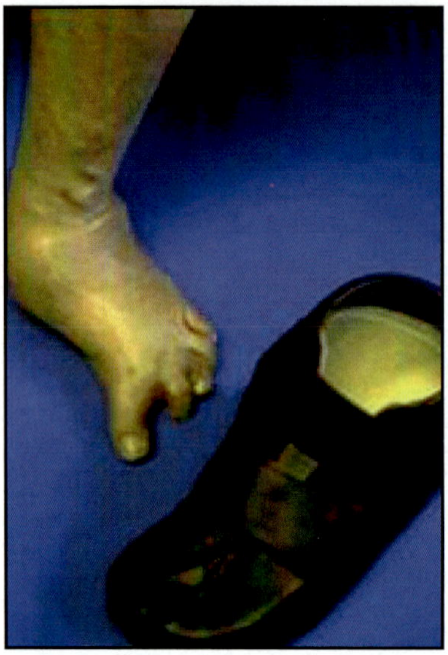

FIGURE 18: ***Custom orthotic shoe with insert.***

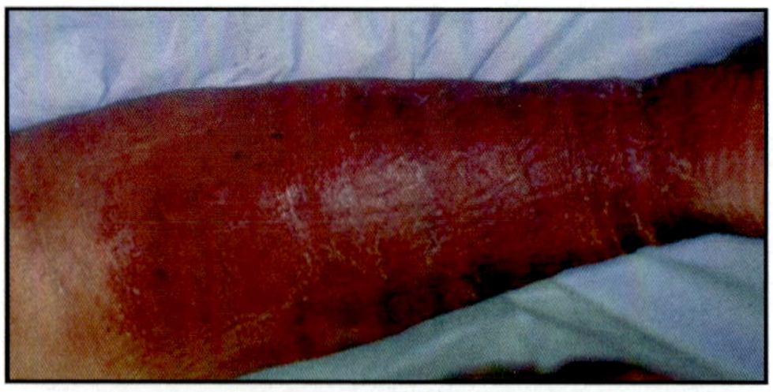

FIGURE 19: ***Inflammatory dermatitis.***

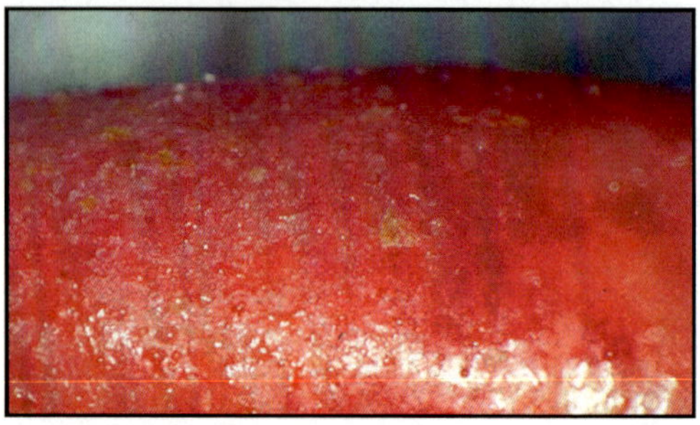

FIGURE 20: ***Reactive inflammation.***

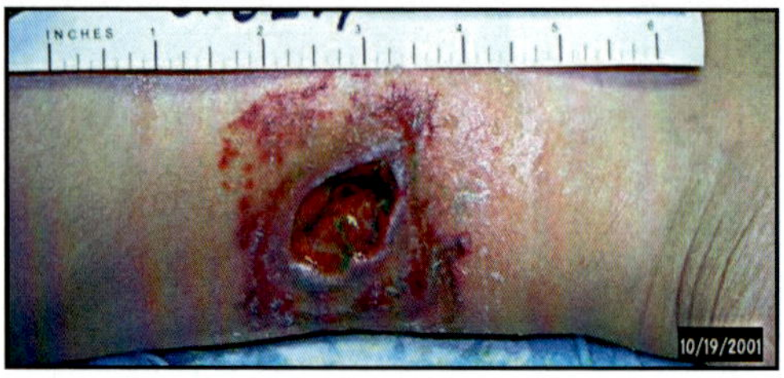

FIGURE 21: ***Vasculitis ulcer.***

ESSENTIAL 6: REDUCING EXCESSIVE INFLAMMATION

Excessive or prolonged inflammation, no matter what the cause, disrupts the normal healing cascade and stalls or stops healing. Inflammation is one of the end consequences of every inhibitor of wound healing. Infection, bioburden, necrotic tissue, trauma, and edema all contribute to wound bed and periwound inflammation. Active management of these wound inhibitors will ultimately resolve the majority of destructive wound inflammation. If excess inflammation persists on subsequent wound evaluations, then something has been missed or treatment was insufficient, and the wound should be carefully reassessed.

Sometimes, chronically inflamed wounds will fail to come into balance even after a comprehensive management plan has been put into action. These outliers often have developed an inflammatory vasculitis presenting as a persistently inflamed and unusually painful wound bed. These patients often have a history of a collagen vascular disease, rheumatoid disorder, reactive airway disease or allergies which may be acting as a sensitizer for the development of vasculitis in the face of chronic wound inflammation. A brief, high dose, tapering regimen of corticosteroids (Medrol dose pack) along with topical periwound steroids will often break this cycle of persistent vasculitis and inflammation. In short, inflammation must be successfully controlled to succeed in healing any problem wound.

ESSENTIAL 7: MAINTAINING THE HEALING ENVIRONMENT

Too often wound care is thought of as only "changing dressings." The knowledgeable clinician understands that picking the best dressing is only one step in the successful management of the problem wound. Wound dressings serve an important function: to support and maintain a proper healing environment. Dressings should never be a replacement for knowledgeable and needed active wound management.

Once evaluated and managed, the problem wound will best be supported by picking a dressing that will maintain a moist, clean, and protected healing environment. Simple and dependable dressing regimens are usually the best, with selective use of complex or interactive dressings when the wound has a specific problem or need. Dressing details are well covered in Modern Wound Dressings: Creating a Healing Milieu, by Rios and Larson-Lohr. It is important for the wound specialists to be familiar with the general classes of dressings, their function and use, and to be able to select the best dressing to support healing of the managed problem wound. As the wound bed responds to treatment and the wound returns to a normal healing cascade, the wound dressing will inevitably change until it finally becomes mostly protective.

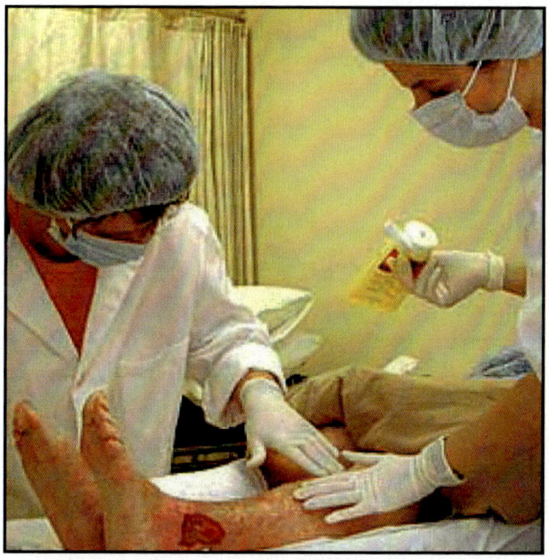

Figure 22: ***Dressing the wound.***

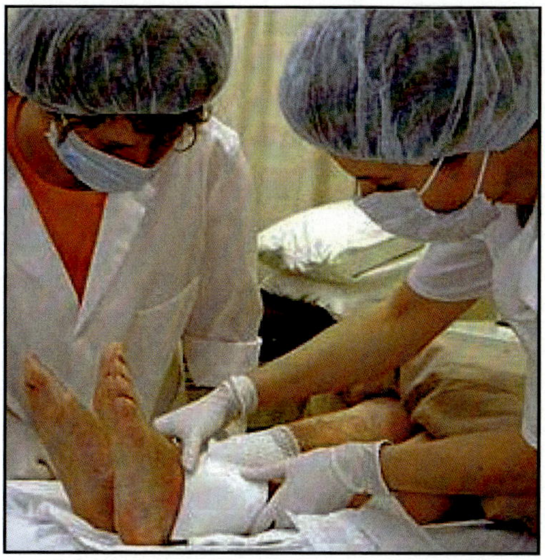

Figure 23: ***Dressing the wound.***

Conclusion

This chapter has served to introduce you to the concept of the Essentials of Wound Management. It can be useful to you, the wound specialist, as a tool, keeping you focused with each patient visit on the most critical factors that contribute to wound failure and limb loss. If aggressively applied, most of your difficult wounds will begin to improve and heal. This allows you time to correct the more insidious negative contributors to wound failure such as glucose control, poor nutrition, smoking, inadequate living conditions, and social support. All of these are important in influencing a longterm and sustainable healed outcome.

REFERENCES

1. Moore K. The scientific basis of wound healing. Advances in Tissue Banking 2001; 5:379-397.
2. Mast BA, Schultz GS. Interactions of cytokines, growth factors and proteases in acute and chronic wounds. Wound Rep Reg 1996; 4: 411-420.
3. Nwomeh BC, Yager DR, Cohen IK. Physiology of the chronic wound. Clin Plast Surg 1998; 25:341-356.
4. Bowler PG, Duerden BI, Armstrong DG. Wound microbiology and associated approaches to wound management. Clin Microbiol Rev 2001; 14(2): 244-269.
5. Gardner SE, Frantz RA, Doebbeling BN. The validity of the clinical signs and symptoms used to identify localized chronic wound infection. Wound Rep Reg 2001; 9:178-186.
6. Lazarus GS, Cooper DM, Knighton DR, et al. Definitions and guidelines for assessment of wounds and evaluation of healing. Arch Dermatol 1994; 130:489-493.
7. Trent JT, et al . Skin and wound biopsy; When, why and how. Adv Skin Wound Care 2003; 16(7):372-375.
8. Hopf HW, Ueno C, Aslam R, et al. Guidelines for the treatment of arterial Insufficiency ulcers. Wound Rep Reg 2006; 14(6):693-710.
9. Hankey GJ, Norman PE, Eikelboom JW. Medical treatment of peripheral arterial disease. 2006; JAMA 295(5):547-553.
10. Percival, SL, Bowler PG. Bio-films and their potential roles in wound healing. Wounds 2004; 16(7): 234-240.
11. Fux CA, Costerton JW, Stewart PS, et al. Survival strategies of infectious bio-films. Trends in Microbiology 2005; 13(1):34-40.
12. Costerton JW, Cheng KJ, Geesey GG, et al. Bacterial bio-films in nature and disease. Annu Rev Microbiol 1987; 41: 435-64.
13. Williams D, Enoch S, Miller D, et al. Effect of sharp debridement using curette on recalcitrant nonhealing venous leg ulcers: a concurrently controlled, prospective cohort study. Wound Rep Reg 2005;13(2): 131-137.
14. Costerton JW, Stewart PS. Battling Bio-films. Sci Am 2001; 285(1):74-81.
15. Steed DL, Donohoe D, Webster MW, et al. Effect of extensive debridement and treatment on the healing of diabetic foot ulcers. Diabetic Ulcer Study Group. J Am Coll Surg 1996; 183(1):61-34.
16. Steed DL. Debridement Am J Surg 2004; 187(5A):71S-74S.
17. Sibbald RG, Williamson D, Orsted HL, et al. Preparing the wound bed – debridement, bacterial balance and moisture balance. Ostomy Wound Manage 2000; 46(11): 14-18, 30.
18. Eming SA, Smola H, Krieg T. Treatment of chronic wounds: state of the art and future concepts. Cells Tissues Organs 2002; 172(2):105-107.
19. Falanga V. Venous Ulceration. J Dermatol Surg Oncol 1993 Aug; 19(8):764-71.
20. Lorimer KR, Harrison MB, Graham ID, Friedber E, Davies B. Assessing venous ulcer population characteristics and practices in a home care community. OWM 2003 May; 19(5):32-43.
21. Callam MJ, Harper DR, Dale JJ, Ruckley CV. Chronic ulcer of the leg:clinical history. Br Med J 1986; 294:1389-91.
22. Nelzen, Berguist D, Lindhagen A. Venous and non-venous leg ulcers:clinical history and appearance in a population study. Br J Surg 1994; 81:182-187.
23. Claudy AL, Mirshahi M, Soria C, Soria J. Detection of undegraded fibrin and tumor necrosis fator-alpha in venous leg ulcers. J AM Acad Dermotl 1991; 25:623-7.
24. Browse NL, Burnand KG. The cause of venous ulceration. Lancet 1982; 2;243-5.
25. Burnand KJ, Clemenson G, Whimster I, Gaunt J, Browse NL. The effect of sustained venous hypertension on the skin capillaries of the canine hind limb. Br J Surg. 1982;69: 41-44.
26. Falanga V, Eaglestein WH. The trap hypothesis of venous ulceration. Lancet 1993;341:1006-8.

27. Reichardt LE. Venous Ulceration: Compression as the mainstay of therapy. JWOCN 1999; 26(1):39-47.
28. Sandeman D, Shearman CP. Clinical aspects of lower limb ulceration. In:Mani J, Falanga V, Shearman CP, Sendeman D. (eds) Chronic Wound Healing, London, WB Saunders, 1999; 4-25.
29. Cordts PR, Hanrahan LM, Rodriguez AA, Woodson J, La Morte WW, Menzolan JO. A prospective, randomized trial of Unna's boot versus Duoderm CGF hydroactive dressing plus compression in the mangement of venous leg ulcers. J Vasc Surg 1992; 15:480-6.
30. Moffatt CJ, O'Hare L. Venous leg ulcerations: treatment with high compression bandaging. Ostomy/Wound Management 1995; 41:16-25.

Notes

CHAPTER

10

Modern Wound Dressings: *Creating a Healing Milieu*

Edna Patricia Rios, RN and Valerie Laron-Lohr, RN

Since the beginning of time, the human body has had to deal with open wounds. Wounds, likely from injury or disease, have even been found on 5,000-year-old mummies in Egypt. Treatment of these wounds was documented on a papyrus dating back to 1400 B.C. The papyrus documents application of a paste of honey, grease, resin, lint, and fresh meat into open wounds to remove dead skin and pus and encourage wound healing. Egyptians invented primitive adhesive bandages by applying gum to linen strips and drawing the wound edges together. Additionally, the Egyptians are credited with introducing the use of mercury as a wound care treatment, and while this treatment would later prove to be toxic, it is credited as being the first introduction of the use of antimicrobial properties in wound care. Evidence also points to the use of green copper pigment and chyrsoedla as antiseptic in open wounds.

Hippocrates (460-377 B.C.) was a Greek physician whose contribution to the advancement of wound care was encouraging hand washing and clean short nails. Hippocrates believed that wounds would heal faster if the edges were brought together and thus allowed to heal by primary intention. While Hippocrates' contributions to wound care were significant, he believed that wounds should be left dry. Any wounds that may have been covered were typically covered with a fat or oiled based ointment. Hippocrates had noted that the wounds of fishermen rarely became inflamed or pus filled; as a result, irrigation of wounds with seawater became common. Hippocrates also encouraged cautious use of bandages, since the 5th century surgeons were already aware that bandaging too tight could risk the development of gangrene.

A Roman physician, Cornelius Celsus (25BC-50 A.D.), was the first to describe classic signs of inflammation: redness, swelling, heat, and pain. Additionally, Celsus is credited with being the first to recognize that healing of acute and chronic wounds differed and each required different management. Claudius Galen (A.D. 130-200) is credited with the theory of "laudable pus," which would influence wound care until the 19th century. The premise of the laudable pus theory was that in order for wounds to heal, wounds would have to produce pus. Wounds would be reopened or have foreign bodies introduced into the wounds, or they were prodded or poked in order to inflame the wound and produce pus. The laudable pus theory was the standard of wound care for over 1000 years until the 19th century, when Pasteur and Lister introduced antiseptic principles.

Treating war-related wounds, specifically those inflicted by firearms, had been a challenge for centuries. With the introduction of gunpowder in the 14th century and cannons during the battle of Crecy in 1346, the challenge of war-related wounds now included smashed bones, torn blood vessels, and the introduction of foreign bodies into the wound, causing contamination that would eventually lead to sepsis. Treatment of these war wounds consisted of cautery in an attempt to stop bleeding. The most common method of cautery during this time was to pour boiling or heated oil into the wound. This painful method of wound treatment was prevalent until 1537 when a French military surgeon, Pare, ran out of oil to treat war injuries during the Siege of Turin. Instead of oil, Pare instructed that wounds be treated with an ointment made of egg yolks, rose oil, and turpentine. Pare was astonished to find that those treated with the ointment not only had less pain, but also had better outcomes. This was pivotal in leading Pare to question the theory of laudable pus, and he altered his practice to include gentler treatment of wounds.

The advent of the industrial revolution during the 19th century had a significant influence on wound care. Until this time wound care was treatment based, but with the industrial revolution came the introduction of cheap materials that were suitable for wound dressings. Until the end of the 19th century, dressing consisted mainly of gauze and lint. The first absorbent dressing consisting of cotton wool with gauze was developed by Gamgee, a surgeon, at the end of the 19th century.

Wound care was advanced further in 1860 when Louis Pasteur discovered anaerobic bacteria. Joseph Lister, a professor of surgery in Glasgow, applied Pasteur's theory to wound infections and the development of septicemia and developed the first antiseptic techniques for surgery. Lister went on to publish an innovative paper, "The Antiseptic Principle," in The Lancet.

During World War I, it was noted that soldiers with wounds who were left on the battlefields until it was safe to retrieve them would return to the trenches with maggots infesting their wounds. These soldiers had fewer infections and lower incidences of septicemia, which was attributed to the maggot's removal of dead tissue in the wound. The use of maggots was brought back to America by Dr. William Baer and utilized as a common wound care treatment until the discovery of sulphonamides, and later penicillin, when the treatment fell out of favor.

Changing Methodology

Finally, in 1962, George Winter published his work on moist wound healing. His publication detailed epithelial cells migrating across the wound bed in the final stage of healing occurring more rapidly in a moist rather than a dry environment. Winter's work is credited with raising the interest in wound care and leading to new wound care dressings. The first hydrocolloid dressing was introduced in the 1970s and became popular in the early 1980s.

During the 1970s and 1980s, the practice of moist wound care became widely accepted. The wound product industry responded to the new practice standard of moist wound care with the introduction of new wound dressings appearing at an astounding pace. For the first time, wound care practitioners had at their disposal several options: alginates, hydrogels, and foams (what we now consider the classics). Then, the new generation of wound dressings was introduced: engineered tissue, growth factors, and biosynthetic collagen, as well as the re-introduction of the old antimicrobial and silver in multiple new delivery forms and dosages. So was born the concept that rather than a dressing being passive in the wound healing process, it would be active in changing the wound milieu.

Today, research is focused at the cellular level and how alteration within the cell can promote wound healing. New ways to manipulate collagen, alter enzymes, and stimulate micro-capillary growth are areas of investigation for new interactive dressings.

The clinician working in chronic wound management today has over 3000 dressings and wound related products to choose from. How to select the appropriate product is becoming a challenge. It is a balance between function, availability, and cost. The 7 classic categories of dressings are no longer adequate to define the product selection that is available, but it is a starting place from which to develop an understanding of dressing function and how to use the classic dressings.

Classic Categories of Dressings

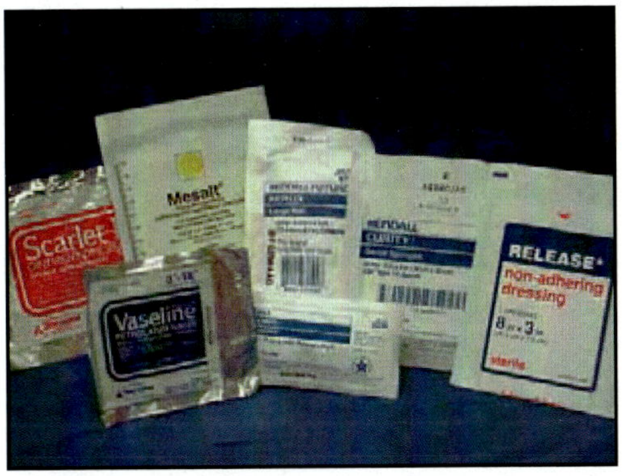

Figure 1: ***Gauze dressings.***

Gauze Dressings: Gauze dressings (see Figure 1) are composed of cotton, polyester, or rayon. They are dry, woven or non-woven, and come packaged as sponges, rolls, pads, ribbons, or strips. Gauze dressings are available sterile or nonsterile, and vary in degree of absorbency according to type. In addition, gauze dressings are available in bulk, with or without an attached adhesive border, and may be impregnated with other products.

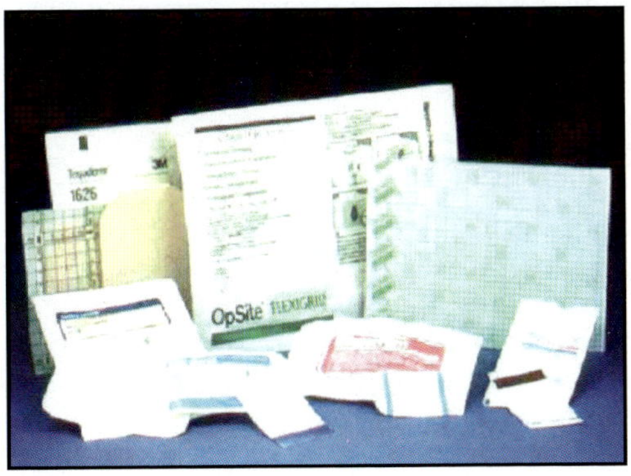

Figure 2: ***Transparent films.***

Transparent Films: Transparent films (see Figure 2) are recognized as the first advanced wound care dressing. Transparent films are adhesive, semi-permeable, polyurethane membrane dressings of varying thickness and size. An adhesive coating on one side allows for adherence to the skin. These dressings provide a waterproof barrier by being impermeable to liquid and microbes, but permeable to moisture vapor and atmospheric gases like oxygen. This clear dressing allows for visualization of the wound and works as a primary dressing for lacerations or skin tears, or as a secondary dressing for dressings needing to remain intact for longer periods of time. Varying sizes of transparent film allows for the correct size to be utilized, allowing for 1 inch of the dressing to adhere to the intact periwound skin. Removal of the dressing must be done carefully to avoid damage to the epidermis. To remove the dressing, gently pull up the edge of the dressing and pull the dressing at a parallel angle to the skin, thus breaking the seal and allowing the dressing to be removed.

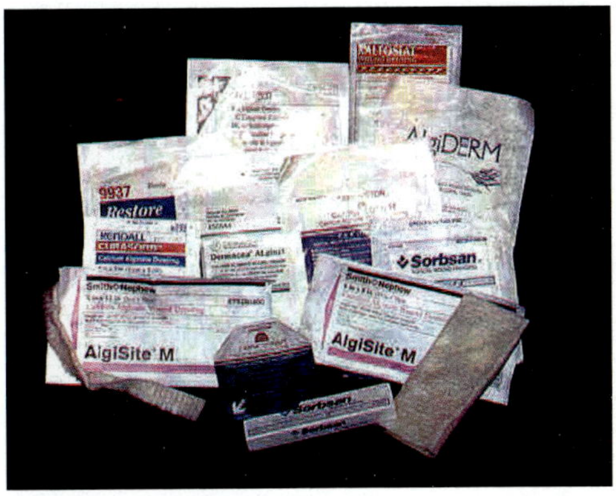

Figure 3: ***Alginates.***

Alginates: Alginates (see Figure 3) are derived from processed seaweed. Alginates include calcium-alginate, calcium-sodium-alginate, and collagen-alginate dressings, all of which are highly absorbent and conform easily to wounds of various shapes and sizes. Exudate from the wound reacts with the dressing to create a gel-like substance. This gel provides a moist environment within the wound that promotes healing. Typically, alginate dressings are capable of absorbing up to 20 times their weight, making them an ideal choice for heavily exudating wounds. Available in both sheet and rope form, a secondary dressing is required to secure them in place.

Hydrogels: Hydrogels (see Figures 4 and 5) are primarily water and/or glycerin based amorphous gels, impregnated gauze, or sheets. They are by far the most versatile dressing available. The amorphous nature of the product allows for the use of filling space within a wound and keeping the wound hydrated. Hydrogels have a high water content, limiting the ability of absorbing large amounts of exudates. They are a good option for maintaining a moist wound environment, allowing for granulation and epithelialization. Additionally, hydrogels facilitate autolytic debridement and can

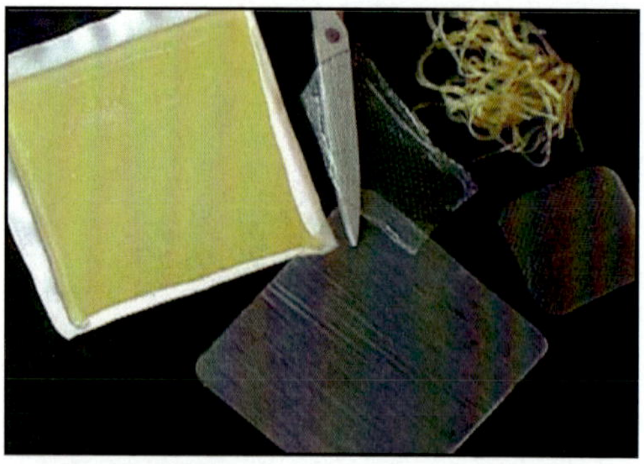

FIGURE 4: ***Hydrogels.***

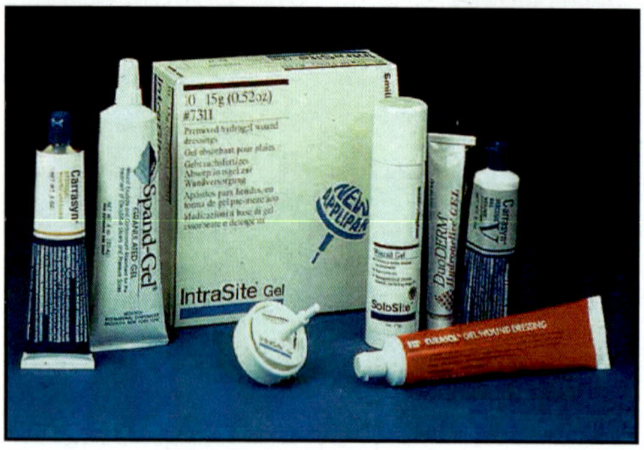

FIGURE 5: ***Amorphous hydrogels.***

be used as a substitute for moist gauze. Hydrogels offer a soothing, cooling relief and may help in reducing pain that can be associated with wounds.

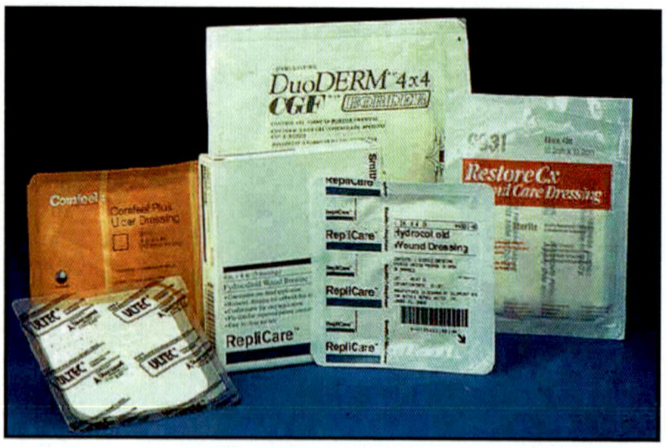

FIGURE 6: ***Hydrocolloids.***

Hydrocolloids: Hydrocolloids (see Figure 6) are significant for being among the first advanced wound care dressing available to practitioners. Hydrocolloids may be occlusive or semi-occlusive and are composed of carboxymethycellulose, pectin, or gelatin. The ability of the dressing to absorb exudates will vary on the thickness and composition of the dressing. As exudate is absorbed by the dressing, a thick colloidal gel develops in the wound bed. This colloidal gel provides a moist healing environment, allowing for granulation, epithelialization, and autolysis of the wound.

Hydrocolloids are available in a variety of sizes and shapes. Newer product designs such as tapered, low profile edges and smooth, satin-like outer coating decrease the incidence of the dressing rolling up, and help reduce friction and shear to the area. While no longer considered an advanced wound care product, use of hydrocolloids remains widely utilized in some care settings.

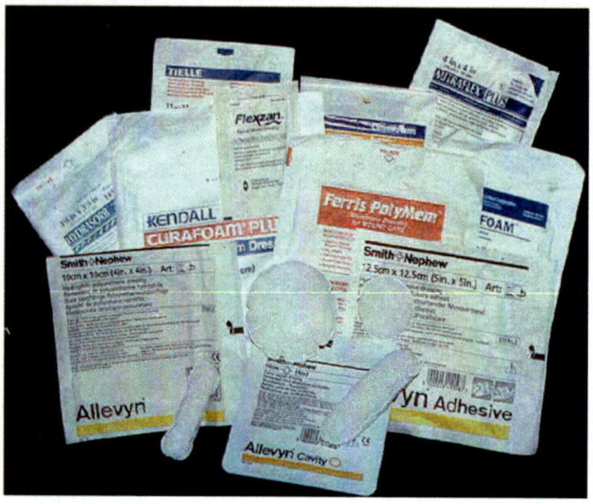

FIGURE 7: ***Foams.***

Foams: Foam dressings (see Figure 7) are non-adherent and non-linting. Available in a variety of thicknesses, the non-adherent layer allows for non-traumatic removal. Foams are composed of polymers that contain small open cells capable of holding fluids and wicking drainage away from the wound. Foams provide moist wound healing, thermoregulation, and protection of partial and full thickness wounds. Additionally, foam's low adherence to the wound bed provides for deceased pain and disruption of healing.

Composite: Composite dressings (see Figure 8) are manufactured as a single dressing that can address different needs, but are composed of a combination of 2 or more physically distinct products. Composite dressings can be utilized as a primary and/or a secondary dressing for partial and full-thickness wounds. An absorptive layer, adhesive border, and strike-through barrier allow for versatility and convenience, offering a simple "Band-Aid" type application and removal, often used in areas prone to increased moisture, due to its waterproof nature

INTERACTIVE DRESSINGS

Interactive dressings interact with the wound bed components to assist in producing an improved wound healing milieu. They can accomplish this via reducing colonization count, reducing the level of exudates, improving wound bed moisture retention, improving wound collagen matrix, removal of cellular products, or providing protection for the epithelializing bed. Interactive dressings come in various forms.

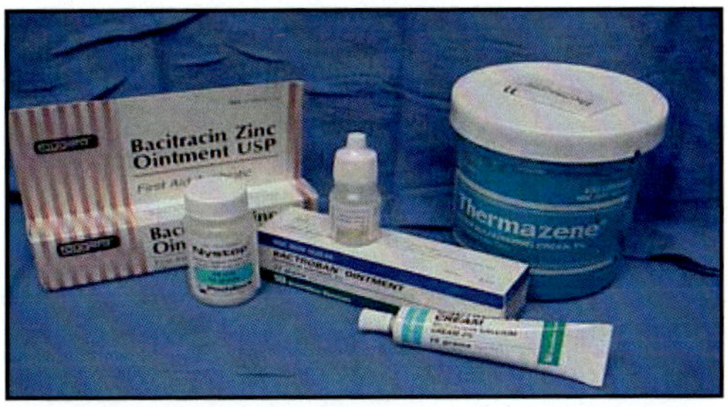

FIGURE 8: ***Antimicrobials.***

Antimicrobials: Safe, broad spectrum antimicrobials or "biocides" (a general term describing a chemical agent, usually broad spectrum, that inactivates microorganisms) and wound dressing products containing these agents (see Figure 8) have been developed to address the needs of chronic wounds with the intent to minimize colonization and prevent local infection, thereby enhancing healing. Both in vitro as well as clinical observations support the utilization of various biocide and antimicrobial products. Several of these products are outlined below.

Silver: The use of silver has been documented for its broad-spectrum antimicrobial activity and compatibility with humans throughout history. The present recognized antimicrobial properties of silver have been empirically evident for more than 3000 years. A plethora of literature has reviewed its historical use, antimicrobial properties, and toxicity. In 1881, a German obstetrician named Dr. Crede used a 1% silver nitrate solution to eliminate congenital blindness (Ophthalmia neonatorum) in newborns caused by post-partum infection of Neisseria gonorrhea. In 1887, von Behring used the same compound to treat typhoid and anthrax. In 1964, Moyer first used silver for the care of burns. In 1968, Fox introduced silver sulfadiazine (SSD), still used today.

Silver dressings are some of our most advanced antimicrobial wound care dressings currently on the market. They are effective not only against microbes such as MRSA and VRE, but also provide a hostile environment to fungus and viruses, with the added benefit of decreasing inflammation. Ionic silver kills detrimental gram positive and gram negative, is safe, and to date has no known clinical resistance. This is because of silver's multifaceted mode of action on pathogenic metabolic pathways. Silver ions attack the cell membrane, the membrane transport system, the RNA and DNA function, as well as the protein function, rendering it difficult for bacterial mutation to occur. Antibiotic resistant bacteria such as MRSA and VRE are eliminated in dressings that have silver ions present in proper dosage. The longevity of silver ion presence in the dressings, through their controlled release mechanisms, ensures that the wound environment is hostile to bioburden for relatively long periods of time.

While clinical resistance at this time has not occurred, resistance has been created in the laboratory when bacteria have repeatedly been exposed to bacterial static levels of silver in place of bactericidal levels. In fact, Levy is quoted as saying, "The current widespread and uncontrolled use of silver may result in more bacteria developing resistance, analogous to the emergence of antibiotic- and biocide-resistant bacteria." One of the questions the clinician should ask when choosing a silver dressing is whether the dose of silver is bacteriostatic or bactericidal, and we should heed the lessons of the past when making our silver choices. While silver ions are bactericidal at low concentrations in water, when exposed to complex, organic biological fluids such as wound exudate, a higher concentration is needed. In complex organic fluids, concentrations greater than 40 ppm and as high as 60.5 ppm are required for the silver to be bactericidal.

Currently, there is a plethora of silver products on the market with a wide range of silver delivery. Thomas, et al., examined the silver content and antimicrobial activity of 10 common silver dressings on the market. They found significant differences in the activity of the products. There was a clear relationship between the silver content of the dressing and the ability of the dressing to be bactericidal, but other factors were also identified. The other factors included: whether the silver was a surface coating or dispersed within the structure of the dressing; what form of silver (ionic, metallic, or bound); and the dressing's affinity for moisture. Dressings that had surface silver, silver in ionic form, and retained moisture performed the best. The challenge for clinicians is to critically examine the wide selections of silver products and choose those that will do the best for the patient.

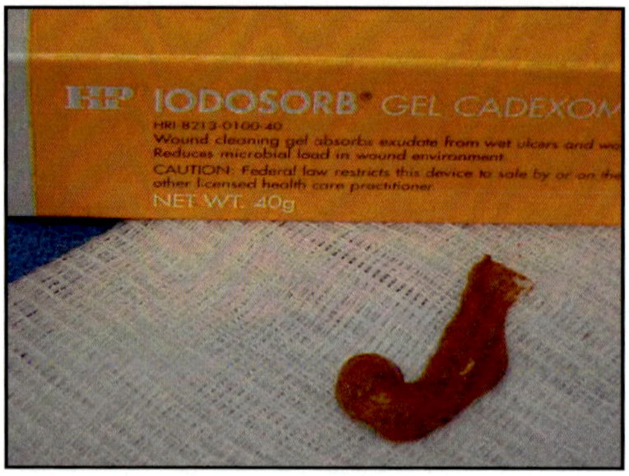

FIGURE 9: *Cadexomer iodine.*

Cadexomer Iodine (Figure 9): Iodine is a potent broad-spectrum antiseptic agent with a controversial past, since it has been shown to impair the function of cells involved in wound healing in vitro. Improved formulations of iodophors or "iodine carriers" provide a release of low levels of iodine over a longer period of time. These present the clinician with a viable iodine-containing product for wound bioburden management. Cadexomer iodine is a slow-release antimicrobial capable of absorbing excess wound exudate while offering a sustained level of iodine in the wound bed. Cadexomer iodine also has established effectiveness in vivo against Staphylococcus aureus and methicillin-resistant Staphylococcus aureus

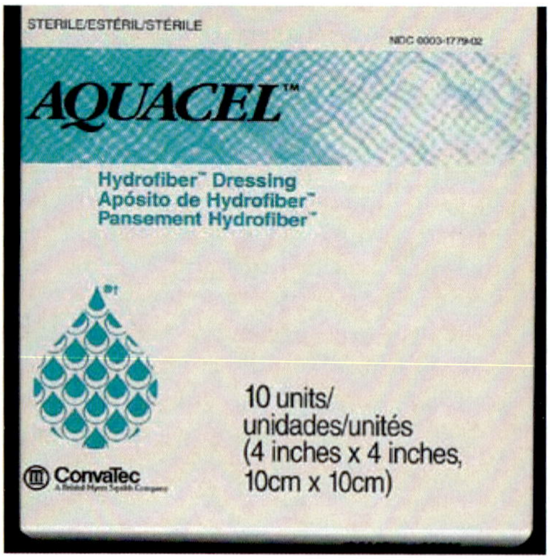

FIGURE 10: *Hydrofiber.*

Hydrofiber Dressings: Nonwoven dressings composed of carboxymethyl cellulose, which forms a gel when exposed to wound fluids. It is indicated for draining partial- or full-thickness wounds and promotes autolytic debridement, but requires a secondary dressing. Hydrofiber dressings (see Figure 10) are nonadhesive, nonocclusive, conformable to the wound, absorb moderate-to-large amounts of wound exudates, and are usually changed every 1-3 days, according to amount of wound drainage.

Polyhexamethylene biguanide (PHMB): PHMB is a broad spectrum antimicrobial agent that impairs the integrity of the outer membrane of bacteria. PHMB is generally saturated at 0.02% into a gauze dressing. PHMB dressings have demonstrated a trend towards effectiveness against gram negative organisms (although not universally true), and gram positive organisms. However, the activity of the PHMB dressing appears dependent on the microbes being in close proximity to the dressings. This has been demonstrated in studies, by the results of the zone of inhibition experiments that indicate that there is little apparent diffusion of the antimicrobial activity away from the dressing.

In some porcine studies, the PHMB dressings have been associated with prolonged bleeding of the wounds, even though hemostasis was achieved prior to dressing the wounds. The bleeding may be due, in part, to the drying and adhering of the dressing to the wound. The PHMB dressing has demonstrated resistance to removal, in spite of attempts to soak the dressing off of the wound bed after contact times as short as 24 hours, and in a continuously moist environment. Additionally, in the same studies, PHMB had been shown to prolong the inflammatory response with a resultant delay in healing of wounds dressed with PHMB dressings. This prolonged inflammatory response may be in part due to the adherent nature of the dressing and the difficulty in removal of the dressing from the wound.

Biologics and Biosynthetics: Bioengineered cellulose provides moist wound healing and versatility, significantly reducing pain and shortening healing time. Other biologics and biosynthetics (see Figure 11) derived from natural sources provide a healing scaffold or matrix, assisting the granulation and epithelialization of partial and full-thickness wounds. These matrix dressings assist in wound closure in the more recalcitrant wounds.

Collagen: Produced by fibroblasts, collagen represents the most abundant protein in the human body and the skin. It is a natural structural protein found in all three phases of the wound healing cascade, stimulates cellular migration, and contributes to new tissue development and wound debridement. Collagen dressings in the form of

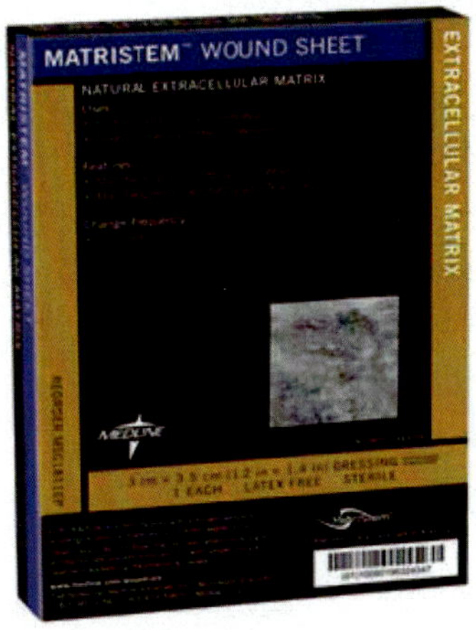

FIGURE 11: ***Biologics and biosynthetics.***

sheets, gels, and particles encourage the deposition and organization of newly formed tissue, creating an environment that fosters healing. These materials are known to stimulate and recruit specific cells, such as macrophages and fibroblasts, to positively enhance and influence wound healing. They can be moisturizing or absorptive, depending on the delivery system, maintaining moist wound healing, are easy to apply and remove, and tend to be conformable.

The collagen in a given collagen dressing can vary in concentration and type. Certain collagen dressings are comprised of Type I (native) collagen; whereas, other collagen dressings contain denatured collagen as well. A given collagen dressing may contain ingredients, such as alginates and cellulose derivatives that can enhance absorbency, flexibility, and comfort, and help maintain a moist wound environment. Collagen dressings have a variety of pore sizes and surface areas, as well. All of these attributes are meant to enhance the wound management aspects of the dressings. Many collagen dressings contain an antimicrobial agent to control pathogens within the wound. Others contain oxidized regenerated cellulose, a plant material that has been combined with collagen to produce a dressing capable of binding to and protecting growth factors, and by binding and inactivating matrix metallo-proteases (MMPs) in the wound environment.

Dressing Selection

For the clinician today, the job of selecting a dressing can be daunting. The first step in selection is to apply the four basic goals of wound healing. You will find that the goals of dressing selection mirror the principles of the "Essentials of Wound Management" chapter.

1. The first goal is to maintain a moist healing environment. Moist wound healing promotes epithelialization, enhances autolytic debridement, prevents wound desiccation, and decreases pain.
2. The second goal is to remove eschar and debris from the wound bed. This will decrease bioburden, improve epithelialization, and decrease inflammation.
3. The third goal is to control exudate. Increased exudate can cause periwound maceration and contributes to an increased bioburden in the wound.
4. The fourth goal is to prevent further wounding. Patients may unknowingly traumatize their wounds due to neuropathy, or a dressing or product may be chosen that actually traumatizes the wound or surrounding skin.

If we take the 4 principles of dressing selection and expand upon Ovington's methodology, the practice of dressing selection using goals, form, and function, we will have a systematic way to select the proper dressings. A nursing assessment of the wound, patient, and setting must occur prior to selecting the dressing. It is essential that the dressing match the patient, the wound, and the setting in order to obtain the optimal result

Ovington gives an all purpose performance-based approach to using wound dressings by asking six basic assessment questions when deciding on a wound dressing:

- What does the wound need? Determined by a complete assessment of the wound and surrounding tissues. Assessment is performed at each dressing change, including the initial. Apply the goals. Anticipate that the needs of the wound will change as the tissue envelope normalizes and the healing process progresses.
- What does the product do? This is the function. Read the product literature and clinical data available.
- How well does it do it? Examine clinical studies and laboratory comparisons to other products in the same category. Talk with other clinicians. Evaluate it on your patients. Does the dressing perform as it is stated? Not all dressings are equal.
- What does the patient need? Comprehensive assessment of the patient, including psycho-

Table 1: *Dressing Categories*

Category	Advantages/Disadvantages	Examples
Gauze Mechanically debride Permeable to gases Fills dead space Economical Readily available Absorptive	Can damage granulation tissue on removal May dehydrate the wound Permeable to fluid and bacteria May require more frequent dressing changes	Kerlix Kling Nu-Gauze Sof-wick Tendersorb Mirasorb
Impregnated Gauze Less adherent to wound bed May keep wound moist	Requires secondary dressing Less absorptive than plain gauze	Xeroform Vaseline gauze Adaptic DermAssist
Films Semi permeable Retain moisture Waterproof Allow wound visualization	Do not use on infected wounds May tear fragile skin May dislodge in high friction areas	Bioclusive Flexfilm Tegaderm Opsite Polyskin II Cutifilm
Hydrocolloids Impermeable to bacteria Facilitates autolytic debridement Conformable Water resistant Self adhesive Reduces pain Can be used under compression dressings	Can not be used in moderate to heavy exudate Do not use on infected wounds Softens and looses shape with heat and friction Caution if there is fragile skin surrounding wound Minimal absorption	Duoderm Replicare Restore Tegasorb Cutinova
Hydrogels Soothing and reduces pain Rehydrates wound Extends period of time between dressing changes Can fill dead space Comes in amorphous gels, sheets, freeze dry forms	Requires secondary dressing Sheets may be difficult to secure Can cause periwound maceration Minimal absorption	NU-GEL Curasol Safe-gel Carrasyn Hypergel Gentell Vigilon Cearsite
Foams Highly absorptive Non-adherent Conformable Protects wound and periwound against trauma Thermal insulation Can be used under compression dressing	May require secondary dressing May macerate wound edge if dressing becomes saturated Not effective for wounds with dry eschar	Allevyn Flexan Lyofoam PolyMem

social. Do they need a dressing that does not require daily changes, do they need protection from trauma, or is there a large amount of exudate?

- What is available? Health insurance coverage, facility formulary, and reimbursement?
- What is practical? Examine the goals of wound management. Does the dressing choice satisfy the goals? Is the dressing easy to apply (patient/family), easy to obtain, and cost-effective?

Cost effectiveness of the product will need to be considered during the selection process. This means understanding indirect costs as well as the

Category	Advantages/Disadvantages	Examples
Alginates Form moist gel in wound Highly absorptive Fills dead space Controls heavily exudative	Can not be used in dry wounds or wounds with minimal exudate Can dehydrate wound bed Reports of burning sensation on application with certain products Requires secondary dressing	Sorbsan Kaltostat Curasorb Algisite Tegagen HG AlgiDERM Seasorb Melgisorb
Composites Combines 2 or more physically distinct products for better outcomes	Can be expensive Provider must have good understanding of properties of dressing Generally requires intact skin border for anchoring dressing	Fibrocol (collagen & alginate) Versiva (foam & hydrofiber) Tielle (foam & polyurethane covering) Safe-Gel (hydrogel & alginate)
Biologics & Biosynthetics Combats bioburden and superficial infection	Wide variety, need to look at effectiveness and appropriate use	Silverlon Silver Cel Aquacel AG SilvaSorb Argales Acticoat Cadexomer Iodine AMD
Collagen Employs a variety of carriers/combining agents such as gels, pastes, polymers, oxidized regenerated cellulose (ORC), and ethylene diamine tetraacetic acid. Stimulate and recruit specific cells to enhance wound healing	Require secondary dressing	Medifil particles/pads BGC Matrix Celerate Gel & powder Fibracol Oasis Promogram Integra

direct cost involved in wound care. Direct cost examples include, but are not limited to the primary and secondary dressings, pharmacy, caregiver time, and diagnostic procedures. Indirect costs are similar to overhead costs, and include examples such as increased length of stay, treatment complications, and litigation. The clinician should read published studies critically to take cost-per-unit outcome into account to determine if treatment measures are indeed cost effective. Sometimes the most expensive product can be less expensive in the long run because it leads to faster healing with a reduced amount of complications.

Managing wound pain with dressings

Dressing removal can be a time of considerable pain to a patient with a sensitive wound. Dried dressing and adherent products are likely to cause pain and trauma at dressing changes. Minimizing the degree of sensory stimulus to the ultrasensitive wound area is important to consider in selecting a dressing that will aid in diminishing wound pain.

Any dressing that sticks to the wound bed, such as gauze, or dries within the wound bed and is then pulled away, stimulates receptors in the skin, which causes pain. The dressing that easily rinses away or slides off inflamed tissue does not provide the same stimulus and is not as painful. Dressings, such as sheet and amorphous hydrogels, hydrofibers, alginates, soft silicones, and cellulose dressings match the goals of wound healing and decrease wound bed stimulus.

Dressings that allow for increased time between changes will help with pain management as the removal stimulus is less frequent and will not aggravate the pain cycle. Contact layers or dressings that remain in close proximity to the wound bed during dressing changes also have proven beneficial in the pain arena. They prevent rubbing or stimulation to the skin that can trigger the pain cycle.

When cleansing the wound, use fluids at body temperature (98 to 100 F) to assist in keeping discomfort lower, cold fluids can trigger a pain response. Avoid the cytotoxic solutions, such as povidone iodine or hydrogen peroxide, when cleaning the wound as these can cause discomfort as well as being lethal to fibroblasts and keratinocytes. Care should be taken when removing a dressing, making every effort to avoid unnecessary manipulation of the wound and prevent further damage to the delicate granulation and healing tissue within the wound bed and to periwound tissue. If the dressing has become dried out, moisten it with an isotonic solution before removing. These simple actions can have a tremendous impact upon the pain felt by the patient during dressing change episodes.

Reimbursement

Healthcare is like any other business; it must generate revenue to remain viable. When considering how to best care for a patient, wound care clinicians need to keep cost in mind and have a good understanding of "what dressing, for how long, on which wounds" to assist in not only obtaining the best outcomes for the patient, but also being mindful of cost. In addition, an understanding of reimbursement and payment procedures of Medicare and Medicaid is essential to contain cost and remain viable. Medicare and Medicaid coverage for wound care dressings varies by healthcare setting and state. Most wound product/device manufacturers have extensive reimbursement guides that can easily be found on their company websites or by contacting the local company representative.

Category and HCPCS Codes

All dressing types, regardless of manufacturer, are classified into generic descriptive categories. Each of these categories is listed in the Common Procedure Coding System, more commonly known as HCPCS. This system is used by Medicare, Medicaid, and other insurers. The codes represent non-physician services that may include wound dressings. Each HCPCS code is assigned an allowable fee amount, regardless of the manufacturer of the product. The allowable fee may vary by regional carrier. A fee schedule is available from each regional carrier.

Utilization Guidelines

In addition to the fee scale Medicare has established, utilization guidelines are also established for each dressing category. If a higher quantity of dressings or supplies are used or required above the utilization guideline, a statement of medical necessity will be required from the physician. This statement will provide physician documented justification of product utilization above the established guideline.

Documentation Support

The importance of wound documentation cannot be underestimated in regard to claim coverage. Every dressing order requires that the physician specify the dressing type, amount used with each dressing change, dressing change frequency, and expected length of need. It is essential that documentation include a diagnosis with a wound description, including the wound stage or grade. If more than one wound is present, each wound needs to be described separately. Wound descriptions need to include how long the wound has been present, the history of the wound thus far, including a description of the wound, how long the wound has been present, and expected healing time. Each wound requires regular evaluation that should include type, location, size, and drainage amount, in addition to any other significant findings.

Table 2: *Companies Providing Wound Dressings*

Company	Telephone / Web Address	Example of Product
3M Wound Care Products	(800) 228-3957 http://solutions.3m.com/wps/portal/3M/en_US/SH/SkinHealth/solutions/skin-wound-care/	Coban 2 layer compression Tegaderm Tegaderm Ag Mesh
AcryMed, Inc.	(503) 624-9830 http://www.acrymed.com	Silversorb FlexiGel OxygeneSys Dissolved Oxygen
Advanced BioHealing, Inc.	(877) 422-4463 or (877) 337-6247 http://www.advancedbiohealing.com	Dermagraft
Afassco, Inc..	(800) 441-6774	Aquaskin
Ambra Le Roy Medical Products	(704) 392-7080 (866) 203-4760	Short Stretch Bandages
AmeriDerm Laboratories	(973) 279-5100 (800)455-7211 www.ameriderm.com	Dermafix Ointment Wound Gel Calcium Alginate
Amerx Health Care	(800) 448-9599 http://www.amerigel.com	AmeriGel gauze dressings AmeriGel wound dressings
Anacapa Technologies	(800) 489-2591 http://www.anacapa-tech.net	Anasept Silver-Sept
Argentum Medical LLC	(630) 232-2507 (888) 551-0188 http://www.silverlon.com	Silverlon: Calcium Alginate, Island Wound and Surgical dressings, Negative Pressure dressings
B. Braun Medical, Inc.	(800) 227-2862 (610) 691-5400 www.bbraunusa.com	Protoscan wound Gel
Beiersdorf, Inc	(800) 227-4703 (203) 563-5800 www.beiersdorf.com	Aquaphor
Beiersdorf-Jobst, Inc.	(800) 537-1063 (704) 554-9933 www.jobst-usa.com	Comprilan Gelcast unna boot Artiflex
Brennen Medical, LLC	(800) 328-9105 (651) 429-7413 www.brennenmed.com	BGC Matrix Glucan II Glucan Silver Matrix MacroPro Gel

BSN Medical, Inc.	(800) 552-1157 (704) 358-4558 www.bsnmedical.com	Cover-Roll Cuticell Elastomull Gelocast
Calmoseptine, Inc	(800) 800-3405 (714) 840-3405 www.calmoseptineointment.com	Calmoseptine ointment
Carrington Laboratories, In	(800) 358-5205 www.carringtonlabs.com	CarraSmart film, gel, & foam
Coloplast Corporation	(800) 533-0464 (612) 337-7800 www.us.coloplast.com	SeaSorb alginate Contreet Silver Biatain foam Comfeel
ConvaTec	(800) 422-8811 www.convatec.com	Aquacel Aquacel Ag Duoderm Versiva
Covidien includes Kendall brand	(800) 962-9888 www.covidien.com www.kendallhealthcare.com	Aquaflo hydrogel Curafil Curasorb alginate Kerlix Telfa
DermaRite Industries LLC	(800) 337-6296 (973) 569-9000 www.dermarite.com	DermaFilm DermaGinate SilverDerm 7
Derma Sciences	(800) 825-4325 (609) 514-4744 www.dermasciences.com	Dermagram Medihoney Algicell
DeRoyal	(800) 251-9864 (865) 362-1357 www.deroyal.com	CovaDerm Aquasorb Kalginate Multidex
Ferris Mfg. Corp.	(800)765-9636 (630) 887-9797 www.polymem.com	PolyMem products
Gentell	(800) 840-9041 (215) 364-3600 www.gentell.com	Dermatell Gentell Hydrogel Gentell Alginate
HEALTHPOINT	(800) 441-8227 www.healthpoint.com	Oasis Wound Matrix Collagenase Santyl Curasol Hydrofera Blue

Hollister	(800) 323-4060 (847) 996-6000 www.hollisterwoundcare.com	Restore alginate Restore Duo & Triact Restore hydrogel
HY-Tape International	(800) 248-0101 www.hytape.com	Hy-Tape, the original pink tape
Integra LifeSciences Corp	(877) 444-1122 (609) 275-9004 www.integra-ls.com/products	Integra, Bilayer Wound Matrix
Medline Industries, Inc.	(800) 633-5463 www.medline.com/wound-skin-care/	Silvasorb Matristem Maxsorb Optifoam
Milliken Healthcare Products, LLC	(866) 491-6556 (864) 503-1323 www.selectcare.milliken.com	AFM Ag AFM Ultra
MPM Medical, Inc.	(800) 232-5512 (972) 893-4090 www.mpmmedicalinc.com/	GelPad ExcelGinate ExcelGinate Ag SilverMed
Noble Biomaterials, Inc.	(877) 978-2842 (570) 955-1800 www.noblebiomaterials.com	SilverSeal contact dressings with X-static
Organogenesis	(888) 432-5232 (781) 575-0775 www.organogenesis.com www.apligraf.com	Apligraf
Smith and Nephew, Inc., Wound Management	(800) 876-1261 (727)392-1261 www.global.smith-nephew.com/us/	Acticoat Profore Allevyn Replicare Biostep
TEI Biosciences	(866) 524-0022 opt 1 (617) 268-1616 www.teibio.com	PriMatrix
UDL Laboratories	(800) 848-0462 http://www.udllabs.com/wound_care/ default.aspx	Sorbsan Proderm Flexzan Hydrocol II Granulex

References

1. Zimmerman, LM, Veith I. Great Ideas in the History of Surgery. Baltimore, MD: Williams and Wilkins, 1961.
2. Forrest RD. Early history of wound treatment, Journal of Royal Society Medicine 75: 198-205, 1982.
3. Sinclair RD, Ryan TJ. A great war for antiseptics. Wound Management, 1993; 4(1), 16-18
4. Winter GD, Scales JT. The effects of air-drying and dressings on the surface of the wound. Nature; 1963; 197:91-92.
5. Ayello EA, Baranoski S, Kerstein MD, Cuddigan J. Wound treatment options, Chapter 9, in Wound Care Essentials Practice Principles, Baranoskin S, Ayello EA (eds) 2004, Lippincott Williams and Wilkins, Philiadelphia, p. 135.
6. Ovington L. Hanging wet to dry dressings out to dry. Home Health Nurse, August 2001, volume 19, number 8, page 477.
7. Ovington LG. The well-dressed wound: an overview of dressing types. WOUNDS 1998;10:1A-11A.
8. Turner TD. The development of wound management products. In: Krasner DL, Rodeheaver GT, Sibbald RG (eds). Chronic Wound Care: A Clinical Source Book for Healthcare Professionals, Third Edition. Wayne, PA: HMP Communications, 2001:293-310.
9. Baranoski S. Skin tears: The enemy of frail skin. Advances in Skin and Wound Care, May/June 2000; 13(3 part 1):123-26.
10. Turner TD. The development of wound management products. In: Krasner DL, Rodeheaver GT, Sibbald RG (eds) in Chronic Wound Care: A Clinical Source Book for Healthcare Professionals, Third Edition. Wayne, PA: HMP Communications, 2001:293-310.
11. Ayello EA, Baranoski S, Kerstein MD, Cuddigan J. Wound debridement, Chapter 8, in Wound Care Essentials Practice Principles, Baranoskin S, Ayello EA (eds) 2004, Lippincott Williams and Wilkins, Philiadelphia, p. 146.
12. Turner TD. The development of wound management products. In: Krasner DL, Rodeheaver GT, Sibbald RG (eds). Chronic Wound Care: A Clinical Source Book for Healthcare Professionals, Third Edition. Wayne, PA: HMP Communications, 2001:293-310.
13. HPIS Quarterly Market Intelligence Update, 2005.
14. Percival SL, Bowler PG, Russell D. Bacterial resistance to silver in wound care. J. Hosp. Infect. 2005; 60-7.
15. Parsons D, Walker M, Bowler P. Silver: Clarifying the claims, OstomyWound management, 52 (6), 2006, 12-13.
16. Howler P. "The science behind silver availability in wounds: John A. Boswick. Burn and Wound Care Sumposium, Maui, Hawaii, Feb 20-24, 2006, page 35 of conference syllabus.
17. Innes M, Umraw N, Fish J, Gomez M, Carlotto R. Burns, 27, (2001), 621-627.
18. Parsons D, Bowler PG, Myles V, Joens S. Silver antimicrobial dressings in wound management: a comparison of antibacterial, physical and chemical characteristics, Wounds. 2005; 17 (8): 222-232.
19. Maple PA, Hamilton-Miller JM, Brumfitt W. Comparison of the in-vitro activities of the topical antimicrobials azelaic acid, nitrofurazone, silver sulphadiazine and mupirocin against methicillin-resistant Staphylococcus aureus. J Antimicrob Chemother 1992; 29: 661-68.
20. Walker M, Cochrane D, Bowler P, Parsons D. Silver deposition and tissue staining associated with wound dressings containing silver, Ostomy/Wound Management 2006: 52 (1): 42-50.
21. Alvarez OM, Patel M, Booker J, Markowitz L. Effectiveness of a biocellulose wound dressing for the treatment of chronic venous leg ulcers: results of a single center randomized study involving 24 patients. WOUNDS 2004;16(7)224-233.
22. Demling R, Neizgoda J, Haraway D, Mostow EN. Small intestinal submucosa wound matrix and full-thickness venous ulcers: preliminary results. WOUNDS 2004;16(1):18-22.

23. Etris M, Cutshall WD, Hiles MC. A new biomaterial derived from small intestine submucosa and developed into a wound matrix device. WOUNDS 2002;14(4):150-66.
24. Ayello EA, Baranoski S, Kerstein MD, Cuddigan J. Wound treatment options, Chapter 9, in Wound Care Essentials Practice Principles, Baranoskin S, Ayello EA. (eds) 2004, Lippincott Williams and Wilkins, Philiadelphia, p. 138.
25. Cullen B, Smith R, McCulloch E, Silcock D, Morrison L. Mechanism of action of PROMOGRAN, a protease modulating matrix, for the treatment of diabetic foot ulcers. Wound Rep Reg 2002;10:16-25.
26. Paustian C, Stegman MR. Preparing the wound bed for healing: The effect of activated polyacrylate dressing on debridement. Ostomy/Wound Management, 2003;49(9):34-42.
27. Konig, et al. Enzymatic versus autolytic debridement of chronic leg ulcers; a prospective randomized trial. J of Wound Care; 14(7), July 2005.
28. Bruggisser R. Bacterial and fungal absorption properties of a hydrogel dressing with a super absorbent polymer core. J Wound Care; 14(9), October 2005.
29. Ovington L. Bacterial toxins and wound healing. Ostomy Wound Management, July 2003;49(7A):8-12.
30. Lipman RDA. Avery Dennison Medical, Odor absorbing hydrocolloid dressing for direct wound contact, Poster Number 82, Wound Healing Society (WHS) 15th Annual Meeting, Chicago, May 18-21, 2005.
31. Lipman RDA. Avery Dennison Medical, Odor absorbing hydrocolloid dressing for direct wound contact, Poster Number 82, Wound Healing Society (WHS) 15th Annual Meeting, Chicago, May 18-21, 2005.
32. European Wound Management Society Position Document: Pain at Wound Dressing Changes. London, UK: Medical Education Partnership Ltd., 2002:2, 8.
33. Briggs M, et al. Minimizing pain at wound dressing-related procedures. A consensus document (A World Union of Wound Healing Societies' Initiative), Medical Education Partnership, Ltd., London, 2004.
34. Alvarez O. Ease the pain of wound care: better choices in debridement and dressing options. Oral presentation at the Symposium on Advances in Skin and Wound Care in San Antonio, TX, 29 April 2006.
35. Reddy M, Kohr R, Queen D, Keast D, Sibbald RG. Practical Treatment of Wound Pain and Trauma: A Patient-Centered Approach. An Overview. Ostomy/Wound Management; 49(4A)April 2003:2-15.
36. Van Rijswijk L, Braden BJ. Pressure ulcer patient and wound assessment: An AHCPR clinical practice guideline update. Ost Wound Manag 1999; 45(Suppl 1A):56S.
37. Rodeheaver GT, Sibbald RG. (eds). Chronic Wound Care: A Clinical Sourcebook for Healthcare Professionals, Third Edition. Wayne, PA: HMP Communications, 2001:369–83.
38. Sibbald RG, Campbell K, Coutts P, Queen D. Intact skin--an integrity not to be lost. Ostomy/Wound Management. 2003;49(6):27-33.
39. Queen D, Woo K, Shulz VN, Sibbald RG. Addressing the pain: Chronic wound pain and palliative cancer care. Ostomy/Wound Management, October 2003;49(10):16-18. October 2003.
40. Dykes PJ, Heggie R, Hill SA. Effects of adhesive dressing on the stratum corneum of the skin. Journal of Wound Care 2001;10(1):7-10.
41. Rolstad BS, Ovington LG. Principles of Wound Management in Acute and Chronic Wounds Current Management Concepts, Third Edition, Bryant RA, Nix DP, eds., Mosby/Elsevier, St. Louis, MO, 2007.
42. Ovington LG. Wound Care Products: How to Choose. Advances in Skin & Wound Care: The Journal for Prevention and Healing. September/October 2001 Vol. 14, No. 5 p. 259.
43. Van Rijswijk L, Braden BJ: Pressure ulcer patient and wound assessment: an AHCPR clinical practice guideline update, Ostomy Wound Management 45(suppl 1A):56S, 1999.

44. Bucknall T. The effect of local infection upon wound healing: An experimental study. Br J Surg 1980;67:851.
45. Wright JB, Lam k, Olson ME, Burrell RE. Is Antimicrobial Efficacy Sufficient? A Question Concerning the Benefits of New Dressings. Wounds 5, 2003
46. Stadelmann WK, Digenis AG, Tobin GR. Impediments to wound healing. Am J Surg 1998;176(Suppl 2A):39S–47S.
47. Kjolseth D, Frank JM, Barker JH, et al. Comparison of the effects of commonly used wound agents on epithelialization and neovascularization. J Am Coll Surgeons 1994;179:305–12.

NOTES

Notes

CHAPTER

11

Hyperbaric Oxygen and the Diabetic Lower Extremity Wound

Craig Broussard, PhD, RN

PERHAPS MANAGEMENT OF DIABETIC lower extremity wounds would better be termed amputation prevention. The 5-year mortality rate is nearly 50% for persons with a diabetic ulcer and nearly 50% for diabetics with a lower extremity amputation.[1] Thus, it is imperative that prompt treatment be instituted. Adjunctive to standard wound care, revascularization, bioengineered tissues, matrix materials and off-loading, is hyperbaric oxygen for the treatment of diabetic ulcers. On August 30, 2002, the Centers for Medicare and Medicaid Services posted approval for reimbursement for the adjunctive use of hyperbaric oxygenation in the treatment of diabetic ulcers.[2]

A number of studies and technical assessments were used to assess the role of hyperbaric oxygenation in the treatment of diabetic ulcers that led to the determination of CMS to approve reimbursement for adjunctive HBOT for diabetic lower extremity wounds. An abstract by Abidia, et al. reported results of 18 diabetics with ischemic, non-healing lower-extremity ulcers where patients were randomized in this double-blind study to evaluate hyperbaric oxygenation in the treatment of diabetic ulcers. Chi-square analysis of wound surface areas found that 13 of 19 ulcers in the hyperbaric treated group healed, compared to only 4 of 14 in the non-hyperbaric treatment group ($p = 0.024$). A mean decrease in wound area was 83% for the treatment group versus 56% for the control ($p = 0.021$). No differences in major amputation rates were found. The study concluded that hyperbaric oxygenation enhanced healing of the diabetic ulcer and that it was a valuable adjunctive therapy in persons when reconstructive surgery was not feasible.[3]

Zamboni, et al. evaluated the effect of hyperbaric oxygenation on chronic non-healing wounds in patients with insulin dependent diabetes. This was a nonrandomized, blinded, and controlled prospective study with a sample size of 10. Five patients were placed into a control group due to either claustrophobia or their lack of proximity to a treatment facility. All patients received standard wound care that consisted of debridement, topical silver sulfadiazine twice daily for 5 days, followed by twice daily moist saline dressings. Antibiotics were administered to patients with infection. Planimetry measures were obtained and wound surface area measurement were compared to the baseline measurement. Patients treated with hyperbaric oxygen showed significantly greater reductions in wound size throughout the 7 weeks studied ($p<0.05$). All patients were followed for up to 6 months following the completion of the study. 4 of 5 (80%) of the control group remained with non-healing wounds, whereas 4 of 5 (80%) of the treatment group had spontaneous healing of their wounds. No subject in either group underwent an amputation. The study demonstrated that adjunctive HBO significantly reduced wound size and concluded that hyperbaric oxygenation was efficacious in the healing of chronic diabetic foot wounds.[4]

Faglia, et al., evaluated the effectiveness of the addition of hyperbaric oxygenation to a comprehensive protocol in decreasing major amputations with severe diabetic foot ulcers in an unblinded, randomized, and controlled trial. The experimental group included 35 subjects and the control group consisted of 33 subjects. Both groups received a diagnostic and therapeutic protocol that included glycemic control, wound care, debridement, antibiotic therapy, angioplasty or bypass graft, and off-loading. In addition, the experimental group received a protocol of hyperbaric oxygenation. This study found 11 (33.3%) subjects in the non-HBO group versus 3 (8.6%) subjects in the HBO group received a major amputation ($p = 0.016$). The relative risk for the treatment group was 0.26 (CI 0.08 – 0.84). Thirty-two limbs were salvaged in the HBO group vs. 22 in the non-HBO group ($p = 0.016$). This study also found that hyperbaric oxygenation had a protective role against amputation (OR 0.084, $p = 0.033$, 95% CI 0.008-0.821) when compared to prognostic indicators for amputation of a low ankle-brachial index (OR 1.715, $p = 0.013$, 95% CI 1.121-2.626) and a high Wagner classification grade (OR 11.199, $p = 0.022$, 95% CI 1.406-89.146). The study concluded that hyperbaric oxygenation in addition to aggressive, multidisciplinary therapy was effective in decreasing major amputations.[5]

Ciaravino, et al. evaluated the efficacy of HBO in problem wounds in a retrospective review of 54 patients including 17 subjects with diabetic ulcers, 8 with arterial insufficiency ulcers, 13 subjects with dehisced amputation stumps, 6 subjects with gangrenous toes, and 10 subjects with non-healing operative wounds. Hyperbaric oxygenation was administered according to an established protocol at 2.0 ATA for 90 minutes, twice daily. Treatment outcomes did not differentiate the various wound types. All wound types were grouped together for treatment outcome. 43 (80%) showed no improvement, 6 (11%) demonstrated some improvement, and 5 (9%) had inconclusive results and none went to complete healing. This case series concluded that it is difficult to justify an ineffective, expensive, and complication-prone treatment for problem lower extremity wounds; however, other studies refute these findings.[6]

Doctor, et al. in a non-blinded, randomized controlled trial assessed 30 patients with diabetic foot lesions with an average duration of 10 years. 15 were placed in the treatment group and 15 in the control group. The purpose of the study was to evaluate the effect of hyperbaric oxygenation in diabetic foot lesions and its use as an adjunctive treatment. Both the control group and the experimental groups received standard wound care that included surgical debridement, incision and drainage, topical dressing care, antibiotics, and insulin administration. The experimental group received four sessions of oxygen breathing at 3 ATA for 45 minutes over a 2-week period. The study found a relative risk reduction for major amputation of 72% (95% CI 6-100%), an absolute risk reduction of 0.334 (95% CI 0.029-0.639), and the number needed to treat to realize this reduction of 3 (2-35). This study concluded that there was a significantly reduced rate of major amputation in the experimental group.[7]

Baroni, et al., studied strict metabolic control, daily debridement, and daily HBO in 28 hospitalized patients presenting with gangrenous lesions of the foot in a small nonrandomized, nonblinded controlled study. Patients were divided into two groups. The first group consisted of 18 subjects; the second consisted of 10 subjects. The first group was treated with HBO, metabolic control, and daily debridement. The second group was treated the same but without HBO. 16 of the 18 subjects treated with hyperbaric oxygenation healed with 2 requiring an amputation versus 1 patient in the non-hyperbaric group healed, 4 required amputation and 5 remained unchanged ($p = 0.001$). This study concluded that leg amputations were decreased in patients who received HBO treatment compared to those who did not receive hyperbaric oxygenation.[8]

Technical assessments have also addressed the efficacy of hyperbaric oxygenation in the treatment of diabetic ulcers. Technical assessments are a methodology used to assess the clinical suitability of a medical intervention based on a systematic review of the literature. Qualitative and quantitative synthesis of data from multiple studies is utilized to reach a conclusion regarding an interventions clinical utility.[9] The Blue Cross Blue Shield technical assessment reviewed a variety of treatment indications for hyperbaric oxygenation. This assessment concluded that there is adequate evidence to support the use of adjunctive hyperbaric oxygenation in the treatment of adequately perfused, non-healing wounds of the lower extremities with a program of standard wound care. In addition, this report concluded that patients with chronic, refractory wounds that are treated with hyperbaric oxygenation have fewer amputations and better heal rates than those not treated with hyperbarics.[10]

The Medical Services Advisory Committee technical assessment completed in Australia also found that persons with diabetic ulcers were less likely to receive an amputation if they were treated with hyperbaric oxygenation. It concluded that there is evidence to support hyperbaric oxygenation improving heal rates in diabetic ulcers and decreasing hospital length of stay.[11]

Subsequent to the determination for reimbursement, evidence continues to mount that HBOT is an effective treatment for diabetic lower extremity wounds. Londahl, et al. in a single site, randomized, double-blinded, placebo controlled study (he Hyperbaric Oxygen Therapy in Diabetics with Chronic Foot Ulcers (HODFU study) randomized 94 patients with Wagner 2, 3, and 4 ulcers into treatment groups receiving either hyperbaric oxygen or air. Results of the trial demonstrated that the group receiving hyperbaric oxygen had significantly better healing at one year than the air group (25 vs. 12 healed, P=0.03). Further sub-analysis demonstrated that using ulcer index, i.e., the largest area and duration ulcer covered with epithelial tissue or gangrenous tissue that had separated and epithelialized, demonstrated that the oxygen treated group had significantly higher healing than the air treated group (23 vs. 10, P=0.009). Adverse reactions were minimal with hypoglycemia within six hours of treatment occurring in only 6 patients in 3,225 treatment sessions. The conclusion of the study demonstrated that HBOT facilitated healing in diabetic foot ulcers.[12]

The Cochrane Library reports a review of literature looking at the effect of hyperbaric oxygen therapy in increasing the rate of healing of diabetic foot ulcers. Pooled data demonstrated that the risk of a major amputation was reduced by hyperbaric oxygen (RR 0.31, 05%CI 0.13-0.71, P=0.006). The author concluded that hyperbaric oxygen in diabetic patients may be justified as a treatment choice.[13]

A Turkish study of 100 patients who were admitted to the emergency surgical department, meeting inclusion criteria of at least age 18 with a foot wound present for at least 4 weeks, were randomly assigned to receive standard treatment or standard treatment plus HBOT. Standard treatment included daily wound care of dressing changes, local debridement, and amputation when indicated. Infection was treated with culture specific antibiotics. Findings in the study revealed that no patients who received standard treatment alone healed without operating room surgical interventions, compared to 33 (66%) of the patients receiving HBOT not requiring operating room interventions. In addition, 24 (48%) of the standard treatment group required a distal amputation, compared to 17 (34%) of the hyperbaric treated group. The authors concluded that HBOT in the treatment of diabetic foot ulcers improved healing and diminished the prevalence of amputation.[14]

A systematic review by Hinchliffe, et al., identified 114 studies related to hyperbaric oxygen in a Medline search. Of these, 4 RCTs[3-6] were identified that provided evidence suggesting that hyperbaric oxygen therapy may reduce the rate of major amputation with one study[7] reporting reductions in ulcer area.[15]

Diabetic Wound Patient Selection for Hyperbaric Oxygenation

Under CMS guidelines, the patient must have Type I or Type II diabetes and have a wound of the lower extremity due to diabetes. The wound must be a Wagner grade III or higher and must have failed treatment using standard wound care. Standard wound care is defined as assessment of vascular status with the correction of vascular problems; maximization of nutritional status and optimization of glycemic control; debridement of non-vital tissue, maintenance of moist wound healing with the use of topical dressings; appropriate off-loading of the wound; and finally, the resolving infection. Failed standard treatment must include no measurable signs of wound healing for at least 30 days following standard wound care, as evidenced by no decrease in wound size as measured by surface area or volume, no decrease in the amount of exudates, AND no decrease in the amount of necrotic tissue (see Figure 1).[2]

In addition to criteria for reimbursement, another consideration in patient selection should include transcutaneous oximetry. Transcutaneous oxygen measures (TCOM) are quantitative measures of oxygen availability to tissue.[16] A demonstration of periwound hypoxia with baseline TCOM measurements of < 40 mmHg that rise to > 100 mmHg while breathing 100% oxygen at 1 ATA is an indication for adjunctive hyperbaric oxygenation.[17] There should also be a demonstration of therapeutic transcutaneous oxygen values during hyperbaric oxygen treatments. A therapeutic value of 200 mmHg or greater in a non-diabetic and 400 mmHg in a diabetic is the minimum value necessary to predict a successful outcome.[18] Fife, et al., found that a minimum of 200 mmHg was 74% reliable in predicting success with hyperbaric oxygenation.[19] A TCOM of < 15 mmHg with an in-chamber TCOM of < 400 mmHg was found to be predictive of failure of hyperbaric oxygenation in diabetic lower extremity ulcers.[19] It should be noted, however, that TCOM measurement in itself is neither a qualifying or disqualifying parameter for treatment under current guidelines, but should be considered as part of patient selection for appropriate use of HBOT.

Treatment Protocols

Once hyperbaric oxygen has been determined to be an appropriate treatment for a person with a diabetic lower extremity wound and the patient has been determined to meet criteria for safe treatment, the patient is typically treated at 2.0 ATA for 90 minutes in the monoplace chamber. A decision to treat at 2.0-2.5 ATA in the multiplace chamber may also be considered. Treatment is typically 5 days per week.[20] Utilization review should be completed after 20 dives or after 30 calendar days. If the patient has demonstrated improvement, an addition 20 treatments may be considered. If after the additional 20 treatments the patient continues to show improvement, up to 20 more treatments may be considered. Generally, treatment should not exceed 60 total dives.

Managing Complications

Aside from complications seen in the general hyperbaric population including such things as barotrauma and claustrophobia, the diabetic patient may be at more risk for episodes of hyperbaric induced hypoglycemia. A search of PubMed, OVID, and CINAHL revealed no research related to the incidence, prevalence, severity, or prevention of hypoglycemia induced in hyperbarics in the diabetic population. However, hyperbaric practitioners do report its occurrence.

In order to minimize the potential for hypoglycemia, all patients with diabetes should have a pretreatment assessment of their blood glucose level by finger stick. Carbohydrates convert to blood glucose within 5 minutes of ingestion and will continue to convert for up to 3 hours.[21] High glycemic foods consist of simple carbohydrates with little or no fiber and have the potential to raise blood sugar much quicker, as there is little need to digest these foods to convert to glucose. Low glycemic index foods consist of more complex carbohydrates and fiber and require digestion to convert to glucose. 1 carbohydrate serving is equal to 15 grams of carbohydrate. 15 grams of carbohydrates is approximately 80 calories. 1 serving of high glycemic carbohydrates should rapidly raise the blood glucose between 45 and 80 mg/dl depending upon weight of the patient.[22] A glucose finding of <120 mg/dl should be treated with dietary carbohydrates prior to treatment. Figure 2 presents an approach to minimize complications of hypoglycemia during the hyperbaric treatment:

Examples of carbohydrate servings and amounts are in the following table:

In addition to routine blood glucose testing prior to the hyperbaric treatment, the astute clini-

Table 1: ***Carbohydrate Serving Equivalent Amounts (15 Gm/Serving)***

Bagel	½ medium	Apple	1 small	Milk	1 cup
Bread	1 slice	Applesauce	½ cup	Fruit Juice	4 oz (1/2 cup)
Graham Crackers	1 ½ pieces	Grapes	½ cup	Hard Candy	2 pieces
Muffin	½ medium	Orange	1 medium	Glucose Tablets	3 tablets
Pretzels	¾ oz	Pineapple	¾ cup cubed	Yogurt, low-fat	6 oz.
Cheese Crackers	4 crackers	Cantaloupe	1 cup cubed	Pudding, regular	4 oz.

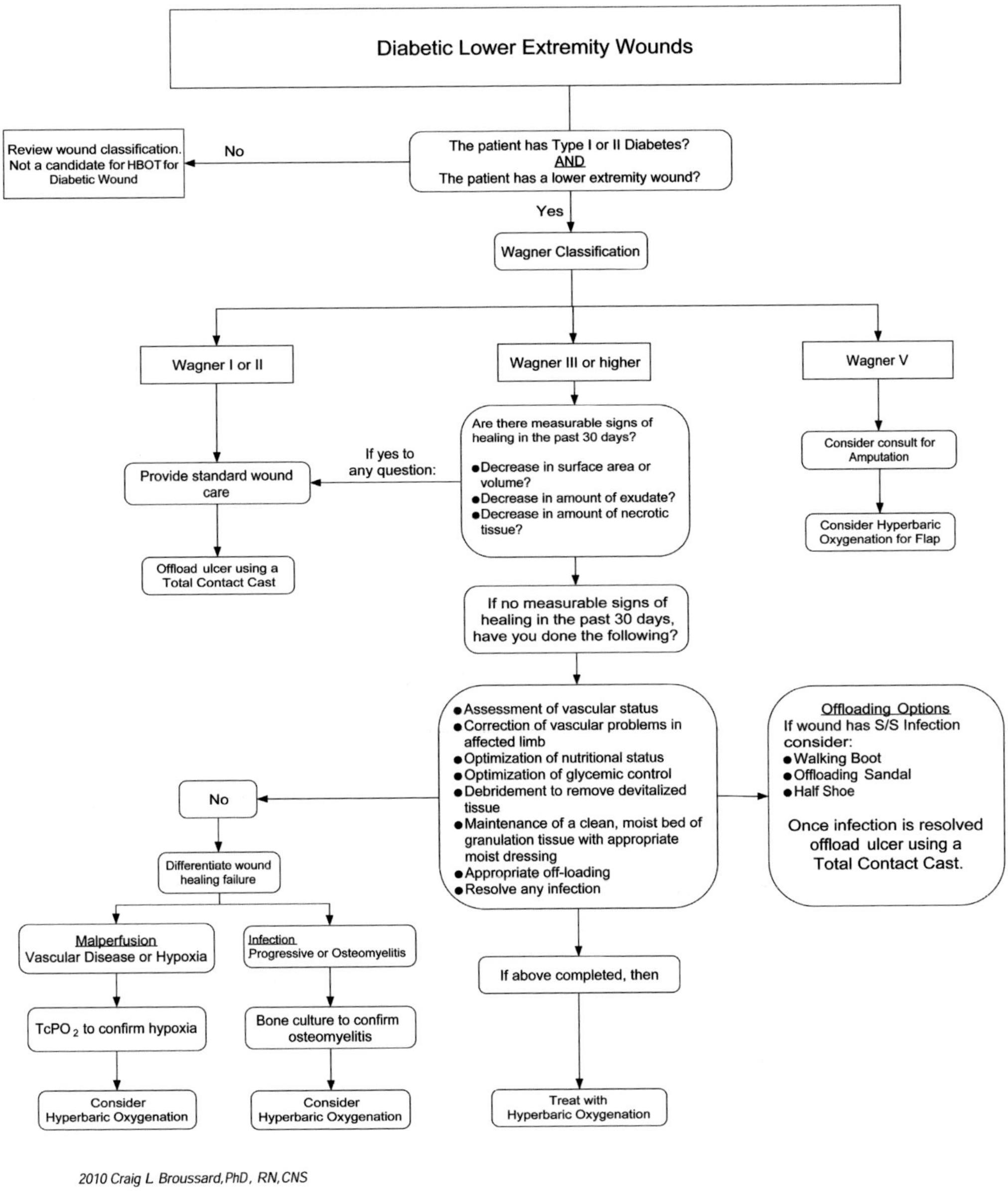

FIGURE 1: ***Diabetic lower extremity wounds.***

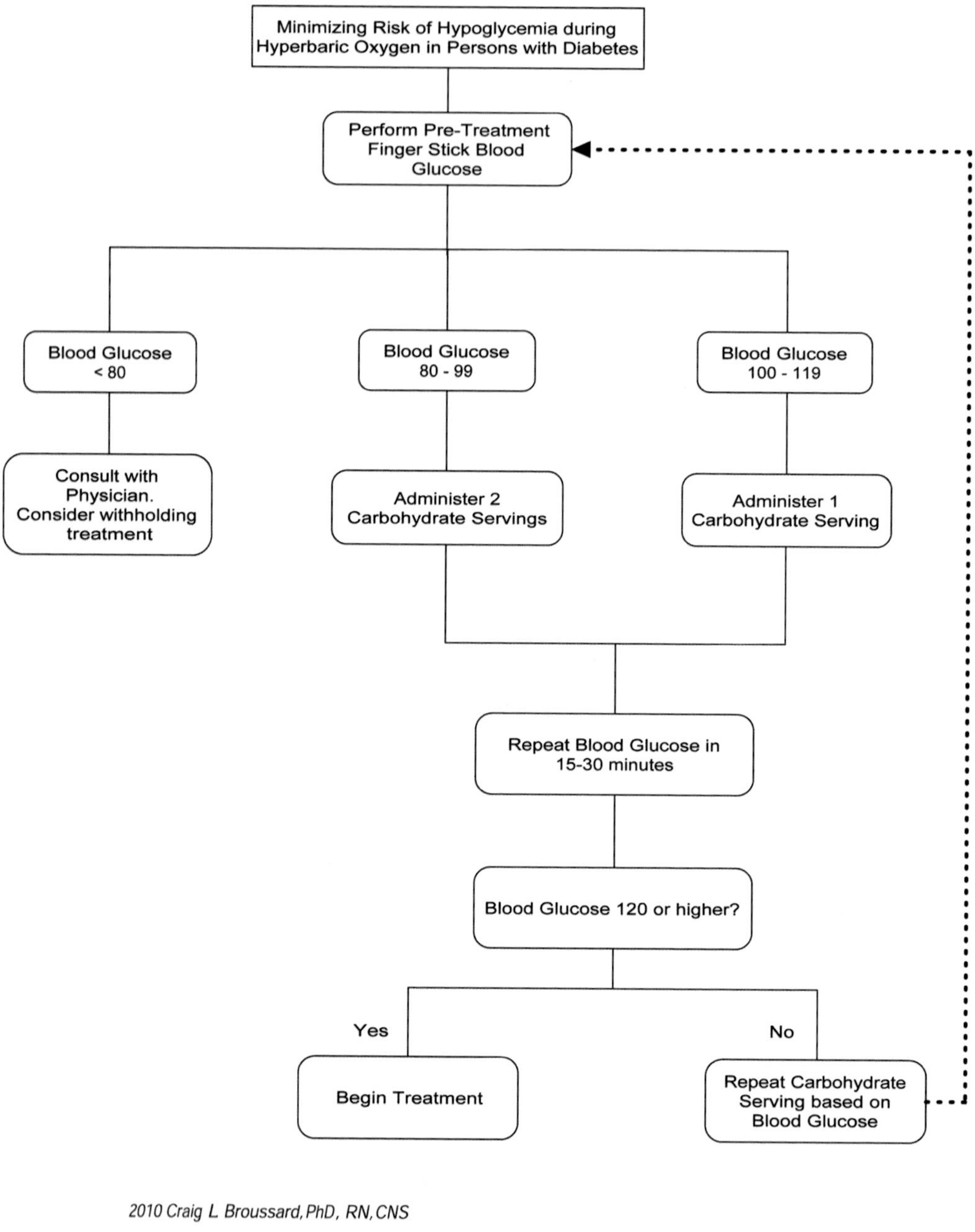

Figure 2: *How to minimize risk or hypoglycemia during hyperbaric oxygenation.*

Table 2: *Insulin Onset, Peak Effect, and Duration*[23]

Insulin Type	Onset	Peak Effect	Duration
Lispro (Humalog)	1 – 15 mins.	30 – 90 mins.	< 5 hours.
Insulin Aspart (Novolog)	15 mins.	45 – 90 mins.	3 – 5 hours
75/25 (Lispro protamine/Lispro)	15 – 60 mins.	1 – 6.5 hours	10 – 16 hours
70/30 (NPH/Regular)	15 – 30 mins.	2 - 3 hours / 8 – 12 hrs.	18 – 24 hours
50/50 (NPH/Regular)	15 – 30 mins.	2 – 3 hours 8 – 12 hours	18 – 24 hours
Regular	30 – 45 mins.	2 – 4 hours	6 – 8 hours
NPH	2 – 4 hours	4 – 10 hours	14 – 18 hours
Lente	3 – 4 hours	4 – 12 hours	16 – 20 hours
Ultralente	6 – 10 hours	Minimal peaking	20 – 30 hours
Lantus	1 hour	No Peak	24 hours

(Adapted from Lehne, RA. (2007). Pharmacology for Nursing Care (6th ed.).

cian will be aware of medication that the diabetic patient is receiving. Anecdotal experience suggests that the insulin dependent diabetic is more prone to hyperbaric induced hypoglycemia. The clinician would be wise to be familiar with both the type of insulin, dose, onset, peak effect, and duration of insulin. Table 2 lists insulin types, onset, peak effect, and duration:

For example, a patient receiving 70/30 NPH/regular insulin at 7 a.m. would be expected to have a peak effect between 9-10 a.m. and again between 3-7 p.m. In addition, if the patient is being dosed on a twice daily schedule again at 7 p.m., it would be expected that he would have another peak effect between 9-10 p.m. and again, for the NPH portion, between 3-7 a.m. the following morning. Thus, a patient receiving evening doses of insulin may peak during an early morning hyperbaric treatment. Should the peak effect occur during the hyperbaric treatment, the patient is more likely experience a hypoglycemic episode. It should be noted that withholding insulin prior to treatment will result in "stacking of insulin" and may result in serious hypoglycemic episodes either during a treatment or at other times during the day.

Post treatment blood glucose findings of < 100 mg/dl should receive treatment with 1-2 carbohydrate servings to prevent a continuing drop in blood sugar, especially in those patients who experience hypoglycemic unawareness.

Ensuring Best Outcomes: Off-loading the Ulcer

It is well established in the literature that optimal results in diabetic foot wounds are achieved by removing pressure, stress, and repetitive trauma to the wound. [24, 25, 26] It is known that continued pressure on an ulcer delays healing and increases the risk for further complications that may lead to wound healing failure and ultimately amputation.

Historically, numerous off-loading techniques have been employed in order to reduce pressure including bed rest, wheelchairs, crutches, and walkers. Most of these techniques, while in theory advantageous, are impractical. Placing a patient on bed rest will not necessarily completely off-load the foot as the patient may be ambulatory for bathroom privileges, and may ultimately result in further deconditioning the patient. Wheelchairs in homes are cumbersome, as homes are not designed for ease of movement in a wheelchair. Practitioners often speak of finding the wheelchair behind hallway doors or behind furniture, not being used by the patient. Crutches are often difficult to maneuver due to the general health and condition of the patient and increase risk of pressure in the axilla. Walkers require transferring pressure to the feet to move the walker forward.

Half shoes are relatively inexpensive to use and often become the means of off-loading ulcers due

TABLE 3: *Indications and Contraindications for TCC Use*

Indications	Contraindications
Non-infected neuropathic plantar foot lesions	Infected wounds
Medial or lateral foot lesions	Gangrene
Heel or digit lesions	Ulcer wider than deep (ulcer should be saucerized)
Post-operative delayed primary closures of wounds	Non-compliance/adherence with follow up care
Pre-ulcerative wounds	Dermal conditions precluding use such as eczema
Acute stages of Charcot neuropathy	Contact allergies
Edema reduction to improve wound healing	Atrophic skin
Reduction of stress on granulating tissue	Severe peripheral vascular disease (Ankle/toe index <0.5
Trauma protection of the foot	Morbid obesity
Non-compliant/adherent patients	Ataxia

to their ease of use and economics. The design of the half shoe is to theoretically remove pressure from the forefoot; however, the act of propulsive walking may increase pressure to the forefoot. Healing sandals are designed to limit gait and off-load an ulcer; however, they may require very specialized training to create a custom insert. The walking boot has been shown to be an effective off-loading device.[27] Concern in the use of the walking boot has been patient compliance, as the device can be removed. By using materials to make the removal more difficult, such as a simple wrapping material, locking straps, or fiberglass strips, compliance may be enhanced. This strategy has become known as the instant total contact cast (iTCC). The advantage of the walking boot and iTCC is the ease of use and that a wide range of clinician experience allows for its use.[28] While this may be an effective strategy, reimbursement for a walking boot is sometimes limited, requiring the patient to pay out-of-pocket for what can be an expensive device.

The gold standard for off-loading the diabetic foot ulcer has been and remains to be the total contact cast.[29, 30, 31] A TCC is a minimally padded cast that is well molded, or in total contact, to the lower leg and foot, allowing for redistribution of the weight bearing forces along the entire surface of the cast, effectively redistributing weight bearing to the entire surface of the foot, reducing unit area vertical forces, and promoting an apropulsive gait to minimize shear forces on an ulcer. The TCC can be used on plantar, medial, and lateral wounds, as well as heel and digit wounds. A major advantage of the TCC is that it allows for healing of an ulcer by pressure reduction of the ulcer while the patient remains ambulatory, reducing the potential of deconditioning the patient. In addition, it eliminates propulsive gait, shortening stride length, thereby effectively reducing shear forces on the ulcer, further minimizing trauma.[32] A review of several TCC studies revealed an average healing time for diabetic foot ulcers of 43.7 days with 88.9% heal rate.[33, 34, 35, 36] One study compared the TCC, the removable cast walker, and the half shoe, and found a heal rate of 89.5% in 33.5 days for the total contact cast. For the removable cast walker, the heal rate decreased to 65% and the time to heal increased by 17 days to 50.4 days. The half shoe had a heal rate of only 58.3% with a time to heal of 2 months or 61 days.[37] It is clear from this randomized, prospective study, that optimal outcomes are achieved with the TCC.

Historically the gold standard for off-loading, the TCC, has been a challenge due to the skill required for appropriate and safe application. One device, relatively new to the market, is the TCC-EZ™ made available by MedEfficiency, Inc. The TCC-EZ uses a fishnet meshed cast technology that is easy to apply and is supported by an outer boot system to provide stability. This tubal, mesh fiberglass, allows for a quick application that can be accomplished in any setting in a short period of time. Application, based on time studies, took less than 8 minutes. In addition, the time to dry for the patient to be ambulatory is less than 14 minutes.[38] This timeframe would equate to a typical application of a multilayered compression wrap for a venous insufficiency ulcer, a doable procedure in a busy wound care or hyperbaric clinic. In terms of hyperbarics, the fiberglass TCC does not pose an increased fire safety hazard. It is recommended that the cast be applied following the hyperbaric treatment so it can dry overnight. It is also recommended that the cast be covered with a pillow slip, towel or sheet to prevent the potential of scratching an acrylic chamber hull.

The procedure for applying the TCC-EZ is relatively straightforward.

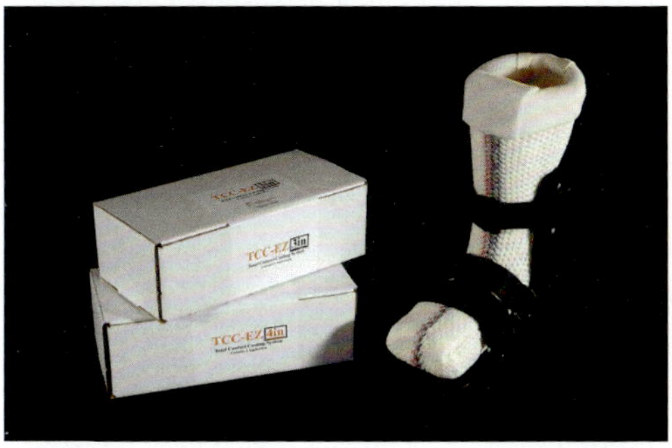

1. Assemble supplies.
2. Debride wound as necessary including paring any hyperkeratotic tissue.

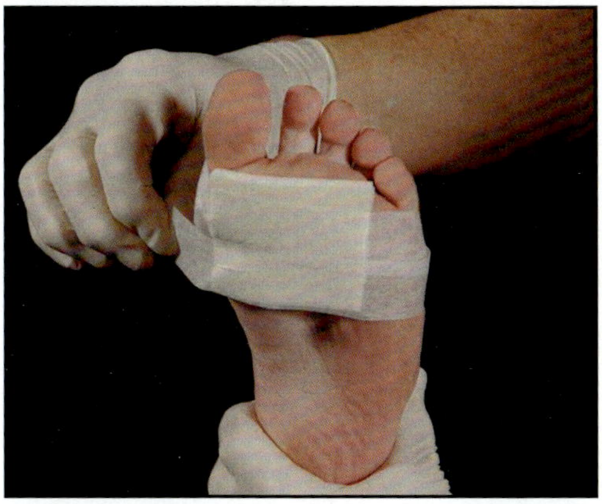

3. Apply foam dressing to absorb any exudate. Silver foam may be used.
4. Foam may be cut to a size just larger than the wound.
5. Anchor dressing using hypo-allergenic paper tape. A liquid film protective barrier may be applied prior to adhesive.

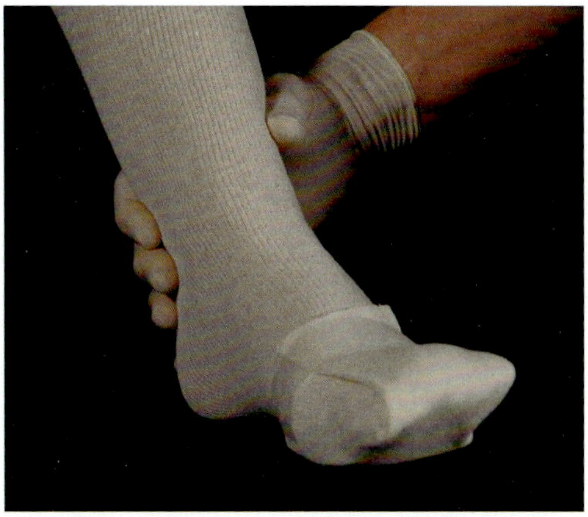

6. Apply stockinette to just below the knee.
7. Tape across the top of the foot to secure stockinette in place.
8. Trim any excess stockinette.

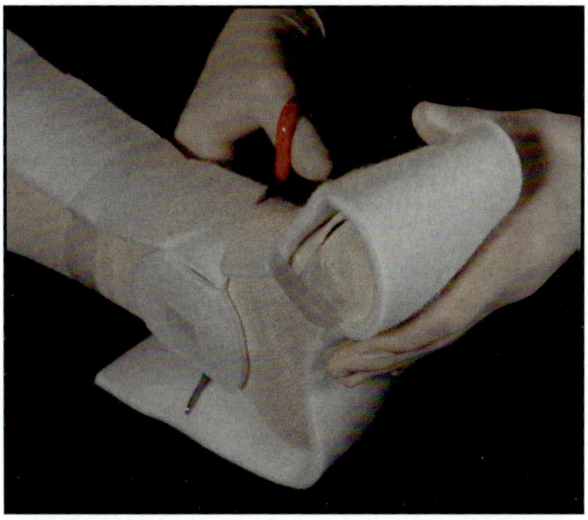

9. Align the felt pad with the short end toward the knee and the long end toward the foot.
10. Align the round disks with the maleoli and tape to hold in place.
11. Tape across the tibia and foot using a plastic tape.
12. Fold the long end of the pad around the foot ensuring enough excess to prevent crowding of the toes.
13. Secure with plastic tape behind the heel and trim any excess.

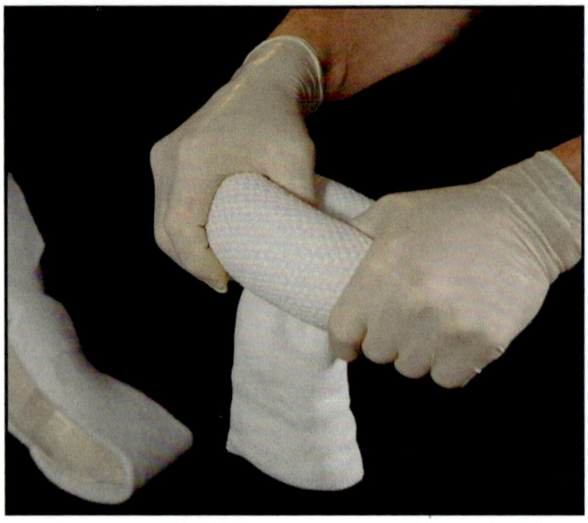

14. Roll the white protective sleeve into a doughnut shape.
15.Leaving 2-3 inches of excess at the toes, apply by rolling over the foot and leg.
16. Protective sleeve should be just below the level of the stockinette.

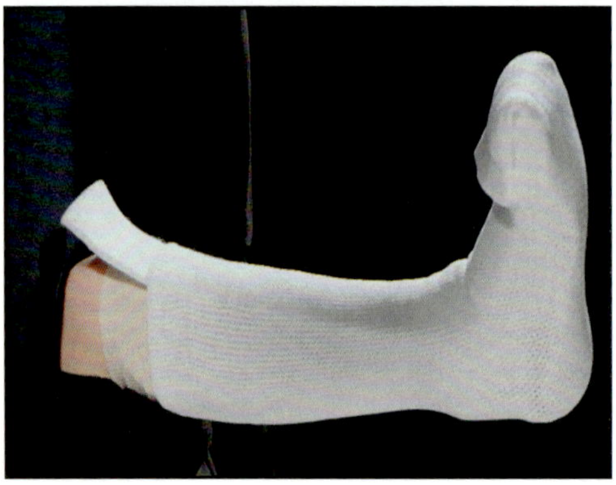

17. Fold the excess sleeve over the top of the toes and trim any excess.
18. Trim any excess felt pad near the knee to be even with the white protective sleeve.
19. Fold the tan stockinette over the edge of the white protective sleeve.

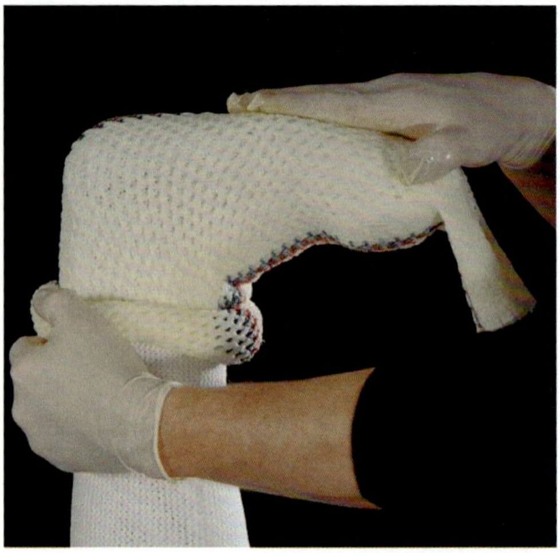

20. To activate the fiberglass, use water at room temperature or just cooler. Water that is too cold will allow the fiberglass to harden too quickly. Water that is too warm will delay hardening of the fiberglass.
21. Roll the tube of fiberglass into a doughnut shape, stretching and moving one's hands around the roll to create an even roll.
22. Allow 2-3 inches of excess.
23. Roll the patient into a prone position.
24. Dip fiberglass roll into water, shaking off any excess water.
25. Apply by unrolling over toes, ankle and leg to just below the edge of the protective sleeve.

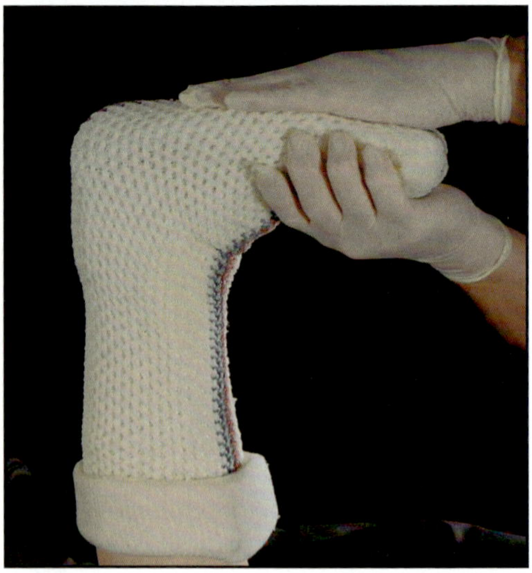

26. Roll the edge of the cast back to the widest part of the leg.
27. Capture the edge of the protective sock and stockinette into the fold.

28. Fold the fiberglass at the toes and hold at foot at a 90° angle until firm.
29. Rub along ankle and heel to contour fully to the extremity.
30. Gently rub along the leg to remove any bubbles.
31. Advise patient that casting material will become warm as it hardens.

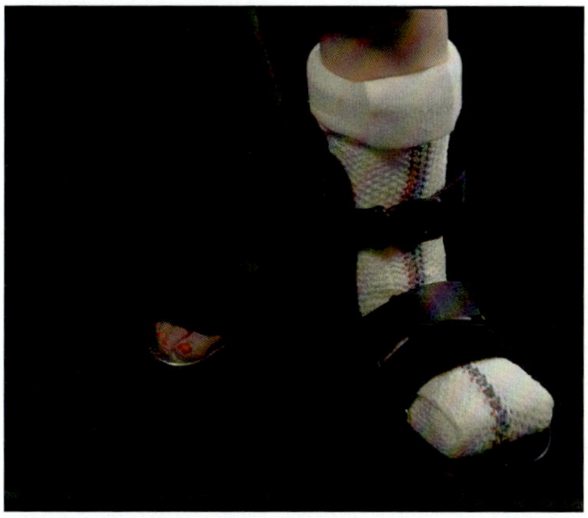

32. Once the fiberglass is firm, the patient may return to a sitting position.
33. Allow the cast to dry for another 10 minutes before applying the outer boot.
34. Apply the boot by aligning the leg with the upright struts.
35. Secure the boot using the toe, ankle and top straps.
36. Patient may now weight bear.

Photographs courtesy of MedEfficiency, Inc. [38]

First application of the TCC-EZ is removed in 3-4 days to ensure that no injury to the patient has occurred and to allow for appropriate reapplication due to edema reduction and potential loosening of the cast. Subsequent to the first removal, the cast is replaced on a weekly basis.

The procedure for removing the cast is straight forward, but does require the use of a cast cutter.

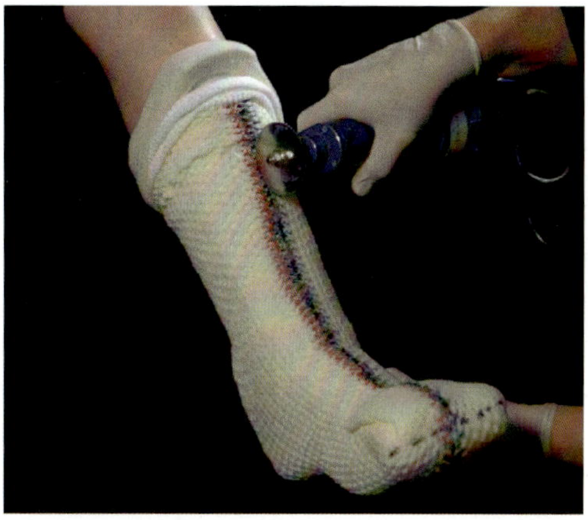

1. Remove the boot from the cast.
2. Cut the stockinette and move the protective padding near the knee.
3. Using a cast saw, cut along the tibia and dorsum of the foot.
4. Make a second cut across the toes

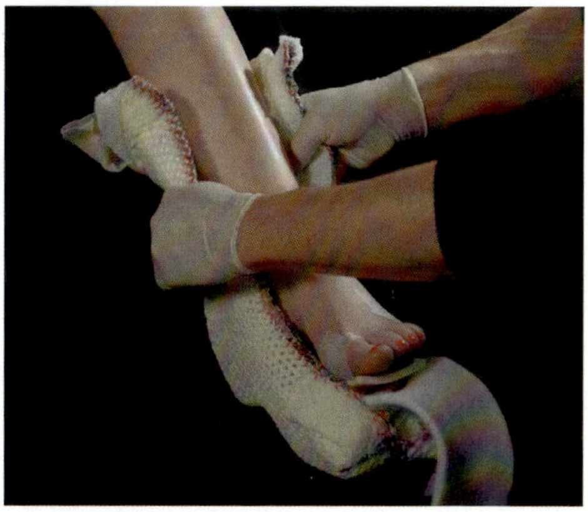

5. Using bandage scissors, cut the white protective layer.
6. Pull the felt pad away from the leg toward the toes.
7. Cut the tan stockinette.
8. Spread the cast with your hands.
9. Remove the cast from the foot.
Photographs courtesy of MedEfficiency, Inc. [38]

An economic advantage of using the TCC is that there is reimbursement under most third party payers, including Medicare. In addition, the TCC can be used with other advanced modalities of care such as bioengineered tissues and dermal matrix materials. The clinician should verify with third party payers if both application of bioengineered tissues, matrix materials, and TCC can be billed and reimbursed during the same visit.

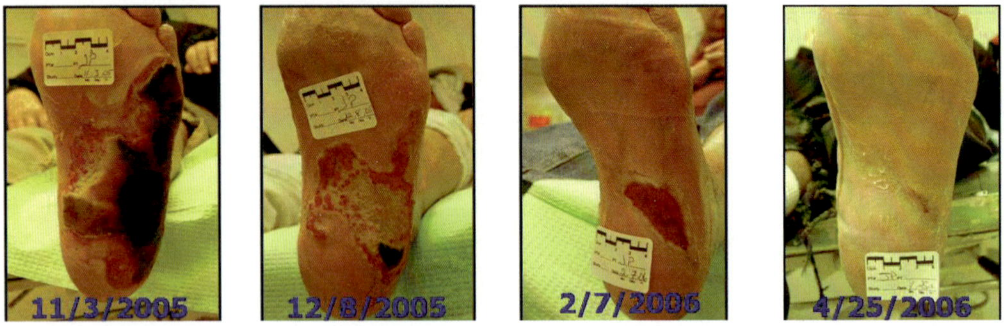

Figures *3a, 3b, 3c, 3d.*
Case study and photographs used with the permission of Diabetic Foot and Wound Center, Denver, CO.

There are disadvantages to TCC; however, with appropriate application and follow up, these can be minimized. Disadvantages include joint stiffness, atrophy of muscles from disuse, chafing, additional skin breakdown, the risk of new ulcerations, and instability of gait.[39]

Two exemplars to TCC will be presented. The first is a case of a 55-year-old diabetic, blind male on renal dialysis who presented with an extensive ulcer on the plantar aspect of the left foot of unknown cause wrapped in a soiled T-shirt. Cultures were obtained and appropriate antibiotics were coordinated with dialysis. A TCC was changed twice weekly along with debridement of the wound. The patient healed in 5 months and 3 weeks after initial presentation.

The second case is of a 66-year-old man with a history of noninsulin dependent diabetes, neuropathy, and a Wagner Grade II wound below the second metatarsal on the right foot. Following debridement, the wound measured 1.5 x 1.0 x o.2 cm. The wound was placed into a TCC-EZ. The first cast change was in three days after initial application, then weekly thereafter. The wound was healed in three weeks with four TCC-EZ applications.

A decision tree is offered in Figure 5 to guide in the selection of off-loading techniques based on Wagner Classification; however, it should be noted that goals of care, patient characteristics, and parameters for safe and appropriate use of off-loading should also be considered.

Summary

Hyperbaric oxygen treatment is an adjunct to the treatment of diabetic lower extremity wounds. Evidence suggests that the use of hyperbaric oxygen will improve healing rates and implies that mortality and morbidity will be decreased, effectively improving the quality of life of persons who experience diabetic ulcers. Hyperbaric oxygen does pose some risk; however,

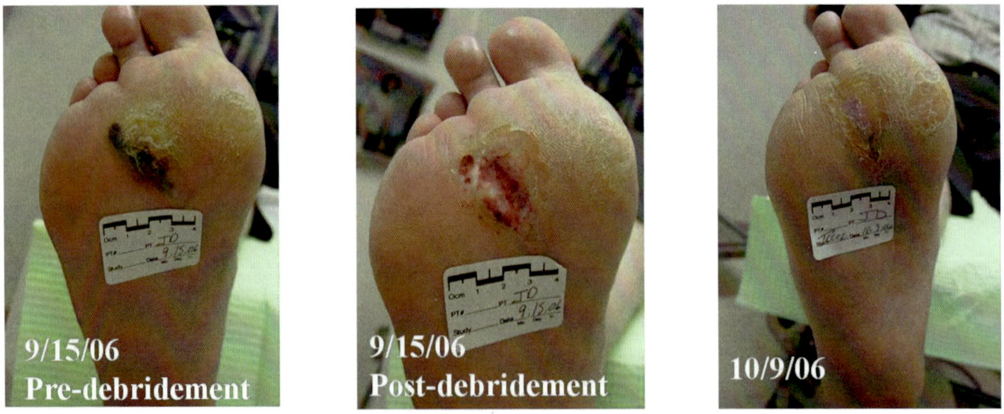

Figures *4a, 4b, 4c.*
Case study and photographs used with the permission of Diabetic Foot and Wound Center, Denver, CO.

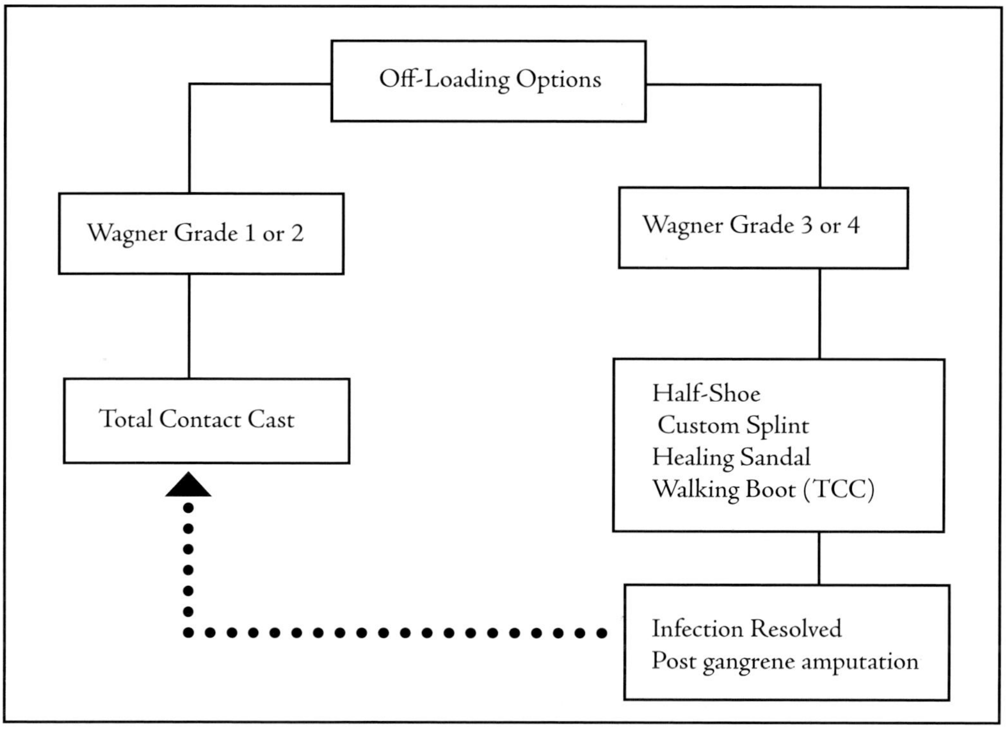

Figure 5: ***Off-loading options.***

with appropriate patient selection and consideration, treatment can be rendered safely. Hyperbarics alone is not the answer to the diabetic lower extremity wound. It is one aspect of a comprehensive plan of care that should include glycemic control, control of infection, improvement or correction of ischemia, debridement, the use of advance wound products such as bioengineered tissues, matrix materials and growth factors, the use of appropriate topical care and off-loading. In addition, modalities of care such as electrical stimulation and ultrasound should be considered in the overall plan of care. A comprehensive approach including hyperbarics will ensure the best outcomes and decrease time to heal for the person with a diabetic lower extremity wound.

References

1. Armstrong DG, Wrobel J, Robbins JM. Guest editorial: are diabetes-related wounds and amputations worse than cancer? Int Wound J: 4(4):286-287, 2007.
2. Centers for Medicare and Medicaid Services. Decision Memorandum. Administrative File: CAG-00060N. Hyperbaric Oxygen Therapy (HBO) in the Treatment of Hypoxic Wounds and Diabetic Wounds of the Lower Extremities. Available at: http://cms.gov/coverage/8b3-mm3.pdf
3. Abidia A, Kuhan G, Laden G, Bahia H, Johnson B, Wilkinson A, et al. Role of hyperbaric oxygen therapy in ischaemic, diabetic, lower-extremity ulcers: double-blind randomized controlled trial [Surgical Research Society Abstracts]. Brit J Surg 2001; 88:744.
4. Zamboni WA, Wong HP, Stephenson LL, Pfeifer, MA. Evaluation of hyperbaric oxygen for diabetic wounds: a prospective study. Undersea Hyper Med 1997; 24:175-179.
5. Faglia E, Favales F, Aldeghi A, Calia P, Quarantiello A, Oriani G, et al. Adjunctive systemic hyperbaric oxygen therapy in treatment of severe prevalently ischemic diabetic foot ulcer. Diabetes Care 1996; 19:1338-1343.
6. Ciaravino ME, Friedell ML, Kammerlocher TC. Is hyperbaric oxygen a useful adjunct in the management of problem lower extremity wounds? Annals Vasc Surg 1996; 10:558-562.
7. Doctor N, Pandya S, Supe A. Hyperbaric oxygen therapy in diabetic foot. J Postgrad Med 1992; 38:112-114.
8. Baroni G, Porro T, Faglia E, Pizzi G, Mastropasqua A, Oriani G, et al. Hyperbaric oxygen in diabetic gangrene treatment. Diabetes Care 1987; 10:81-94.
9. Agency for Healthcare Research and Quality. Technology Assessments. Available at: http://ahrq.gov/clinic/techix.htm
10. Hyperbaric Oxygen Therapy for Wound Healing: Part I. Blue Cross Blue Shield Association TEC, Technology Assessment, August 1999. USA
11. Hyperbaric Oxygen Therapy. Australian Medicare Service Advisory Committee (MSAC). Technology Assessment. April 2000. Canberra, Australia.
12. Londahl M, Katzman P, Nilsson A, Hammarlund C. Hyperbaric oxygen therapy facilitates healing of chronic foot ulcers in patients with diabetes. Diabetes Care 2010; 33(5): 998-1003.
13. Kranke P, Bennett MH, Debus SE, Roeckl-Wiedmann I, Schnabel A. Hyperbaric oxygen therapy for chronic wounds. Cochrane Database of Systematic Reviews 2004, Issue 1. Art. No.: CD004123. DOI: 10.1002/14651858.CD004123.pub2.
14. Duzgun AP, Satir HZ, Ozozan O, Saylam B, Kulah B, Coskun F. Effect of hyperbaric oxygen therapy on healing of diabetic foot ulcers. J Foot Ankle Surg. 2008 Nov-Dec;47(6):515-9.
15. Hinchliffe RJ, Valk GD, Apelqvist J, Armstrong DG, Bakker K, Game FL, Hartemann-Heurtier A, Löndahl M, Price PE, van Houtum WH, Jeffcoate WJ. A systematic review of the effectiveness of interventions to enhance the healing of chronic ulcers of the foot in diabetes. Diabetes Metab Res Rev. 2008 May-Jun;24 Suppl 1:S119-44.
16. American Diabetes Association. Consensus development conference on diabetic foot wound care. Diabetes Care 1999; 22:1354-1360.
17. Sheffield PJ. Measuring tissue oxygen tension: a review. Undersea Hyper Med 1998; 25:179-188.
18. Warriner R. The rationale for hyperbaric oxygen treatment in problem wounds. Introduction to Hyperbaric Medicine and Problem Wound Management; Praxis Clinical Services; 2002 August 18-24; Conroe, TX.
19. Fife, CE, Buyukcakir C, Otto GH, Sheffield P, Warriner RA, Love TL, Mader J. The predictive value of transcutaneous oxygen tension measurement in diabetic lower extremity ulcers treated with hyperbaric oxygen therapy: a retrospective analysis of 1144 patients. Wound Rep Reg 2002; 10:198-207.
20. Gesell LB. Hyperbaric Oxygen Therapy Indications. The Hyperbaric Oxygen Therapy Committee Report (12 ed.). Durham, NC: Undersea and Hyperbaric Medical Society, 2008.

21. Lifeclinic. (n.d.). Carbohydrates. Accessed on June 10, 2010 from http://www.lifeclinic.com/focus/nutrition/carbohydrate.asp?printpage=true
22. Diabetes Network. (n.d.). Low Blood Sugars (Hypoglycemia). Accessed on June 10, 2010 from http://www.diabetesnet.com/diabetes_control_tips/hypoglycemia_treatment.php#axzz0qeVwSGsa
23. Lehne RA. Pharmacology for Nursing Care. 6th ed. St. Louis (MO): Saunders Elsevier; 2007.
24. Boulton AJ. Pressure and the diabetic foot: clinical science and off-loading techniques. Am J Surg 187: 17S-24S, 2004.
25. Pinzur MS, Slovenkai, MP, Trepman E, et al. Guidelines for diabetic foot care: recommendations endorsed by the Diabetes Committee of the American Orthopaedic Foot and Ankle Society. Foot Ankle Int, 26: 113, 2005.
26. Brem H, Sheehan P, Rosenberb, HJ, Schneider JS, Boulton AJM. Evidence-based protocol for diabetic foot ulcers. Plastic and Reconstructive Surgery:117:193S-209S, 2006.
27. Lavery LA, Vela SA, Lavery DC, Quebedeaux TL: Reducing dynamic foot pressures in high-risk diabetic subjects with foot ulcerations: a comparison of treatments. Diabetes Care 19:818–821, 1996
28. Armstrong DG, Lavery LA, Wu S, Boulton, AJM. Evaluation of removable and irremovable cast walkers in the healing of diabetic foot wounds: a randomized controlled trial. Diabetes Care:28(3):551-554, 2005.
29. Armstrong DG, Nguyen HC, Lavery LA, van Schie CHM, Boulton AJM, Harkless LB. Offloading the diabetic foot wound: a randomized clinical trial. Diabetes Care 24:1019-1022, 2001.
30. Brand PW. The diabetic foot. In Ellenberg M, Rifkin H, eds. Diabetes mellitus, theory and practice. 3rd ed. New York: Medical Examination Publishing, pp. 803-828, 1983.
31. American Diabetes Association. Consensus development conference on diabetic wound care. Diabetes Care 22:1354-1360, 1999.
32. Martin N, Oldani T, Claxton MJ. A guide to offloading the diabetic foot. Podiatry Today: 18(9), 67-74, 2005.
33. Mueller MJ, Diamond JE, Sinacore Dr, et al: Total contact casting in treatment of diabetic plantar ulcers: a controlled clinical trial. Diabetes Care 12: 384-388, 1989.
34. Sinacore DR, Mueller MJ, Diamond JE, et al: Diabetic neuropathic ulcers treated by total contact casting: a clinical report. Phys Ther 67: 1543-1549, 1987.
35. Helm PA, Walker SC: Total contact casting in diabetic patients with neuropathic foot ulcerations. Arch Phys Med Rehabil 65: 691-693, 1984.
36. Myerson M, Papa J, Eaton K, Wilson K: The total contact cast for management of neuropathic plantar ulceration of the foot. J Bone Joint Surg 74A: 261-269, 1992.
37. Armstrong DG, Nguyen HC, Lavery LA, et al: Off-loading the diabetic foot wound. Diabetes Care 24(6): 1019-1022, 2001.
38. Medefficiency, Inc. TCC-EZ. Accessed on June 10, 2010, from http://www.medefficiency.com/company.html
39. Snyder RJ, Lanier KK. Diabetes: offloading difficult wounds. Lower Extremity Review. Accessed on June 15, 2010, from http://www.lowerextremityreview.com/index.php/article/diabetes-offloading-difficult-wounds

Notes

CHAPTER

12

Role of Transcutaneous Oxygen Monitoring for the Chronic Wound Patient

VALERIE LARSON-LOHR, RN AND HELEN NORVELL, RN

TRANSCUTANEOUS OXYGEN MEASUREMENT (TCOM) is a tool used within the chronic wound environment to assess the patient's ability to heal from an oxygen standpoint. The TCOM is useful in the hands of skilled technicians and healthcare providers who understand both the strengths and the weaknesses of this test. In this chapter, we will review the physiology and equipment, discuss the challenges, and review the role of TCOM in assessment and treatment of the chronic wound patient.

THE EQUIPMENT

The modified Clark electrode is the key to the ability to perform tissue oxygen measurements. In the 1950s, Clark took the elementary electrode developed by Davies and Brinks and combined the anode and cathode together behind a single membrane. It wasn't until Huch modified the electrode to include a heating element and a thermistor that it could be used outside of a laboratory setting. Today, the modified Clark electrode, with a heating element and thermistor, is able to maintain a preset temperature between 42 and 45 degrees centigrade. In the United States there are two TCOM machines that employ the Radiometer TINA sensor: Radiometer (Copenhagen, Denmark) and PeriMed (Stockholm, Sweden). This allows a TCOM study to be done within the 100% oxygen environment of a monoplace hyperbaric chamber. The

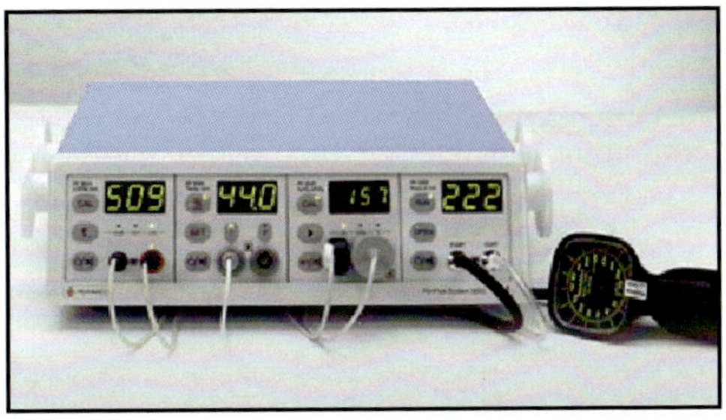

FIGURE 1: *PeriFlux System 5000 by PeriMed.*

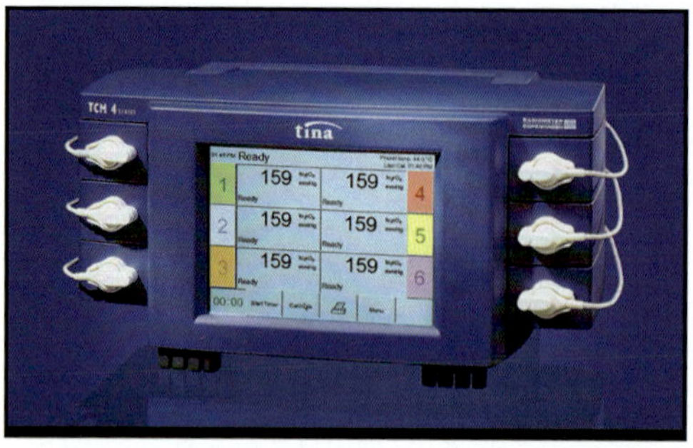

Figure 2: *TCM 400 by Radiometer.*

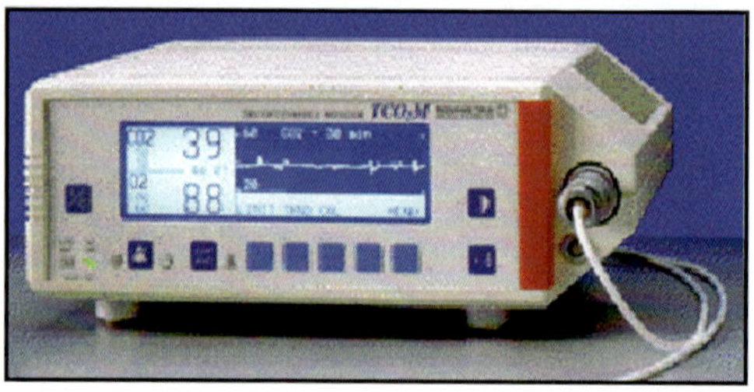

Figure 3: *TCO2M by Novametrix.*

third machine, Novametrix (Wallingford, CT) does not employ the Radiometer TINA sensor and cannot be used within a pressurized oxygen environment (Figures 1,2, and 3).

Accurately measuring tissue oxygen with a modified Clark electrode is very technically dependant. The ability to produce and reproduce reliable results is directly related to understanding how the oxygen is measured. The oxygen that is measured is what is directly seen below the electrode head. It is through arterialization of the capillaries and the release of oxygen to diffuse through the skin that the electrode has the oxygen to measure. Maximum arterialization occurs at 45°C, but in patients with compromised skin or who are elderly, this temperature can blister and damage skin that has already been wounded. The majority of centers performing TCOM commonly use 44°C, which is less damaging to the skin. The electrode is applied to the skin through a fixation ring. Contact fluid is placed in the fixation ring and the modified Clark electrode is secured to the fixation ring. The skin is heated by the electrode, which dilates the capillaries, shifting the oxyhemoglobin curve to the right. This causes the hemoglobin molecules to release oxygen, and the gas is able to diffuse through the skin and into the contact fluid. The oxygen that is dissolved in the contact fluid is then reduced to a measurable current, transmitted to the machine module where the electrical current is interpreted, and converted to mmHg. It takes 10 to 15 minutes for oxygen to equilibrate in the contact fluid and is representative of the level of oxygen in the tissue.

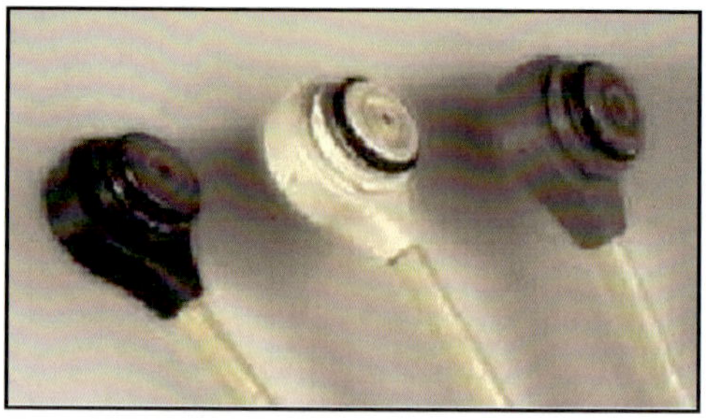

Figure 4: *Modified Clark Electrodes.*

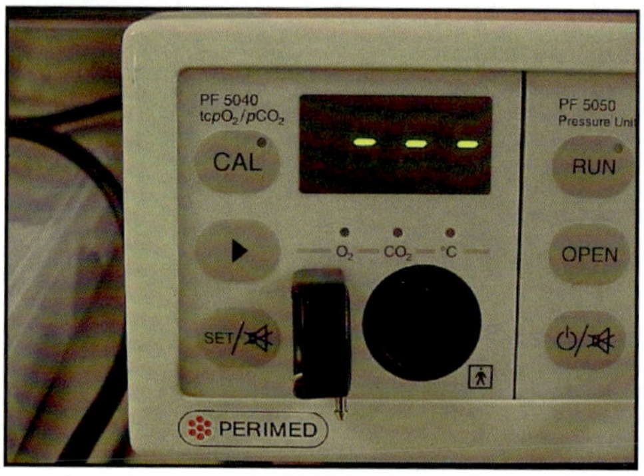

Figure 5: ***Perimed Module showing CAL button and electrode holder.***

Practical Application

Preparing the Equipment

Turn the unit on. Calibrate the electrode and set parameters using the manufacturer's guidelines. Connect the electrode plug to the electrode connector on the unit. Insert the membrane electrode into the electrode holder and turn clockwise until it clicks into place. Push the CAL button on the equipment module to initiate the calibration procedure. The entire calibration procedure should take between 2 to 4 minutes. If your calibration takes longer than this, you may error out and be required to change the membrane on the electrode. Most machines now utilize a two-point calibration. Two-point is a low calibration to zero and the high calibration is to ambient oxygen at current barometric pressure (barometric pressure x 20.9). The majority of TCOM machines today are equipped with an internal barometer allowing the high point calibration to be performed automatically.

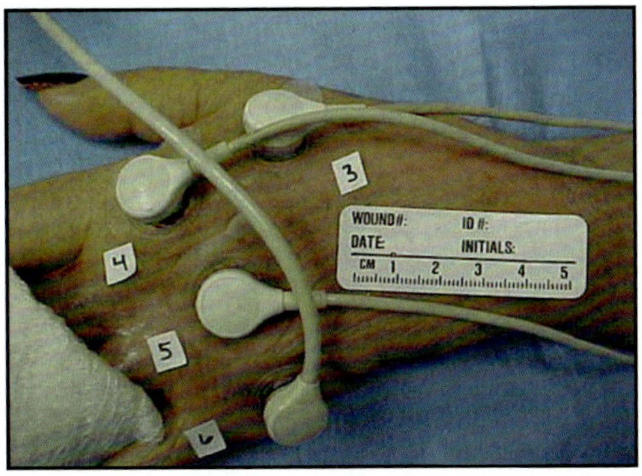

Figure 6: ***TCOM electrodes in place on a patient.***

Preparing the Patient

Provide a position of comfort while maintaining the patient supine with legs horizontal. Limit activities of the patient during the test. Keeping the patient warm, calm, controlling pain and decreasing any anxiety aids in obtaining reliable results. If the patient is a smoker, ask that the patient not smoke 2 hours before the exam. Nicotine is a powerful vasoconstrictor and can decrease results by 10%. Explain to the patient what to expect during the exam, emphasizing that it is painless and requires minimal extremity movement during the testing period. The length of time to perform the test will be approximately 1 hour.

Site Selection

Site selection should take into account anatomical structures, wound location, and condition of surrounding tissue. Bony prominences, large superficial vessels and pulse sites, callous areas, areas with significant edema, soles of feet, and palms of hands should be avoided as they can falsely lower or elevate the TCOM reading. The best electrode contact will be on flat or slightly convex areas. The number of electrodes to be used is largely determined by what is available. Remember that the electrode sees virtually only what is below it, so in order to do a complete evaluation of tissue oxygen levels, a minimum of 6 electrode leads is recommended. A reference of baseline oxygenation will need to be obtained. Commonly this is done with a lead placed on the chest, mid-clavicular, third intercostals space. Many centers have chosen to use all their leads for placement on the extremity in question and obtain a reference oxygen level utilizing oximetry.

Skin Preparation

In preparing the extremity for the electrode sensor, the skin will need to be free of oils or lotions, hair, and dry, loose skin. Wash the extremity and dry. Shave any hair present. Exfoliate the skin with micropore tape using caution on skin that is fragile so as not to cause additional wounds. Skin Prep has been used to aid in the adherence of the fixation ring to the skin. If Skin Prep is used, care should be taken not to coat the skin that will be directly under the sensor, as the Skin Prep will not allow the oxygen to diffuse freely through the skin into the fluid. As the fixation rings are placed on the skin, assure there is a good seal so oxygen cannot leak into the fluid. The first step in assuring a good seal is by running a cotton tip application around the circumference of the ring. Follow this with the use of overlay rings or placing tape over the fixation ring in a "window pane" method. Do not place tape directly over the electrode/sensor head as it will alter the oxygen reading.

Electrode Equilibration

It is important that a standardized procedure be utilized in order to obtain reliable, reproducible results. The TCOM evaluation is performed in three phases. The first phase is the baseline at room air. Research has shown in patients with compromised circulation, 15 to 20 minutes is required for the oxygen to equilibrate in the fluid. When the sensor is initially connected to the fixation ring, the technician will see a drop in the oxygen value as the tissue oxygen has not had time to diffuse through the skin into the fluid. The technician should observe all the sensor readings and evaluate if the readings are what is expected. If a sensor suddenly shows a high oxygen value, a leak to room air would be suspected. The readings from all sensors should be stabilized at 15 minutes. The purpose of baseline testing is to determine if the tissue is hypoxic in a normal resting state of the patient.

Phase 2 is elevation. Degree of elevation should be determined by protocol of the facility with a minimum elevation of 30 degrees. Many texts will state 45 degrees, but in practical application this degree of elevation is difficult to achieve with most patients. Care should be taken with elevation so as not to impinge on arterial flow with the device used to elevate the leg(s). A large foam wedge is commonly used to achieve this and also aids in providing consistency in providing the 30 degree elevation. The elevation challenge is to determine if there is adequate vascular reserve during extremity elevation and can be indicative of large or small vessel disease. The total elevation time is 10 minutes. During the first five minutes, the technician will see an initial drop in the oxygen reading. If there is adequate vascular reserve to maintain normoxic or baseline oxygen levels, then in the final 5 minutes the tissue oxygen reading should return to the initial room air resting values. If the oxygen level is 10% or less when compared to baseline oxygen readings, this is indicative of large or small vessel disease and should be evaluated further to determine a correctable cause.

Phase 3 is the oxygen challenge. During this phase, 100% percent oxygen is delivered to the patient with a tight-fitting mask, such as a Scott's Aviator Mask or other mask designed to fit snugly against the face. Many wound centers performing TCOM evaluations do not have a tight-fitting facemask and may be forced to look for an alternative. A non-rebreather mask has been used as a substitute, though not ideal. If a non-rebreather mask is utilized for the oxygen challenge, oxygen should be delivered at high flow rates (10 to 15 liters/minute), and every effort should be made to seal the mask to the patient's face so ambient air is not entrained. Even with these steps, the non-rebreather mask does not deliver 100% oxygen, depending on the fit of the mask to the patient; best delivery of oxygen would be in the 90 percentile. Under no circumstances should a nasal cannula be utilized. The duration of the oxygen challenge is 10 minutes. The purpose is to look for reversible hypoxia and to aid in determining if hyperbaric oxygen would be of use in healing the wounded tissue. Our process is to record values at 3, 5, and 10 minutes, looking for rate of rise. At the conclusion of the 10-minute oxygen challenge, the TCOM evaluation is complete (see Table 1).

Hyperbaric Oxygen Challenge: With the information obtained from the TCOM evaluation, the physician may determine a hyperbaric oxygen challenge is needed. In order to perform this test, extension cables and TCOM pass-throughs are required as the actual machine will remain outside of the chamber. In this scenario, the extension cables are connected to the TCOM machine and then to the TCOM passthrough. The sensor cable is then connected to the inside part of the TCOM pass-through. The calibration of the sensor is performed as previously discussed. Our practice is to use 3 to 4 leads during the in-chamber TCOM to obtain a good sample of response data from which to determine efficacy of hyperbaric oxygen treatments. The patient is prepared for the hyperbaric oxygen chamber, and in a monoplace setting, the gurney is connected to the chamber. Leads are placed and baseline 15 minute readings are performed. The patient is then placed inside the chamber and compression is started. When the patient reaches the desired depth (our centers use 2.0 ATA), the first reading is obtained. Subsequent readings are taken at 10, 20, and 30 minutes, once again looking for rate of rise. At this point, if the patient is only in the hyperbaric chamber for a TCOM challenge, decompression is started and the TCOM machine is turned off. If the patient is to receive a full hyperbaric oxygen treatment, the machine is turned off and the treatment completed. It is important that the TCOM machine not be left on for the entire treatment due to the potential of the heated sensor to cause blister to skin.

TABLE 1: ***TCOM Evalutation***

Obtained response on 100% oxygen at surface	Guidelines
>300 mmHg	Excellent response
>200 mmHg	Good response
100 -200 mmHg	Adequate response, non-limb threatening ischemia
51-99mmHg	Significant ischemia

CONDITIONS AFFECTING VALUES

Conditions that cause falsely high values: The most common condition that results in a false elevation in oxygen reading is an air leak to the fluid in the fixation ring. A large leak will be demonstrated by the oxygen reading going to that of the ambient oxygen. A smaller leak can be detected by observing all the leads during the equilibration time period and noting any that are not producing a reading that you would expect and not congruent with surrounding leads.

Placing a sensor directly over a large vessel will give a falsely high tissue oxygen level. During mapping lead placement, care should be taken to identify large vessels and avoid sensor placement.

Conditions that cause falsely low values: In placing sensor leads, any tissue that is calloused or thick should be avoided, such as soles of feet, palms of hands, and lateral aspects of heels. Callous will not allow oxygen to diffuse normally into the fluid in the fixation ring. Close to the surface bones and tendons will also result in inaccurate readings.

In the patient with vascular compromise of their extremities, even mild edema can have an impact on the transcutaneous readings. With edema, fluid occupies space between cells and most importantly between the capillary loops and the surface tissue. This results in oxygen not readily diffusing through the fluid and tissue into the fixation ring fluid. When placing the sensors, it is better to avoid areas of edema, or if this is not possible, account for the edema in the documentation and notify the physician doing the interpretation of the presence of edema.

The TCOM sensor uses oxygen during the measurement period. This can result in a reading of zero in a severely compromised extremity that still has viable tissue. The sensor's use of oxygen can impact the readings on tissue that has had its vessels severed and no constant resupply of oxygen, such as a newly placed skin flap. A related phenomenon is reaction of the carotid body during the oxygen challenge phase. The carotid body, sensing an elevation in oxygen, causes systemic vasoconstriction that results in a lower value at the sensor site than was obtained at baseline reading. If this occurs, it is indicative of a proximal occlusions or severe arterial disease.

Recording Results

Results should be recorded on a form that allows the physician to clearly see the anatomical position of the electrode, flow of readings from stabilization, elevation, and oxygen challenge. The technician should record any problems that occur during the test, condition of the sites, and status of the patient. The technician should not record an interpretation. Only the physician or other provider who is credentialed to interpret should do so. A simultaneous flow recording should be printed and attached to the documentation.

Research and Application in the Clinical Wound Care and Hyperbaric Setting

With the discovery of oxygen-related blindness in premature infants in the early 1950s, TCOMs were first used to monitor neonatal arterial oxygenation. Other medical specialties began to look at TCOMs to determine if there was any applicability within their area of practice. Vascular surgery used TCOMs to evaluate peripheral circulation; orthopedic surgeons to determine level of amputation best suited for healing; plastic surgery to monitor viability of skin flaps; anesthesiology to monitor early signs of hypoxia; and wound care and hyperbaric medicine to determine wound healing from an oxygen standpoint and selection of patients for hyperbaric oxygen therapy. But what was the foundation for the use in hyperbaric medicine and wound care? What conclusions can be drawn from the research?

- Dowd, et al., compared 161 volunteers to 62 patients with ischemic skin due to peripheral vascular disease. Results showed that TcpO2 was related to degree of ischemia and, in many cases, a more accurate guide to skin viability than clinical assessment. Measurement at the site of amputation in 24 patients demonstrated that a TCPO2 level of ≥ 40 mmHg was necessary for healing.
- White and Klein reviewed studies of transcutaneous oximetry involving 260 amputees who did not receive hyperbaric oxygen, and found that a TcpO2 value of 40 or greater was predictive of spontaneous healing. Levels below 35 mmHg were predictive of healing failure.
- Bacharach, et al., studied TcpO2 levels in 90 amputation sites to determine if it could be used to predict healing in lower limbs with arterial occlusive disease. Values were measured supine and elevated. The results were a TcpO2 of > 40 mm Hg was associated with primary or delayed healing, <20 mm Hg was associated with failure.
- Pecoraro, et al., set out to characterize the chronology and identify factors affecting healing in diabetic ulcers, since what determines faulty healing is obscure. They found that the periwound TcpO2 measurements were significantly associated with initial rate of tissue repair. Their conclusion was that periwound cutaneous perfusion is a critical physiological determinant of diabetic ulcer healing, indicating a 39-fold increase risk of healing failure when TcpO2 is <20 mmHg.
- Ballard, et al., did a prospective evaluation of transcutaneous oxygen monitoring to see if it could accurately predict severity of foot ischemia and be used to select appropriate treatment for patients with diabetes and tissue necrosis or ischemic rest pain. They studied 66 limbs and found a TcpO2 value ³ 30 mm Hg, the patient's foot problem could

be managed with conservative wound care, debridement or a minor foot amputation. When the TcpO2 value was < 30 mm Hg, then arteriography was performed with an anticipated need for vascular reconstruction. They concluded TCOM can prospectively determine severity of foot ischemia, aid in selecting appropriate treatment, decreasing total cost of diabetic ischemic foot care.

• Workman and Sheffield produced the first known TcpO2 data under hyperbaric conditions in early 1983. Their study included 18 normal subjects and 4 patients. In the normal subjects, TcpO2 values exceeded 1,000 mmHg at 2.4 ATA. With the 4 patients, initial values > 30 mmHg healed (2 patients) and initial values < 30 mmHg did not heal.

• Smith, et al., studied 26 patient transcutaneous oxygen measurements to evaluate the use in predicting the response of wounds to hyperbaric oxygen therapy. Periwound measurements were obtained before the initial treatment and after 10 hyperbaric treatments. If the patient's wound had a 5% reduction in wound score, they were identified as responders. Nine patients were responders. Periwound measurements correlated directly with an improvement in wound score per treatment ($p=0.03$). An elevated periwound TCOM at 2.4 atm and reduced a periwound TCOM at surface were associated with a more rapid response to HBO treatments

• Mathieu, et al., studied 23 patients with major vascular trauma of the limbs. Evaluation was by clinical examination and TCOM. 16 patients had arterial repair and seven had evidence of peripheral ischemia without an arterial lesion. On surface air, TcpO2 values between the traumatized limb and the non-traumatized limb were significantly lower, but neither the absolute TcpO2, nor the ratio between the values could predict an outcome of amputation. What was found to be predictive was the TcpO2 value at 2.5 atm abs in predicting a need for amputation or not.

• In 2002, Fife, et al. did a retrospective analysis of 1,144 patients to determine the reliability of transcutaneous oxygen tension measurement in predicting the outcomes of diabetics who were treated for lower extremity wounds. An overall improvement of 75.6% of the patients improved after receiving hyperbaric oxygen therapy. The best single way to make a distinction between success and failure of hyperbaric oxygen therapy was a TcpO2 measured in chamber using a cut-off score of 200 mmHg. The dependability of in-chamber TcpO2 as an isolated measure was 74% with a positive predictive value of 58%. When combining information about sea-level air and in-chamber oxygen, results are better. A normobaric air TcpO2 < 15 mmHg combined with an in- chamber TcpO2 < 400 mmHg, predicts failure of hyperbaric oxygen therapy with a reliability of 75.8% and a positive predictive value of 73.3%.

In 2009, Undersea Hyperbaric Medicine published a consensus statement based upon the proceedings of a workshop on Transcutaneous Oximetry: art, science, and practice. Consensus was reached on 9 issues.

1. Normal Extremity Values- > 50 mmHg

2. Definition of Hypoxia- < 40 mmHg, in diabetes and renal failure, wounds behave as hypoxic £ 50 mmHg.

3. Prediction of Healing- It is easier to determine a value below which a wound will not heal, than to find a value above which a wound is reliably predicted to heal.

4. Arterial Disease- Critical limb ischemia will almost always have a TcpO2 < 30 and usually < 20 mmHg. There are variables that can cause low TcpO2 levels that need to be considered in conjunction with clinical history and conditions during testing.

5. Normal Oxygen Challenge at Sea Level- Normal subjects during oxygen challenge of testing on the extremity always increase to a value > 100 mmHg. Values between <30 mmHg on air and > 100 mmHg on 100% oxygen suggests adequate arterial inflow, but a local barrier to oxygen diffusion. A 100% normobaric oxygen TcpO2 level < 30 mmHg is consistent with severe arterial disease.

6. Amputation Healing- TcpO2 <40 mmHg on normobaric air is associated with a lower than normal chance of amputation healing. If TcpO2 increase is <10% on 100% normobaric oxygen, this is at least 68% accurate in predicting failure of healing after an amputation in which wound oxygenation is not or can not be increased.

7. Predicting Response to Revascularization- TcpO2 that increases >40 mmHg during normobaric air after revascularization is a significant improvement, usually associated with subsequent healing. TcpO2 values can increase for as much as 28 days after revascularization.

8. Predicting Lack of Response to Oxygen- When testing from normobaric air to normobaric oxygen, if the increase in TcpO2 is < 10 mmHg, or if it decreases, then benefit from HBOT is highly unlikely.

9. Predicting Benefit from HBOT- If the

wound is hypoxic while breathing normobaric air, and TcpO2 values on 100% normobaric oxygen increases to above 35mmHg with a significant rise of >50% above the normobaric air value, there is a likelihood of benefiting from HBOT. In the diabetic foot ulcer, in-chamber TcpO2 values are the best way to predict benefit from HBOT. If the wound is hypoxic on normobaric air, and a TcpO2 of >200mmHg is achieved breathing hyperbaric oxygen, it is a 75% predictor for success with the diabetic foot ulcer. Conversely, an in-chamber TcpO2 <100 mmHg has an 89% chance of failure. A single study by Mathieu and associates suggests that an in-chamber TcpO2 > 50 mmHg in pedicle musculocutaneous flap transplantation was predictive of a successful outcome.

At the conclusion of the consensus workshop, a number of suggestions were made concerning best practice, but it is summed up best by one of the authors, "A thorough assessment of the patient must be done prior to acceptance for hyperbaric oxygen therapy, and the decision to treat should not be based on the TcPO2 alone."

A transcutaneous oxygen measurement is a tool that can aid in decision-making, but decisions should not be based only on this tool. It is technically sensitive and requires skill not only of the technician performing the test, but of the physician interpreting the test. In 25 years, we have come long way in understanding the strengths and the limitations of this tool, in understanding the oxygen tension values and what they mean to the healing potential of the wound, or if the extremity will be saved. It will be interesting to see what the next 25 years will tell us.

References

1. Clark CL, Wolf D, et al. Continuous recording of blood oxygen tensions by polarography. J Appl Physiol, 6:189-193 1953.
2. Davis PW, Brink F. Microelectrodes for measuring local oxygen tension in animal tissues. Rev SCI Instru. 13:524-533 1942.
3. Huch R, Lübbers DW, Huch A. Quantitative continuous measurements of partial oxygen pressure on the skin of adults and newborn babies. Pflugers Arch 337:185-198 1972.
4. Sheffield PJ. Measuring tissue oxygen tension, a review. J Undersea Hyperb Medicine. 1998. 179-188.
5. Fife CE, Buyukcakir C, Otto GH, et al. The predictive value of transcutaneous oxygen tension measurement in diabetic lower extremity ulcers treated with hyperbaric oxygen therapy: A retrospective review of 1144 patients. Wound Rep Reg 10:198-207; 2002.
6. Dowd GSE, Linge K, Bentley G. Measurement of Transcutaneous Oxygen Pressure in Normal and Ischemic Skin. Journal of Bone and Joint Surgery. Vol 65-B, No 1: January 1983.
7. White RA, Klein SR. Amputation level selection by transcutaneous oxygen pressure determination. In: Lower Extremity Amputation, Moore WS, Malone JM (eds.) W.B. Saunders, Philadelphia, 1989, 44-49.
8. Bacharach JM, Rooke TW, Osmundson PJ, Gloviczki P. Predictive value of transcutaneous oxygen pressure and amputation success by use of supine and elevation measurements. J Vasc Surg. 15:558-563, 1992.
9. Pecoraro RE, Ahroni JH, Boydo EJ, Stense VL. Chronology and determinants of tissue repair in diabetic lower extremity ulcers. Diabetes Oct; 40(10): 1305-1313, 1991.
10. Ballard JL, Eke CC, Bunt TJ, Killeen JD. A prospective evaluation of transcutaneous oxygen measurements in the management of diabetic foot problems. Journal of Vascular Surgery. 22, 4:485-492, 1995.
11. Workman WT, Sheffield PJ. Continuous transcutaneous oxygen monitoring in patients undergoing hyperbaric oxygen therapy. In: Huch R, Huch A, eds. Continuous transcutaneous blood gas monitoring. New York: Marcel Decker 1983: 667-672.
12. Smith BM, Desvigne LD, Slade JB, Dooley JW, Warren DC. Transcutaneous oxygen measurements predict healing of leg wounds with hyperbaric therapy. Wound Repair Regen. Apr-Jun;4(2):224-229, 1996.
13. Mathieu D, Wattel F, Bouachour G, Billard V, Defoin JF. Post-traumatic Limb Ischemia: Prediction of Final Outcome by Transcutaneous Oxygen Measurements in Hyperbaric Oxygen. Journal of Trauma-Injury Infection & Critical Care 30:3, 1990.
14. Fife CE, Smart DR, Sheffield PJ, Hopp HW, Hawkins G, and Clarke D. Transcutaneous Oximetry in Clinical Practice: Consensus statements from an expert panel based on evidence. UHM 2009, Vol. 36, No. 1, pp 43-53.

CHAPTER

13

Assessment and Documentation of the Nursing Process

LAURA JOSEFSEN, RN

THE SPECIALTY OF NURSING IS A MULTIFUNCTIONAL PART in the medical model that pulls together all the pieces for the cohesive whole. Nursing is the profession representing patient rights, and functions as the multidisciplinary person in the medical model who coordinates patient care and activities. Nurses provide management for the quality, education, intervention, and nursing assessment of patient care.

Through the nursing process, nurses manage and place into operation the interdisciplinary team's plan for the patient, as well as record the care and the progression of that care toward the patient specific goals. Documentation is becoming increasingly interdisciplinary and moving toward the goals to decrease duplication in charting, better utilization of nursing time, and enhance patient outcomes through better communication with all members of the team.

Documentation is a vital part of the nursing care; indeed, it is as essential as the nursing process. Documentation is defined as the written or electronic patient specific assessment and treatment that identifies the care or service, interventions, and outcomes for that patient

The documentation tool is critical to the evaluation and communication of clinical care given. It is no longer "just a place to write information," it is THE TOOL by which we are held accountable. We no longer have the luxury of saying "charting is taking away from the time I could be using for patient care."

This tool is the mechanism to communicate current and accurate information in a way that can be understood by everyone involved with the patient. The accuracy of this information will guide the treatment of the patient, as well as set the stage for the potential safety or risk of the patient.

"THE BEST ADVICE TO ANY NURSE IS TO THINK BEFORE YOU CHART"

— *Lanette L. Anderson MSN, JD, RN*

Documentation has been a source of frustration for nurses, with the two main issues being redundancy and excessive time spent on documentation. It is estimated that for every hour nurses spend doing patient care, there is at least one half hour of paperwork generated. Studies have looked at not only the documentation, but the process of how the present documents can be improved.

Keenan, et al., looked at the issues that nurses revealed regarding attitudes toward documentation. She reviewed 18 studies associated with Recordkeeping Quality (completeness and time), and 22 studies reviewing Improved Documentation and Care Planning Process. [1] Examples of the main issues include:

- Time spent documenting patient care is generally not regarded by nurses as being patient care.[1]
- Studies indicate that document focus, rather than patient-centric focus of the medical record, does little to support shared understanding by the clinicians in the care and the communication needed to ensure the continuity, quality, and safety of care.[1]

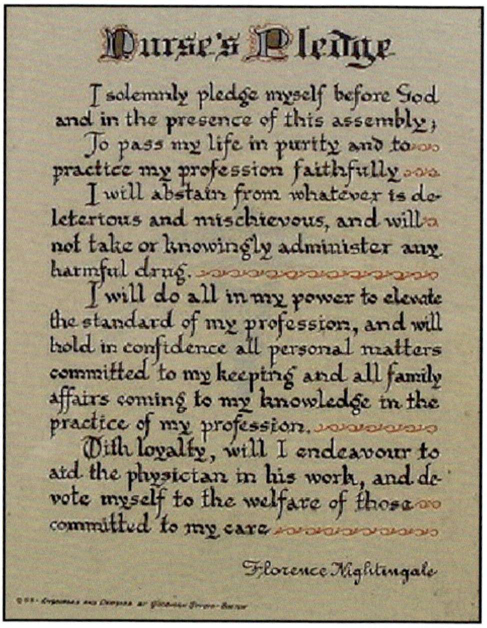

Nurse's Pledge

I solemnly pledge myself before God and in the presence of this assembly;
To pass my life in purity and to practice my profession faithfully.
I will abstain from whatever is deleterious and mischievous, and will not take or knowingly administer any harmful drug.
I will do all in my power to elevate the standard of my profession, and will hold in confidence all personal matters committed to my keeping and all family affairs coming to my knowledge in the practice of my profession.
With loyalty, will I endeavour to aid the physician in his work, and devote myself to the welfare of those committed to my care.

Florence Nightingale

Figure 1: *Nurse's Pledge.*

- Keenan, et al., summarizes that medical records that provide little clinical value not only waste nurse's time, but also limit the time available to engage in value-added care activities.[1]
- Karklainen, et al.,[1] completed a pre-and post intervention study, which involved educational intervention to promote a more patient-focused documentation. The major change observed was more attention by nurses to patient views and increased recording of these in the care plan.

She states in summary,[1] "there is a significant need for improvement in the process of documentation of patient care by nurses, and that by putting more substantial and sustained effort into improving the process of documentation of patient care by nurses holds the potential to decrease healthcare costs."

What do we need to know?

Healthcare is a business. Third party payers evaluate the documentation and medical necessity of treatment to determine appropriateness of payment. Financial reimbursement may be affected by the quality of the documentation. Chart audits are performed regularly by clinicians, other medical personnel, Centers for Medicare and Medicaid Services (CMS), insurance companies, regulatory agencies, corporations, and the companies that gather huge quantities of data nationwide. The auditors may or may not have clinical backgrounds or experience. The documentation needs to be clear enough to be understood by everyone involved with that chart.

How does your documentation stand up to all of these reviews? **The perception is that the quality of the documentation equates to the quality of care.** The appearance of your chart, whether electronic or paper, gives the impression of whether you are organized and if the documentation is comprehensive.

The first part of the process is nursing assessment to determine the baseline for patient treatment, including the nursing plan of care.

The second part of the process evaluates what was documented. This provides the data to compare this information to the current standard of practice and whether the current practice is effective, provides for optimal outcomes, and is cost effective.

Does the documentation include the components of:

- Information to validate the billing charges
- Changes in the patient condition
- Evidence of patient participation in the treatment plan
- Patient specific education
- Patient compliance
- Assessment and evaluation (initial and ongoing)
- Determine patient understanding and willingness to follow instructions
- Patient outcome
- Effective time management

Transparency

Data is being collected on a nationwide basis more than ever before. Comprehensive documentation is as critical as a complete assessment. We are no longer functioning within small communities or just in "our own hospital" setting, but because of increased technology, we are part of a nationwide/worldwide organization. Report cards are available to the public on-line. Medicare has adopted a Pay for Performance system of reimbursement.

What is different now?

What do we already know?

Everything we do is being looked at.

- Is it relevant?
- Is it the right treatment plan?
- Is the patient receiving appropriate follow-up care?
- Is it orderly, comprehensive and concise?
- Is it cost effective?
- Does it communicate well?

Whether you are using a paper form or electronic medical record, a comprehensive history, examination, and clinical decision-making is the basis from which everything else follows.

Documentation should meet or exceed hospital, state, federal, private industry, CMS, and the Joint Commission Requirements as well as the Undersea and Hyperbaric Medical Society recommendations.

What is being reflected in your documentation? The first recommendation is to have a summary sheet or form that provides an instant overview of the history, medications, tests, and ongoing treatment of the patient. The perception by the reviewer is that the patient care is more thorough and comprehensive, as well as gives the appearance

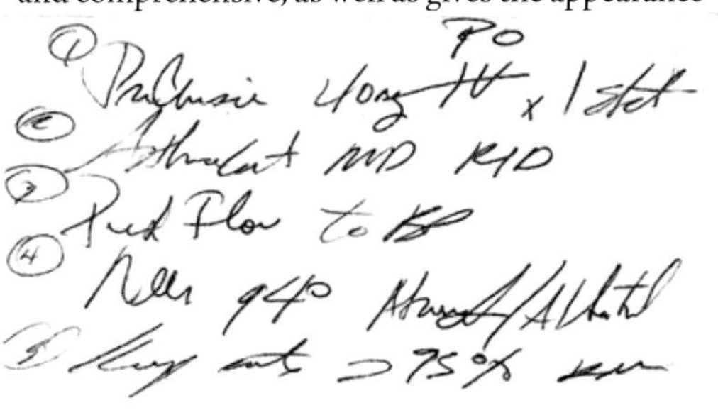

Figure 2: ***Illegible handwriting.***

of being organized. The summary sheet is a Joint Commission documentation requirement.

Documentation Assessment

Good documentation includes:

- Being accurate
- Using objective information
- Timely documentation
- Use only approved abbreviations

Legibility is critical

1. Basically, if something cannot be read, IT DOES NOT EXIST.
2. Chart reviewers will NOT "guess" at words that are not legible.
3. Clinical staff, pharmacists, home health agencies, insurance carriers, etc., should NOT guess at what is written.
4. If your signature is not legible, print your name - legibly - next your signature.

Forms

All forms should be filled out completely leaving no blank spaces – even if there needs to be just a line in that space. This includes forms that the patient or caregiver fills out.

The patient has the right to give or not give the information, but an area that is blank leaves several questions open:

- Is the information applicable?
- Was the information missed on initial assessment?
- Did the clinician pay attention to it?
- Does the patient not want the information revealed?

A line or note to show that each area was asked about gives the appearance of being more comprehensive with your assessment.

Consistent, accessible, orderly

- The information should be easily accessible and not haphazardly mixed throughout the chart.
- There is cause for concern when a chart is disorganized because it increases the potential for missing information.

Complete and concise documentation

- It is less complicated
- Saves time by being organized
- Documentation is more comprehensive
- Retrieving information is easier and faster
- Documentation is in real time
- Patient information is readily available
- Optimal outcomes are enhanced

- Comprehensive documentation leads to increased reimbursement
- Decreased cost due to better efficiency, and
- Documentation is accomplished in less time.

Incomplete charting raises questions about the quality of care given.

Methods of Documentation

Electronic Health Records

- Electronic documentation allows for easier, organized, and comprehensive input to the medical record.
- Education is a key factor to increase the quality and completeness of the documentation.
- The quality of the documentation increases as nurses become more familiar with the electronic medical process.

Narrative Documentation

- This is the traditional method for recording nursing care provided.
- This is in a story format that documents information in a chronological order without an organized framework.
- The disadvantage to this method is the increased potential for information being missed.

Figure 3: *BNA.*

Problem-Orientated Medical Record (POMR)

The nursing process forms the basis for a single list of patient issues that are generated by the members of the healthcare team

SOAP/IER

A structured way narrative progress notes are written by all healthcare team members:

Subjective: The patient's observations and statements

Objective: The care provider's observations that state the facts

Assessment: The clinician's evaluation of the patient issue

Plans: Patient specific goals and recommendations

Intervention: The action taken to meet the patient's identified needs

Evaluation: Determining the success of the intervention

Revision: Modifying the course of action as needed

PIE

PIE documentation is developed by nurses and is a concise and organized way to assess patient progress:

Problem: Identification of the patient's needs

Intervention: Development of the Nursing Plan of Care

Evaluation: Determining the success of the interventions of the Plan of Care

Focused charting DAR (Data Action Response):

Data, both subjective and objective

Action or nursing interventions

Response of the client.

- Notes are structured according to the patient issues
- Documentation follows the nursing process
- Graphic and flow sheets are used
  - Indicate who performed the assessment or intervention
  - Identify the checkmark or symbol
- Narrative notes are used in this process

Charting by Inclusion:

- Ongoing, regular basis
- Makes note of all assessment findings, nursing interventions, and patient outcomes
- "If it is not charted, then it was not done"

Charting by Exception:

- Makes note of negative findings
- Completed when assessment findings, nursing interventions, or patient outcomes vary from the established assessment norms or standards of care existing within a particular agency
- All standards have been met with a normal or expected response unless documented otherwise

Typically, there are several combinations of systems for each clinical area. There is no one system that fits all areas of practice.

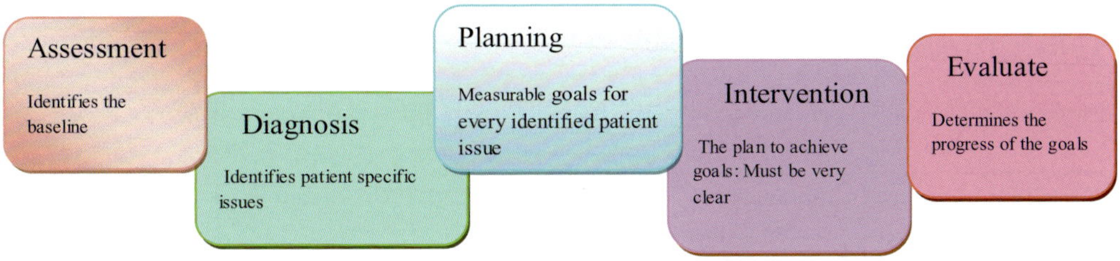

Figure 4: ***Documentation requirements.***

The type, model, or system of documentation selected should be in accordance with the facility and population needs. Regardless of the method used, registered nurses are responsible and accountable for documenting patient care accurately and completely.

Nursing Assessment

The nursing process is ongoing and identifies the patient specific issues that include the patient's physical needs, as well as their psychosocial needs. The nursing process is a holistic approach to patient centered, goal oriented care.

The nursing process identifies the changes in the patient condition and addresses and modifies the nursing plan of care accordingly.

For the patient receiving hyperbaric oxygen therapy, the Baromedical Nurses Association Standards of Care [c] is recommended, at *http://www.hyperbaricnurses.org/*

The nursing process provides for the quality care for the patient, as well as a mechanism for positive impact on clinical practice outcomes. Nursing professionalism, knowledge, insights, and wisdom are important contributions to the healthcare team and provide a positive effect on the action of other health team members.

It has been recognized that nursing documentation does not adequately reflect nursing practice. The documentation process is evolving to integrative documentation systems that involve a collaborative approach with physicians and other disciplines. The nursing documentation needs to clearly identify the nursing assessment, patient specific issues, plan of care, interventions, and evaluations. The documentation should reflect the specialty of nursing as the multifunctional part in the medical model that pulls together all the pieces for the cohesive whole.

Our goal is quality nursing care – it is what we do

Nursing documentation provides an account of the judgment and critical thinking used in the nursing process. Each of these steps depends on how accurate and complete the previous step is.

Quality improvement measures what was stated and compares it to the general standard of practice. One of the parts of the quality improvement process is accomplished by documentation. Quality improvement is an ongoing process of identifying and evaluating practice to provide optimal care. This is an exciting concept because it is an ongoing, ever-changing process.

Documentation is the tool designed to validate what we identify, assess, recommend, treat, and reassess. This tool is critical to our practice, essential for our success, and our success depends on how well we use this tool. Remember, the perception is that the quality of the documentation equates to the quality of care.

TABLE 1: *Documentation Assessment Tool – Example*[14]

Professional Documentation Standards - Queensland Nursing Council Information Sheet # 3

Quality Professional Documentation	Competence, Accountability, documentation	Requires registered nurses...to communicate effectively with individuals and groups	Accountability means that a nurse...must be prepared to answer to others...for their actions, and the responsibilities that are inherent in their positions	Quality professional documentation is the cornerstone of effective documentation. It is also an integral part of accountable practice
Nursing Documentation	Refers to any health record relating to nursing...of a client, family unit. Formal documentation includes all types such as electronic/ computer-held records, paper files and audio or video recordings	Informal communication methods such as communication books and verbal shift reports alert the healthcare team to critical information. They should direct others to the health record where the pertinent, detailed information is recorded	These do not replace the need for formal documentation	
Quality Professional Documentation	Benefits: Ensuring the client is consulted and included in care planning and that their decisions are recorded	Supporting continuity of care by allowing another nurse... to safely take over the client's ongoing care	Giving useful historical information if the client needs future healthcare	Providing a legal record of the care they have received
Benefits the nurse...by	Giving clear and dependable instructions, highlighting their unique contribution to client care	Increasing professional credibility by recording clinical judgment, delegation decisions, and critical thinking	Involving them in a structured reflective reasoning process	Saving time and energy. Despite the common misconception that record keeping is a waste of valuable care-giving time, quality professional documentation saves time, because less energy is spent searching for information or instructions. Conversely, poor documentation wastes time due to lost, incomplete or misleading information

QPD benefits the organization/employer by	Providing complete and reliable data to justify financial expenditure and resource allocation such as staffing levels and equipment	Facilitating research, auditing and quality improvement processes		
Employers and quality practice settings. Employers, nurses...share responsibility to create practice settings that support quality professional documentation. Employers can assist nurses... to meet the standards by	Maintaining a documentation system that promotes pertinent sharing of information among team members while protecting client confidentiality	Providing an appropriate physical environment, reliable equipment, ample storage, and quick retrieval processes	Factoring sufficient time for staff to produce quality professional documentation into workload and staff ratio calculations	Developing documentation policies, procedures, and forms in conjunction with nursing...staff: regularly monitoring and evaluating the quality of documentation
Professional misconduct and documentation – examples:	Failure to keep records as required, inappropriate destruction of records	Falsification of a nursing license or job application	Falsification of clinical records including medication administration, observations, and incident forms	May include: documenting care that never occurred or occurred at another time, signing a document that is known to contain false or misleading information, falsely signing for care when it was actually carried out by another person, signing as a witness to the disposal of controlled drugs when the act was not witnessed

Table 2: *Documentation Standards F.A.C.T.U.A.L.*[15]

Focus on the client	Must be personalized to reflect the client's needs, values, rights, and their involvement in care decisions	TIP Recording client's comments supports understanding of their needs	However, identify subjective information by framing it in quotation marks for example, Jeanne says that the pain is "excruciating"
Accurate	Must give a true and clear picture of the client's perspective of their health and wellbeing, the plan of care, the care provided and the effects of that care	TIP Be accurate when recording times. Remember to include the date and time that you make the record and print your name and position with your signature. Electronic signatures are valid	Only sign or initial YOUR observations, assessments or reports. Exceptions are emergency situations where a person is given the roll of designated recorder. Transcribing medication orders is a substandard practice that increases errors Co-signing entries made by other care providers blurs accountability. If you co-sign a health record, you must be very clear about what you are signing for and document the reason. Are you signing as a witness to a signature, or that you confirm that care was given, or that you have read the health record, or some other reason
Complete. Documentation must include all relevant information. Records should be more comprehensive, in-depth and frequent if the client is very ill or exposed to high risk. To identify how often and how detailed documentation should be, consider:	The complexity of the client's health needs. The degree that the client's condition, care, or treatment puts them at risk. The employer's policies and any legal requirements that apply in the practice setting If an unusual event has happened, such as a transfer, refusal of care, accident, or error	TIP When recording information about a referral or exchange of information with someone else, clearly identify them by name. It is often difficult to get a balance between completeness and consciousness. However, avoid duplication of information	In legal proceedings absence of information may be interpreted as an absence of action

Timely. Documentation must record all significant events as soon as possible, to reflect the client's current status	Update changes in a client's care plan as soon as possible.	TIP A chronological entry, that is, information recorded during or immediately after an event, reduces the likelihood of errors or misunderstandings and is more reliable than information recorded later, which is based on memory Never write a report or sign for care, treatment, observations, or medications in advance	Don't record late entries in the margin. Record and sign a late entry after previous entries – remember to include the date and time of the event and the date and time it was written
Understandable: Documentation must be written in plain language and, if abbreviations or symbols are used, must be well understood	TIP Remember to use the full word if the meaning could be misinterpreted, especially when referring to drug administration times or doses	Correct spelling and punctuation aid understanding	
Always objective. Documentation must be based on clear and unbiased statements	TIP: Avoid unfounded conclusions or value judgments and meaningless or vague phrases such as 'up and about' or 'usual day'	Disparaging remarks which criticize clients can bias other staff's perception of the client	
Legible	Documentation must be easy to read and decipherable	TIP If you make an error, draw a line through the entry and include your signature, date and reason. Do not delete computer-based entries but "strikethrough' it	

Table 3: ***Section C Self Audit***[15]

F.A.C.T.U.A.L.	The Standards
1. Focus on the client	Must be personalized to reflect the client's needs, values, rights and their involvement in the care decision
2. Accurate	Must give a true and clear picture of the client's perspective of their health and wellbeing, the plan of care, the care provided, and the effects of that care
3. Complete	Must include all relevant information
4. Timely	All significant events must be recorded as soon as possible so that the record reflects the client's current status
5. Understandable	Must be written in plain language and if abbreviations or symbols are used, they must be well understood
6. Always objective	Must be based on clear, unbiased statements
7. Legible	Must be easy to read and decipherable

REFERENCES

1. Keenan G, Yakel E, Tschannen D, Mandeville M. Chapter 49 Documentation and the Nurse Care Planning Process. This is available at www.ahrq.gov/qual/nurseshdbk/docs/keenang_dncpp.pdf
2. Gugerty, Brian, et.al, Challenges and Opportunities in Documentation of the Nursing Care of Patients. A Report of the Maryland Nursing Workforce Commission, Documentation Work Group, May2007. This is available at http://www.mbon.org/commission2/documentation_challenges.pdf
3. Patient Safety & Quality: An Evidence-Based Handbook for Nurses, AHRQ Publication No. 08-0043, April 2008
4. Good Medical Practice and the Law: Physician Documentation Checklist Offered, Vol 24, No.9, October 2000. This is available at http://med.stanford.edu/shs/update/archives/oct2000/checklist.html
5. Micheletti, Julie, Improving Physician Documentation Enhances Compliance, Journal of Health Care Compliance - Sept- Oct 2005
6. General Documentation Guidelines, State of Missouri Department of Health and Senior Services, March 2007. This is available at http://www.dhss.mo.gov/ -
7. Documentation Guidelines for Registered Nurses, College & Association of Registered Nurses of Alberta, Sept 2006.
8. Nursing Documentation, College of Registered Nurses of British Columbia, pub No 151. This is available at www.crnbc.ca/NursingPractice/Requirements.aspx
9. Documentation Guidelines for Registered Nurses 2005. College of Registered Nurses of Nova Scotia. This is available at http://www.crnns.ca/documents/CRNNS%20Documentation%20Guidelines%202005.pdf
10. Swindle, Jennifer, Good documentation: what it means for your physicians and your revenue cycle: the complexity of E/M coding bedevils medical practices to this day Healthcare Financial Management, Sept 2006
11. Morales, Katie, Nursing Documentation. This is available at http://www.nursetogether.com
12. Cougras, Sheila Benefits of Electronic Hyperbaric Documentation. BNA Update, Vol 23, Issue 2,July 2009
13. ANA Principles for Documentation
14. Professional Documentation Standards, Queensland Nursing Council 2005 available at http://www.qnc.gld.gov.au/home/index.aspx - framework information 03 professional documentation standards - Professional documentation standards 18 October 2007
15. Module 1: Overview of course, introduction to ANMC competencies, introduction to terminology, introduction to documentation, introduction to care plans and clinical pathways http://.cqu.edu.au/eSG/NURS11147eStudyGuide/NURSE11147_1.pdf
16. Gialanella, Kathleen, Documentation- Avoiding the pitfalls of documentation practices, Advance for Nurses June 2004. This is available at www.advanceweb.com.
17. Anderson L. Documentation: Impact on Quality of Care. This is available at http://www.nurseto gether.com

Notes

CHAPTER

14

Patient Education

Monica Skarban, RN

Healthcare today has many facets that bring new technology with the younger generations, while others stray toward more friendly organic principles and therapies for medical cures and prevention. No matter what medicine you lean toward, empowering the patients to find information for their well-being is becoming more cumbersome.

With the common use of today's social connections, patients across the globe utilize the internet to look up medical information specific to their disease entity or medical questions. How can these patients find the most accurate information with so much rubbish lacking quality, research-related studies to validate the claims? Millions can find anecdotal regimes. How can the common patient find reputable patient education to meet their educational needs, and, once they find it, can they understand it?

Patients, friends, and family need information, skills, and support to get through the cycle of illness, health, and wellness. Patients want to know what the disease processes are, symptoms and indications, what tests are needed, what medications should be taken, and how to find the wellness curve back to their normal active lives. Caregivers have tried for years to give patient education specific to their needs. It is a normal human instinct to search out more information and strive to become saturated with information so they can come to a solid conclusion with what their path will be. It is important for today's caregivers to ensure the patient has all the current and up-to-date avenues to getting the right education during their medical education journey. Accreditation agencies are requiring proof through documentation that the healthcare facilities can provide patient education that is understandable and useful specifically for the culture, race, or religion.

> "So never lose an opportunity of urging a practical beginning, however small, for it is wonderful how often in such matters the mustard-seed germinates and roots itself."
>
> —*Florence Nightingale*

The type of information and support the patient needs varies with individuals, as everyone's situation is different. A patient with acute illness requires different one-on-one education than the long-term illness patients and families. The short term illnesses require prompt interactions to get through the temporary adjustments of life, while the long term illness will need ongoing instructional support to continue daily activities depending on how the disease progresses. Therefore, patient education is an interactive process that deserves constant communication between the caregivers and the patients or family members.

Caregivers need to be aware of the interactions, as well as understanding how the patient will react to the education. Knowing the factors that demonstrate an acceptance of the educational efforts go a long way to knowledge integration and comprehension.

Non-Compliant versus non-adherent patient

When a patient comes back to the clinic or medical facility with a deteriorating or failed outcome, the provider or caregiver may imply or document that the patient was non-compliant with the original plan of care, causing the poor outcome or worsening of the disease process. Nurses need to be certain we use the correct terminology for what actually occurred and ensure the patient understood the original plan of care that was given and agreed upon by his medical provider. That is very different than the non-compliant patient, who knowingly chooses to veer from the given plan of care, understanding the potential repercussions.

When a patient is waiting for discharge from an inpatient experience, they may be really sick. They may not be ready to learn. Here are some patient education suggestions to secure an adherent future.

1. Include not only the patient but also the spouse, significant other, and/or other family members to ensure all aspects have been covered. Group discussion stimulates additional questions to create thorough teaching techniques
2. Do not use medical jargon that is hard to understand. Stay away from pharmaceutical company handouts that are hard to read and contain confusing information for the layperson.
3. Use techniques that confirm comprehension of desired information.
   a. Ask open-ended questions to stay away from one-word answers.
   b. Stay away from the statement: "Do you understand?" The patient may not really understand, but recognized the easier option of an affirmative response with a smile.
   c. Use words that mean something to the general public. The word "positive" has a good connotation for most people, but in healthcare issues, sometimes the word "positive" means a bad finding.

> "Education is not a preparation for life; education is life itself."-
>
> —***John Dewey***

4. Keep topics short and concise: patients can only absorb 2-3 things at a time if they are preoccupied with an acute or chronic illness.
5. Make sure written instructions are simple and to the point.
6. Reinforcement:
   a. Teach the one concept you want your clients to truly learn in the first lesson; then teach it again before you finish.
   b. Ask the patient to re-state what you have taught them
   c. Use visual aids, if possible, to describe using multiple senses
   d. Always include written instructions to take home with them for reinforcement

Joint Commission trend on education

In today's medical facilities, nurses are doing more with less because of the financial limitations and disappearing reimbursement encounters. Medical facilities are trying to cut non-productive time to provide excellent care and maintain the time-sensitive administrative details that must be completed during their shift. Joint Commission standards focus on learning outcomes that meet the needs of our growing diverse populations. The question is, are we going to give up essential education at the expense of limited resources, or find ways to give technologically current education with variable characteristics needed for our diverse patient population?

The Joint Commission works to continuously improve the safety and quality of care provided to the public through the provision of healthcare accreditation and related services that support performance improvement in healthcare organizations. As quality healthcare and patient safety

New Joint Commission Standard RI.01.01.03
The hospital respects the patient's right to receive information in a manner he or she understands.
Elements of Performance for RI.01.01.03
1. The hospital provides information in a manner tailored to the patient's age, language, and ability to understand. (See also RI.01.01.01, EPs 2and 5; PC.04.01.05, EP 8)
The hospital provides language interpreting and translation services. (See also RI.01.01.01, EPs 2 and 5; PC.02.01.21, EP 2; HR.01.02.01, EP 1)
Note: Language interpreting options may include hospital-employed language interpreters, contract interpreting services, or trained bilingual staff. These options may be provided in person or via telephone or video. The hospital determines which translated documents and languages are needed based on its patient population.
2. The hospital provides interpreting and translation services, as necessary. (See also RI.01.01.01, EP)
3. The hospital provides information to the patient who has vision, speech, hearing, or cognitive impairments in a manner that meets the patient's needs. (See also RI.01.01.01, EPs 2 and 5; PC.02.01.21, EP 2)
4. The hospital communicates with the patient who has vision, speech, hearing, or cognitive impairments in a manner that meets the patient's needs. (See also RI.01.01.01, EP 2)

are dependent upon effective communication, the Joint Commission encourages healthcare organizations to address the cultural and linguistic needs of our nation's rapidly growing and diverse population. The Joint Commission has developed recognition among those working in the area of cultural competence for its hospitals, language, and culture study and its ongoing related work (http://www.jointcommission.org/AccreditationPrograms/Hospitals/).

In March 2002, the Joint Commission, together with the Centers for Medicare and Medicaid Services, launched a national campaign to urge patients to take a role in preventing healthcare errors by becoming active, involved, and informed participants on the healthcare team. The program features brochures, posters, and buttons on a variety of patient safety topics. The patient-specific education program is called Speak Up™. The description of the acronym Speak Up ™ is:

Speak up if you have questions or concerns. If you still don't understand, ask again. It's your body and you have a right to know.

Pay attention to the care you get. Always make sure you're getting the right treatments and medicines by the right healthcare professionals. Don't assume anything.

Educate yourself about your illness. Learn about the medical tests you get, and your treatment plan.

Ask a trusted family member or friend to be your advocate (advisor or supporter).

Know what medicines you take and why you take them. Medicine errors are the most common health- care mistakes.

Use a hospital, clinic, surgery center, or other type of healthcare organization that has been carefully checked out. For example, the Joint Commission visits hospitals to see if they are meeting the Joint Commission's quality standards.

Participate in all decisions about your treatment. You are the center of the healthcare team.

Visit *http://www.jointcommission.org/AboutUs/Fact_Sheets/about_speakup.htm* for more information.

In a survey conducted in 2008, of the more than 1,900 organizations that responded, nearly 85% reported that campaigns like Speak Up bring value to the accreditation and certification process. They also reported that the program has promoted and increased communication with both patients and staff about safety. This is a free service to the community and should be utilized by all facilities as a reference for communicating with their patients.

Patient-Centered Communication standards were approved by the Joint Commission in December, 2009, and released to the field in January, 2010. The standards are published in the

2011 Comprehensive Accreditation Manual for Hospitals (CAMH): The Official Handbook. Joint Commission surveyors will evaluate compliance with the Patient-Centered Communication standards beginning January 1, 2011; however, findings will not affect the accreditation decision at this time. The information collected by Joint Commission surveyors and staff during this implementation pilot phase will be used to prepare the field for common implementation questions and concerns. Compliance with the Patient-Centered Communication standards will be included in the accreditation decision no earlier than January, 2012.

Visit http://www.jointcommission.org/NR/rdonlyres/26D4ABD6-3489-4101-B397-56C9EF7CC7FB/0/Post_PatientCenteredCareStandardsEPs_20100609.pdf for more information.

Other important published Joint Commission reports

Another initiative developed from the Joint Commission in spring of 2010 includes new recommendations to inspire hospitals to integrate concepts from the communication, cultural competence, and patient- and family-centered care fields into their organizations. The program is entitled Advancing Effective Communication, Cultural Competence, and Patient- and Family-Centered Care: A Roadmap for Hospitals. It is a monograph developed by the Joint Commission and is considered the Roadmap for Hospitals, which provides recommendations to help hospitals address unique patient needs, meet the new Patient-Centered Communication standards, and comply with existing Joint Commission requirements. Example practices, information on laws and regulations, and links to supplemental information, model policies, and educational tools are also included. The Joint Commission website provides self-assessment guidelines and example practices for each of the Patient-Centered Communication standards.

Exploring Cultural and Linguistic Services in the Nation's Hospitals: A Report of Findings was released in March, 2007. The report recommends targeted strategies to address language and cultural needs that currently pose challenges to hospitals seeking to deliver safe, effective care to the diverse American population. Key findings of the report:

- Hospitals face a variety of challenges in meeting the cultural and language needs of their patient populations.
- Efforts to address language are more concrete than those to address culture.
- There are wide ranges of practices for meeting the cultural and language needs of patients, and varied interpretations of "good" versus "poor" practice.
- There is a gap between current practice and desired practice, particularly related to the provision of language services. This may be attributable to missing resources or, in some cases, the resources are available, but are not being used or processes are not being followed.
- Collection of patient demographic data is inconsistent across and within hospitals, and few hospitals use these data to improve services for diverse patients.

One Size Does Not Fit All: Meeting the Health Care Needs of Diverse Populations was released in April, 2008. This report provides a thematic framework that was derived from current practices that hospitals are employing to provide care and services to diverse patients. As the range of practices mentioned in the report illustrates, there is no "one size fits all" solution, and the road map to cultural competence is unique for each organization. However, based on data gathered from the HLC study, this report recommends that organizations:

- Identify the needs of the patient population being served and assess how well these needs are being met through current systems.
- Bring people across the organization together to explore cultural and language issues by sharing experiences, evaluating current practices, discussing barriers, and identifying gaps.
- Make assessment, monitoring, and evaluation of cultural and language needs and services a continuous process.

This report includes a self-assessment tool that organizations can use to initiate discussions about the needs, resources, and goals for providing the highest quality care to every patient served.

When is patient education needed?

For the most part, patient education can be completed in the hospital acute care setting, outpatient clinic area, long care setting, a rehabilitation center, or anywhere a medical caregiver gives care. In the acute care setting, discharge planning carries the weight of home care education that the patient will need when they go home to ensure continuity of care. This is extremely important with the elderly who usually bring multiple disease processes and complex medical needs. Literature review shows that there are critical components to discharge planning of these types of patients. The essential discharge elements include communication, coordination, education, patient participation, and collaboration between medical personnel. Results of a study completed by Lin, et al. (2005) concerning completing these elements justify high attainment in patient satisfaction and quality of life. Appropriate and comprehensive education has become more and more difficult to accomplish. There are multiple reasons for this, including a huge influx of clients from varying cultures, the lack of time available for patient education in tightly scheduled, managed care visits, the lack of educational information written at an appropriate educational level, and/or the readability in the appropriate language other than English, and lack of reimbursement for time spent on patient education. Margaret Freda (2004) has postulated that over the past several decades, the old patriarchal system (in which the client was considered the object of care) has evolved into the current system in which the client is ideally considered a partner in care and has changed the way we provide education. She describes how the goal of teaching has changed from telling the patient the best actions to take, to now assisting them in learning about their healthcare to improve their own health and to actively participate in their own healthcare decisions. This newer view of health education has not been easily accepted by our clients, thus making it difficult to communicate with the patients.

Knowles' Adult Learning Principles were discussed in 1980. These principles remain current and useful today. You can use these principles when planning effective healthcare education. Those principles can be related to today's hyperbaric therapy:

1. Adults learn best when there is a perceived

Figure 1: ***Aurora Health Care intranet patient education website***
Printed with permission from Aurora Health Care, Milwaukee, WI

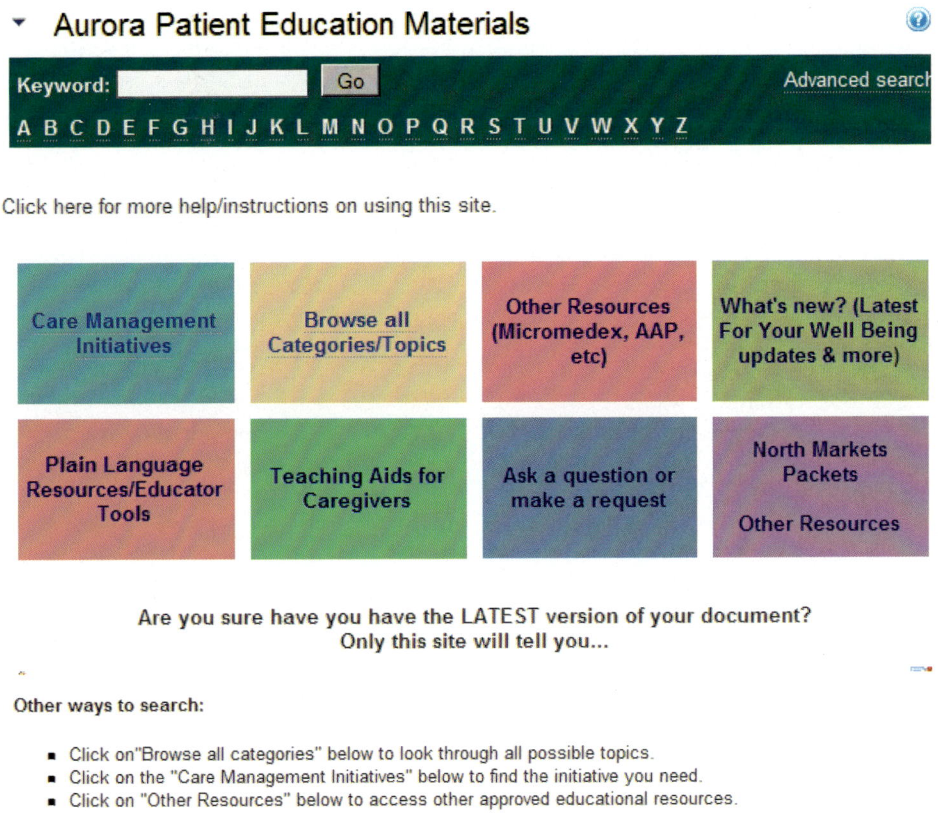

need: patient must understand why they need hyperbaric oxygen and how it will affect their specific disease process.
2. Teaching of adults should progress from the known to the unknown. Always assess what the patient already knows and build off their knowledge base.
3. Teaching of adults should progress from the simpler concepts to more complex concepts. Assess if a patient has ever experienced pressure in their ears from flying or traveling up a mountain before you can teach ear-clearing techniques.
4. Adults learn best using active participation. Give a tour of the department, and if there is a patient that is available to share their hyperbaric pressure experiences, give an opportunity for client-to-client interaction.
5. Adults require opportunities to practice new skills. Provide a glass of water and have the patient swallow water while holding their nose. Ask them if they feel the pressure in their ears. Determine if they can clear their ears appropriately.
6. Adults need the behavior reinforced. Pre- and post-treatment discussions are imperative. Check the ears to ensure there is no barotrauma.
7. Immediate feedback and correction of misconceptions increases learning.

Developing patient education materials

Nurses should be involved in all aspects of patient education, including the development of print or web resources. Patient education is an integral part of the nursing process relating to the patient satisfaction and quality of life outcomes. For years, nurses have not been a part of the development of these brochures or websites. With the increase of nurse specialists and technological expertise, patient education documents, brochures, websites and videos need nursing oversight. The Aurora Health Care Medical Organization in Eastern Wisconsin utilizes intranet resources with a list of all of the system-wide educational handouts that are used in not only the multi-hospital settings, but also with our visiting nurse components. There is a process in place that involves the specialty nurses to update the information for multiple center use. See Figure 1 for a screen shot of what the nurses see as they access various sources of patient education assistance.

Since not all facilities have this technological advantage, let us take a moment to point out the important factors in developing patient education material from scratch or from existing pamphlets.

Guidelines for developing education materials

1. Use what is already available, or develop new material. There is not too much that is commercially written on hyperbaric medicine for patient education. There is basic education that is the same for all hyperbaric patients.
2. Review related, available material online and print it. Utilize website information that is appropriate for your facility-specific scope of care/approvals for hyperbaric- UHMS.org is the most popular and helpful.
3. Evaluate websites systematically. There are various websites that provide guidelines for how to select the best website: look for evaluation tables to include guidelines on how to minimally assess authority, currency, objectivity, accuracy, and structure.
4. Assess available online and printed information for readability. After assessing the web material, consider using some of the updated material. The most recent literature shows that more than 23 million American adults may not understand the instructions or materials provided by healthcare providers. Consider rewriting the material to a lower level readability level.
5. Use tools for assessing readability. There are numerous formulas for determining readability. Some are more complicated than others, but they all share the same common characteristics, examining the difficulty of the vocabulary and the average sentence length.
6. Rewrite materials for easier-to-read levels. Rewrite printed material if the readability is not appropriate for the selected population, see Table

Patient Education Development Guide

Many medical facilities have a team that will review internal patient education and guide the staff with useful examples to build their first patient education tool related to their specialty. If you do not have a patient education center at your facility, you may want to check with your library or the research facility for additional assistance. In development of our clinical patient education, we used

Table 1:
Improving Readability: Simplifying Complex Word

Replace this word	With this word or phrase
Administer	Give
Anemia	Low blood count
Blood transfusion	Receive blood
Catheter	Tube
Contaminated	Dirty
Determine	Find out
Diabetes	High blood sugar
Dialyze, dialysis	Remove fluid and waste
Discontinue, terminate	Stop
Difficulties	Problems
Document	Record, write down
Edema	Swelling
Effluent	Drain fluid
Erythropoietin	Epo
Experience	Have
Hypertension	High blood pressure
Indicate	Show
Injection	Shot
Intravenous	In a vein
Notify	Call
Obtain	Collect
Ointment	Cream
Phosphorus	Phosphate
Physician	Doctor
Procedure	Task, skill
Sodium	Salt
Subcutaneous	Under your skin
Troubleshooting	Problem solving
Ultra filtrate	Remove fluid
Utilize	Use
Venipuncture	Draw blood
Dive	Treatment
Petroleum	Vaseline products
TCOM	Value of oxygen in the skin around your wound site

Note: This table is summarized from the following reference: Aldridge (2004) with additions from this author

these suggested guidelines:

Begin with looking at what you want to include in your patient education:

- Organize your ideas to include three to five main messages that stand out to the reader.
- Write short sentences that state one key point or express one idea in each sentence that are "need to know" information and answers the qestion, "what's in it for me?"
- Avoid complex grammatical sentence structure, write in the active voice.
- Use simple line drawings, charts, or graphs to reinforce text and draw attention to key points. If you wish to use pictures or content from other sources, copyright laws must be adhered to.

How to organize:

- Grab your reader with a catchy title that clearly indicates what the piece is about
- Keep process in order that it happens
- Put most important information first, and least important information last
- Make sure readers can go back and easily locate important information
- Use headers and summaries to introduce new material, reinforce and highlight key points.

How to write it:

- Keep in mind the style, tone, and reading levels
- Clarity and brief comments
- Use bold or italics to emphasize key points
- Use at least 12 font text size (avoid using multiple fonts- it is distracting to the reader)
- Use one or two syllable words and sentences
- Use commonly spoken terms rather than medical jargon
- Avoid stereotypes
- Write in the active voice and use the second person (you) rather than third person (the patient, he/she)
- Make content relative to your reader, sensitive to culture, age, and gender
- Utilize a 5th-8th grade level when possible
- Edit it and try a sample copy with a few patients. Get feedback and revise as needed.

Development of a Hyperbaric Oxygen Therapy and Treatment Patient Education Handout

As hyperbaric specialists, it is our duty to prepare proper education to our patients on this specific medicine and therapy. Attached is an example of what the Aurora Health

Aurora Health Care®
www.AuroraHealthCare.org

For Your Well Being

Hyperbaric Oxygen Therapy and Treatment in the Monoplace Chamber

What is hyperbaric oxygen therapy?
Hyperbaric oxygen therapy is a medical treatment that promotes wound healing. It involves breathing 100% oxygen while sitting or lying in a chamber that is pressurized.

Why hyperbaric treatments?
In the chamber, large doses of oxygen are dissolved into your blood and body tissues. This increased oxygen promotes wound healing by:
- Stimulating small blood vessel growth, or
- Stopping tissue damage from carbon monoxide poisoning, or
- Helping to heal body tissue after radiation therapy.

A hyperbaric doctor will talk with you about the reasons for your treatment. The number of treatments you need depends on your condition and how you respond to treatment.

How often will I have treatments?
Generally, treatments are scheduled daily, Monday through Friday. Plan on being in the department for at least two hours for each treatment. On occasion, you may be treated twice a day. Weekend treatments are rare and are based on patient needs.

Please call the hyperbaric department as soon as possible if you have a cold or flu symptoms (fever of 100° F or higher, cough, runny nose, vomiting, diarrhea or general aching). Your therapy will probably be postponed until the doctor clears you. You may leave a message by calling the hyperbaric department or clinic directly.

Are there restrictions I should follow?
While being treated in hyperbaric you should not use tobacco. Tobacco products of any kind will cause your blood vessels to shrink in size, making treatments less effective. We can refer you to programs that will help you stop smoking. If you cannot stop using tobacco products, your treatments may be stopped.

There are no eating restrictions when receiving hyperbaric treatments. If you are already on a special diet for diabetes, kidney failure, or other reasons, you should continue it.

Do not take any injections within 45 minutes before your hyperbaric treatment. Also avoid taking stool softeners and diuretics (water pills) right before your treatment.

We will review all the medicines you are taking. Hyperbaric treatments should not change the effect of most of your medicines. Please talk with us if you have any questions about taking your medicines.

What will I wear during my treatments?
Breathing 100% oxygen in the hyperbaric chamber results in an increased risk of fire. You must wear only hospital-provided clothing made of 100% cotton or a cotton/polyester blend to reduce static electricity and fire risk. We will give you a gown to change into before your treatment.

For the same safety reasons, no lighters, matches, body warmers, watches, hearing aids, reading, writing, or any battery-operated items are allowed. You will be able to watch TV.

Continued

X19817 (05/09) ©AHC *Wound Care/Hyperbaric Medicine*

Hyperbaric Oxygen Therapy and Treatment in the Monoplace Chamber, Page 2

What should I expect during treatment?

Treatments should be painless. Because of the air pressure changes in the chamber, your ears may have a sense of fullness when the treatment begins. If you feel any pain, please tell the hyperbaric attendant. We will review the steps for "ear clearing" before your treatment.

As with any medical treatment, there are complications that can be a part of hyperbaric treatment. The hyperbaric doctor will discuss these with you and get your consent to start treatments.

We will do dressing changes before or right after the treatment, based on your wound care needs. You will be given an assigned time for care as needed. The hyperbaric doctor will see you as needed, and we will keep the doctor up to date on your progress.

Visual changes can occasionally occur during hyperbaric treatments. Do not buy any new eyeglasses during hyperbaric treatment. In most cases your vision should return to pre-treatment status within 6 to 8 weeks after treatment has stopped.

Other needs

We will notify your primary care doctor when your hyperbaric treatments start.

If dressing changes are needed when the department is closed, we will arrange for home nursing care or instruct someone in your family. If other care arrangements are needed, we may contact our Social Services department.

If you need transportation to or from the hospital, please let us know. We can help arrange for transportation or move your treatment times if needed.

It is your responsibility to verify insurance coverage. We will help you in any way we can through our financial counselor.

The information presented is intended for general information and educational purposes. It is not intended to replace the advice of your health care provider. Contact your health care provider if you believe you have a health problem.
Aurora Health Care is a not-for-profit health care provider and a national leader in efforts to improve the quality of health care.

X19817 (05/09) ©AHC *Wound Care/Hyperbaric Medicine*

Care organization in Eastern Wisconsin has included in one of many patient educational handouts, specifically geared towards the monoplace hyperbaric medicine treatment sites. The subtopics include a description of the needed information at a level that most people can understand. Those subtopics are:

- What is hyperbaric oxygen therapy?
- Why hyperbaric treatments?
- How often will I have the treatment?
- Are there restrictions I should follow?
- Do not take any injections within 45 minutes before your hyperbaric treatment.
- What should I wear during my treatments?
- What should I expect during treatment?

Other Needs:

Follow with hours of operation, phone numbers, voice mail, or 24-hour service, if applicable.

http://www.aurorahealthcare.org/FYWB_pdfs/x19817.pdf

Printed with permission from Aurora Health Care, Milwaukee, WI

Websites and the internet

The worldwide internet, which provides resources for any topic you can think of, did not exist publicly before 1991. For example, input "hyperbaric medicine" in a search engine and you will receive over 448,000 hits from various internet sites. Pew Internet and American Life Project provides information about internet use in 2007; 71% of American adults accessed the internet and 80% of those users searched for healthcare-related information. How do you know you have a reputable internet site when the information you are searching for is potentially a matter of life or death? As medical providers, you can probably sift through the sites to find the ones that have acceptable content. What about our patients who are finding the internet the only way to find answers to their questions before they see their primary provider?

With today's financial insecurities, we are trying to have patients be more responsive to their own financial responsibilities- more choices than ever before. The approved indications received from insurance carriers for care is not a guarantee anymore. Patients also now search out clinical outcomes, patient satisfaction, and physician competency scores online as they decide who and where they prefer to take the medical care.

Barriers to integrating internet education include nurses not feeling comfortable with the computer, lack of training, inadequate time for learning, or lack of online access in the workplace (Lawrence, 2006). Administrative support is essential if nurses are to integrate the online sources into patient education.

Open a hospital-based website for education that is open for all medical areas. Involve the experts of the specialized areas and place protective back-ups to keep the information. Nurses cannot keep in touch with every sub-specialty. They need the experts in that field to design patient information for that specific medical diagnosis/procedure/treatment. Technology for hospital-designed computerized patient education can provide instant handouts that provide up-to-date information for all sites in the organization.

After you have hospital owned, internet web-based patient information handouts, consider proceeding to designing a website specific to your medical technology, hyperbaric medicine and/or wound care. Place all the information that you would share in the patient education handout. Add pictures of the clinic area and website links that your staff has agreed have quality, reputable information as your guide for the patients. Online sources may be used to help patients understand their disease, giving opportunities for asking more questions, and enhance patient confidence by quantifying the internet information with what they have been given by your medical providers.

The internet is a very powerful tool for patient education; however, it may be limited to more affluent populations or members with higher level of education. Patients with low income, less education, understand languages other than English, elderly, or disabled may have more difficulty using computers or getting into the internet (Chaka, et al. 2006). Keep in mind what patients can use and print information for these patients that cannot utilize the internet.

Conclusion

Nurses need to understand the importance of patient education and how to achieve it under the most difficult situations. It is important to recognize that a patient's outcome may be linked to the comprehension of the information that was given to them. No matter whether the nurses share information verbally, with written documents, or if they send their clients to the computer to search out the worst and the best of internet sites, patients are yearning and craving as much medical information as they can get, and it is our job to ensure it is accurate and helpful. Our medical facilities are being forced to move toward complete computerized documentation to maintain patient safety and clarity of documentation. It is time to put your best thoughts on paper and computerize it.

The accrediting agencies have dynamic websites to assist with patient safety and education information. These websites are available 24 hours a day, 7 days a week. It is highly recommended to check these sites frequently to ensure the quality of information that you are giving your patient is updated and current. Don't reinvent the wheel; utilize free information that is given by the government or qualified specialty medicine agencies.

Computer skills are paramount in providing patient information. Get additional classes for you and your staff to be more acquainted with how to work with computers and programs to design proper patient education. Utilize appropriate guidelines to ensure the writing is appropriate for the readers in general.

Lastly and above all, a caregiver's job is to make sure the patient understands: they comprehend what is happening to them so that they may be adherent to their medical plan of care. The hyperbaric community has many similarities that we can share with each other. Use the resources given in the chapter to search out assistance to ensure you maintain quality education for your patients.

Safe Internet Websites for Medical Information

American Nurses Association

The American Nurses Association (ANA) is the only full-service professional organization representing the interests of the nation's 3.1 million registered nurses through its constituent member nurses associations, its organizational affiliates, and its workforce advocacy affiliate, the Center for American Nurses. The ANA advances the nursing profession by fostering high standards of nursing practice, promoting the rights of nurses in the workplace, projecting a positive and realistic view of nursing, and by lobbying the Congress and regulatory agencies on health care issues affecting nurses and the public.

http://www.nursingworld.org/

Baromedical Nurses Association

The BNA provides nurses with a professional organization in order to maintain and promote the status and standards of practice in hyperbaric nursing.

http://www.hyperbaricnurses.org/

Centers for Medicare and Medicaid Centers

http://www.cms.gov/

Health Finder

Welcome to healthfinder.gov, a government Web site offering information and tools to help you and those you care about stay healthy. healthfinder.gov has resources on a wide range of health topics selected from over 1,600 government and non-profit organizations to bring you the best, most reliable health information on the Internet.

http://www.healthfinder.gov/

Medical Library Association

The Medical Library Association (MLA) is a nonprofit, educational organization with more than 4,000 health sciences information professional members and partners worldwide. MLA provides lifelong educational opportunities, supports a knowledge base of health information research, and works with a global network of partners to promote the importance of quality information for improved health to the healthcare community and the public.

http://www.mlanet.org/

Medline Plus

MedlinePlus will direct you to information to help answer health questions. MedlinePlus brings together authoritative information from NLM, the National Institutes of Health (NIH), and other government agencies and health-related organizations. Preformulated MEDLINE searches are included in MedlinePlus and give easy access to medical journal articles. MedlinePlus also has extensive information about drugs, an illustrated medical encyclopedia, interactive patient tutorials, and latest health news.

http://www.nlm.nih.gov/medlineplus/

National Board on Diving and Hyperbaric Medical Technology

The NBDHMT is a non-profit certifying organization designed to meet the clinical, technical, and safety needs of the discipline of undersea and hyperbaric medicine. Opportunities exist for certification as a Diver Medic (DMT), as a Hyperbaric Technologist (CHT), and as a Hyperbaric Nurse (CHRN).
http://www.nbdhmt.org/

National Institute of Health

The National Institutes of Health (NIH), a part of the U.S. Department of Health and Human Services, is the nation's medical research agency—making important medical discoveries that improve health and save lives.

http://www.nih.gov/index.html

NIH Senior Health

This easy-to-use website features basic health and wellness information for older adults from the National Institutes of Health.

http://nihseniorhealth.gov/index.html

Undersea and Hyperbaric Medical Society

The Undersea and Hyperbaric Medical Society (UHMS) is an international, non-profit organization serving over 2,400 members from more than 50 countries. The UHMS is the primary source of scientific information for diving and hyperbaric medicine physiology worldwide.

http://uhms.org/

Joint Commission Speak Up Initiatives

The Joint Commission's award-winning patient safety program

http://www.jointcommission.org/patientsafety/speakup/

References:

1. Abbott SA. (1998). The benefits of patient education. Gastroenterology Nursing, 21(5), 207-9.
2. Aldridge, MD. (2004). Writing and designing readable patient education materials. Nephrology Nursing Journal, 31(4), 373-7.
3. Anderson AS, and Klemm P. (2008). The Internet: friend or foe when providing patient education? Clinical Journal of Oncology Nursing, 12(1), 55-63.
4. Bingham J, Cha J, Magee JD, Puno F, Smith CE, Van Gorp M. (2002). Quality assurance processes for designing patient education web sites. CIN: Computers, Informatics, Nursing, 20(5), 191-200.
5. Bryant, RA, & Nix, DP. (2007). Acute & chronic wounds. St. Louis: Mosby Elsevier. 570-578.
6. Carroll A, and Dowling M. (2007). Discharge planning: communication, education and patient participation. British Journal of Nursing, 16(14), 882-6.
7. Czaja SJ, Charness N, Fisk AD, Hertzog C, Nair SN, Rogers WA, et al. (2006). Factors predicting the use of technology: Findings from the Center for Research and Education on Aging and Technology Enhancement (CREATE). Psychology and Aging, 21 (2), 333-352.
8. Comerford Freda M. (2004). Issues in patient education. Journal of Midwifery & Women's Health, Retrieved from www.jmwh.org doi: 10.1016
9. Freda MC. (2004). Issues in patient education. Journal of Midwifery & Women's Health, 49(3), 203-9.
10. Gerteis M, Edgman-Levitan S, Daley J, and Delbanco TL. (1993). Through the Patient's eyes. San Francisco: Jossey-Bass Inc.
11. Giordan A, Golay A, Jacquemet S. (1999). A new approach for patient education: beyond constructivism. Patient Education & Counseling, 38(1), 61-7.
12. Harrison MB, Logan J, Toman C. (2001). Clinical practice guidelines: necessary but not sufficient for evidence-based patient education and counseling. Patient Education & Counseling, 42(3), 279-87.
13. Health literacy competencies staff should have. (2010, March 1). Retrieved from http://find.galegroup.com/gtx/infomark.do?&contentSet=IAC-
14. Hyperbaric Oxygen Therapy and Treatment in the Monoplace Chamber. (2009, May). Retrieved from *http://www.aurorahealthcare.org/FYWB_pdfs/x19817.pdf*
15. Hubley J. (2006). Patient education in the developing world—a discipline comes of age. Patient Education & Counseling, 61(1), 161-4.
16. Keulers BJ, Welters CFM, Spauwen PHM and Houpt P. (2007). Can face-to-face patient education be replaced by computer-based patient education? A randomized trial. Patient Education and Counseling, 67(1-2), 176-182.
17. Knowles M. (1980). The modern practice of adult education. New York: Cambridge.
18. Leino-Kilpi H, Salantera S, Virtanen H. (2007). Empowering discourse in patient education. Patient Education & Counseling, 66(2), 140-6.
19. Lewis D. (2003). Computers in patient education. CIN: Computers, Informatics, Nursing, 21(2), 88-96.
20. Lin PC, Wang JL, Chang SY, Yang FM. (2005). Effectiveness of a discharge-planning pilot program for orthopaedic patients in Taiwan International. Int J Nurs Stud 42 (7): 723-31.
21. Monsivais D, Reynolds A, (2003). Developing and evaluating patient education materials. Journal of Continuing Education in Nursing, 34(4), 172-6.
22. Nonadherent patients may not understand. (2010, May 1). Retrieved from http://find.galegroup.com/gtx/infomark.do?&contentSet=IAC-
23. Opermann MH. (2003). Using health web sites for patient education. Journal of Wound, Ostomy, & Continence Nursing, 30(4), 217-23.

24. Pew Internet & American Life Project. (2007). Internet activities. Retrieved January 2, 2008, from http://www.pewinterent.org/trends/Internet_Activities_8.28.07.htm
25. Redman BK. (2008). When is patient education unethical? Nursing Ethics, 15(6), 813-20.26. Stromberg A, Dahlstrom U, and Fridlund B. (2005). Computer-based education for patients with chronic heart failure. A randomized, controlled, multicentre trial of the effects on knowledge, compliance and quality of life. Patient Education and Counseling, 64, 128-135.

Notes

CHAPTER

15

Staff Competencies and Training

Linda M. Miller, RN and Laura Josefsen, RN

Safety is the most important issue in the practice of hyperbaric medicine. Safety has to come first in your daily schedule for every patient every day, and for every treatment. Individual patient assessment is performed prior to every hyperbaric treatment, the equipment is checked on a regular schedule (daily, weekly, monthly, semiannually, and annually), safety posters and signs (restricted items, oxygen in use, and no smoking) are in place, and the emergency guidelines are posted by the hyperbaric chamber.

Comprehensive training and clinical competencies are essential to educate and validate the knowledge required to treat patients in the clinical setting. This will decrease the potential for adverse events for the patient, the family, and the staff. The method for evaluation of the staff member needs to be clear, objective and validated by a competent preceptor.

Hyperbaric specific training is essential for safe outcomes. The initial recommended training is to complete an approved Introductory Hyperbaric Course approved by the Education Committee of the Undersea and Hyperbaric Medicine Society (UHMS).

The Safety Director should attend a Safety Director course, since the Safety Director is directly responsible for the safety of the entire hyperbaric facility. It is recommended that the Safety Director become a part of the facility Safety Committee to enhance the awareness of the unique requirements in the hyperbaric unit. Safety and fire drills should be practiced on a regular basis, and it is a good idea to include the local Fire Marshall at least annually.

Monthly in-service training is highly recommended to not only educate the staff, but to maintain an awareness of safety. The hyperbaric facility should have a 12-month education plan for in-services to include specific safety issues.

Hyperbaric conferences, symposiums, and workshops are provided throughout the year and provide up to the minute information on what is new, a review of what has been done, and they are great for sharing ideas with colleagues. These are especially exciting because they bring together the physicians, nurses, and technicians to share information, and each group brings their specific contribution to the process of hyperbaric medicine.

A fun way to receive training is to become a surveyor on the UHMS Accreditation Team. In that venue, the physician, the nurse, and the technician are each given portions of the process to evaluate. It is a two-day process that is busy, fun, intense, challenging, and rewarding.

The Baromedical Nurses Association is a networking nursing organization to provide resources to the hyperbaric nurse (www.hyperbaric-nurses.org). The Baromedical Nurses Association Certification Board works in conjunction with the NBDHMT to provide a certification process for hyperbaric nurses. The National Board of Diving and Hyperbaric Technology at www.nbdhmt.org provides a 480-hour competency guideline in detail for the hyperbaric technician.[1] The nurses should, in our scope of practice, be familiar with these requirements.

To recognize the training that we work so hard to get, clinical competencies are the records to validate that we have met the recommended standards to provide optimum safe nursing care for our patients.

Clinical competencies are performed initially and at least annually. This may be in the form of a checklist as shown below. Typical components include a self-assessment scale, a development plan, and several methods of validation. There may also be a testing component to further evaluate the knowledge base.

The first part of this example includes general clinical knowledge, followed by a wound care module, then the hyperbaric module.

A suggested format will include

- Initial clinical competency assessment
- Facility practice
- Hire start date
- Assessment start date
- Projected end date

Directions for Assessment:

- The Validator may be the preceptor, clinical educator, advanced practice nurse, medical director or chief medical officer.

The Codes:

- **Self-Assesment Scale**

Competency reflects the ability to perform the procedure safely, correctly, effectively, and legally.

1 = I have no prior experience.
2 = I have observed only.
3 = I have performed before, but need more practice.
4 = I can perform without assistance.

- **Development Plan**

Minimum planned activity to facilitate competency achievement

LPV = Learn, Practice and Validate
PV = Practice and Validate
V = Validate only

- **Methods of Validation**

QI = QI Monitor/Chart Audit
D = Discussion
O = Observation of Daily Work
RD/S = Return Demonstration in Simulated Setting
RD/C = Return Demonstration in Clinical Setting
PT = Post Test
E = Exemplar

Competency Statement	Self Assessment Scale	Development Plan	Validation Method

GENERAL ORIENTATION

1. Completes wound program orientation with preceptor.
2. Recognizes and understands organizational and reporting structure.
3. Completes education program as directed by supervisor.
4. Completes facility-specific tours and introductions with preceptor.
5. Reviews, understands, and discusses job description and expectations with preceptor.
6. Reviews and signs acceptance of policies and procedures for practice setting.
8. Reviews and understands employee handbook.
9. Reviews and signs acceptance of ethics policy and compliance policies and procedures.

COMMUNICATION

1. Recognizes and understands reporting structure and communication responsibilities with supervisor and team members.

WOUNDCARE ORIENTATION

PHYSICAL ASSESSMENT

1. Demonstrates knowledge of anatomy of skin and integumentary system.
2. Demonstrates knowledge of physiology and phases of healing.
3. Demonstrates knowledge of pathophysiology, including bioburden and infection.
4. Demonstrates knowledge of diagnostic tests.
5. Demonstrates knowledge of assessment of skin and wound.
6. Demonstrates knowledge of wound types, including atypical wounds

7. Demonstrates knowledge of factors affecting healing.
8. Demonstrates knowledge of medical history and comorbidities.
9. Demonstrates knowledge of assessment of edema and managing edematous lower legs.
10. Demonstrates knowledge of lower extremity and vascular evaluation.
11. Demonstrates knowledge of bioburden and infection control.

PATIENT PREPARATION AND WOUND TREATMENT

1. Demonstrates knowledge of patient comfort and pain management.
2. Demonstrates knowledge of nutritional assessment and intervention.
3. Demonstrates knowledge of standard infection control practices, including hand hygiene.
4. Demonstrates knowledge of safety considerations.
5. Demonstrates knowledge of compression indications and contraindications.
6. Demonstrates knowledge of debridement indications and contraindications.
7. Demonstrates basic knowledge of dressings and wound bed preparation.
8. Demonstrates knowledge of topical agents.
9. Demonstrates knowledge of surgery, including grafting.
10. Demonstrates knowledge of pressure management, support surfaces and offloading.
11. Demonstrates knowledge of casting/splints.
12. Demonstrates knowledge of assistive devices.
13. Demonstrates knowledge of NPWT.
14. Demonstrates knowledge of skin substitutes.

PATIENT/CAREGIVER EDUCATION

1. Demonstrates knowledge of reinforcing purposes and patient participation and adherence.
2. Demonstrates knowledge of psychosocial and cultural issues.

DOCUMENTATION

1. Demonstrates understanding of documentation requirements.
2. Demonstrates documentation relevant to patient history, physical, review of symptoms, impression and plan that is accurate, thorough and timely.

REGULATORY ISSUES AND REIMBURSEMENT REQUIREMENTS

1. Demonstrates understanding of HIPAA requirements.
2. Demonstrates understanding of billing requirements.

MARKETING AND CLIENT RELATIONS

1. Demonstrates knowledge of building and maintaining collaborative relationships with all team members that are included in the care of the patient

COST-EFFECTIVENESS IN WOUND CARE

Demonstrates knowledge and practice of cost effectiveness in wound care, obtaining best result with least cost.Demonstrates knowledge of facility formularies, and restrictions and substitutions available.

HYPERBARIC COMPETENCIES ORIENTATION

1. Documentation of attendance at HBO Introductory Course.
2. Documentation of current licensure as applicable.
3. Review and understands the HBO Safety Manual.
4. Completes HBO facility tour.
5. Identifies location of emergency procedures guidelines.
6. Identifies location of personal protective equipment.
7. Identifies location of HBO log and maintenance books.
8. Lists items allowed/not allowed in HBO chamber.
9. Identifies location of restricted items posters.
10. Identifies location of no smoking/oxygen in use signs.
11. Identify location of HBO reference library.
12. Identifies location of operator breathing source/mask for each chamber.
13. Demonstrates how to access facility fire alarm system.
14. State policy on HBO physician and operator presence during HBO treatment.
15. State role and duties of the Safety Director.
16. State policy on gas handling.

17. State policy on gas storage.
18. State policy on storage of hazardous materials.
19. Demonstrate chamber compression and decompression.
20. State policy for housekeeping in HBO area.
21. Identify lighting requirements for HBO area to include overhead and emergency lighting.
22. Identify backup system for electrical failure.
23. Identify bulk oxygen storage tank and surrounding area.
24. State requirements for fire drills.
25. State requirements for ongoing safety education.
26. State smoking policy for chamber area and patients.
27. Identify patient education for HBO treatments.

COMMUNICATION

1. Understand physician notification of patient issues.
2. State reporting process for defective equipment.
3. State reporting process for HBO risk management.

PATIENT/CAREGIVER EDUCATION

1. Demonstrates knowledge of reinforcing purposes, patient participation, and adherence to plan of care.
2. Demonstrates knowledge of psychosocial and cultural issues.

DOCUMENTATION

1. Demonstrates understanding of documentation requirements.
2. Ensure HBO consent form signed
3. Know and demonstrate knowledge of all forms, electronic medical record, and paperwork used to document patient treatment.
4. Complete pre-treatment patient assessment and treatment protocol forms.
5. Complete ancillary patient chart notes and post treatment documentation.
6. Demonstrates working knowledge of HBO regulatory guidelines to include:
   - American Society of Mechanical Engineers (ASME)
   - Pressure Vessels for Human Occupancy (PVHO)
   - American National Standards Institute (ANSI)
   - Compressed Gas Association (CGA)
   - Code of Federal Regulations (CFR)
   - National Fire Protection Association (NFPA)
   - The Joint Commission (TJC)
   - Undersea and Hyperbaric Medicine Society (UHMS)
   - Food and Drug Administration (FDA)
7. Complete a record of a typical patient HBO treatment.
8. Demonstrate completion of daily, weekly, monthly, semiannual, and annual maintenance logs.
9. Demonstrate completion of daily patient treatment logs per chamber.

CHAMBER EQUIPMENT

1. Know and demonstrate knowledge of the routing of the compressed gas supply.
2. Demonstrate emergency shut-off procedures on chamber and at entrance to HBO room.
3. Demonstrate use of and the reason for adjusting the flow meter during HBO treatment.
4. Show location of exhaust valve on outside wall.
5. Demonstrate use of chamber communication system.
6. List factors that may influence operator/patient communications.
7. Be familiar with applicable forms of voice and visual communications.
8. Demonstrate inspection of valve seats, gaskets, hoses, and lubricants that are oxygen compatible.
9. Demonstrate acrylic inspection and documentation.
10. Identify stamp on HBO chamber per ANSI/ASME PVHO PVHO-1 standard.
11. Identify oxygen level gauge on wall.
12. Verify integrity of chamber ground wire.
13. Verify integrity of patient grounding strap.
14. Verify communication wires protected from physical damage and coming into contact with flammable materials.

GAS HANDLING

1. Contents of compressed gas cylinders are legibly marked on the exterior of cylinder.
2. High pressure gas cylinders are stored in assigned locations and accessible only to authorized personnel.

3. High pressure gas cylinders are not stored near flammable materials.
4. Large gas cylinders are stored in such a manner that they are restrained from being knocked over.
5. Large gas cylinders are transported by the use of a hand truck that provides a means of restraining the cylinder.
6. Protection valves are in place.
7. Pressure reducing regulators are used to reduce the pressure from the cylinder to the supply line.
8. PPE used when handling liquid oxygen cylinders.

Breathing Gas Supply

1. Know and demonstrate knowledge of the source of the breathing gas supply.
2. Demonstrate knowledge of how to use emergency operator mask.

Pressure Safety

1. Know and demonstrate knowledge of correct procedure for operating/securing door of chamber.
2. Know proper set-up and connection of all pass-throughs.
3. List the potential pressure hazards in and around the chamber.
4. Demonstrate operation of all pressure boundary doors.

Fire Extinguishing System

1. Know location of fire extinguishers.
2. Know location of fire alarms.
3. Demonstrate use of portable fire extinguisher.

Fire Safety

1. Demonstrate knowledge of possible ignition sources.
2. List items not allowed in hyperbaric chamber.
3. Demonstrate knowledge for a fire emergency:
   a. in the chamber
   b. in the immediate area of chamber
   c. in the hyperbaric room
   d. in the hallway
   e. in the facility

Chamber Standard Operating Procedures

1. Demonstrate inspection and understanding of chamber console panel layout.
2. Locate and operate automatic controls.
3. Locate and operate manual controls.
4. Demonstrate compression and decompression of chamber.

Checklists, Dive Tables, and Treatment Protocols

1. Demonstrate knowledge of chamber checklists.
2. Demonstrate knowledge of patient checklists.
3. Demonstrate knowledge of decompression tables.
4. Demonstrate knowledge of decompression protocols.
5. Demonstrate knowledge of decompression table computations.

Chamber Emergency Operating Procedures

1. Know console/panel layout as it pertains to emergency and override controls.
2. State reasons to use emergency decompression button.
3. State proper way to use emergency decompression button.

Patient Assessment

1. Know and demonstrate knowledge of current appropriate referral conditions for HBO treatment.
2. List expected benefits for approved conditions.
3. Demonstrate knowledge of treatment plan and know the duties of each staff member involved.
4. Observe an initial consultation.
5. Review patient's reason for referral.
6. Discuss understanding of rationale for treatment plan.
7. Determine patient adherence and cooperation.
8. Demonstrate knowledge of side-effects:
   a. Middle ear/tympanic membrane changes
   b. Blood glucose control
9. Ensure consent form signed prior to HBO treatments

Patient Preparation and Hyperbaric Treatments

(per Baromedical Nurses Association Recommended Standards of Care Guidelines [2])

1. Demonstrates knowledge of anxiety related to knowledge deficit of HBO therapy and treatment procedures.

2. Demonstrates knowledge of potential for injury related to transferring patients in/out of chamber, explosion of equipment, fire, and/or medical support treatment.
3. Demonstrates knowledge of potential for barotrauma to ears, sinuses, teeth, and lungs or cerebral gas embolism related to changes in atmosphere.
4. Demonstrates knowledge of potential for oxygen toxicity related to delivery of 100% oxygen at an increased atmospheric pressure.
5. Demonstrates knowledge of potential for inadequate therapeutic gas delivery related to delivery system and patient needs/limitations.
6. Demonstrates knowledge of anxiety and fear related to feelings of confinement anxiety associated with HBO chamber.
7. Demonstrates basic knowledge of pain related to associated medical problems.
8. Demonstrates knowledge of discomfort related to temperature and humidity changes inside hyperbaric chamber.
9. Demonstrates knowledge of potential for ineffective coping related to stresses of illness and/or poor psychosocial support systems.
10. Demonstrates knowledge of potential for dysrhythmia related to disease pathology.
11. Demonstrates knowledge of potential for fluid volume deficit related to dehydration and fluid shifts.
12. Demonstrates knowledge of altered cerebral tissue perfusion related to:
    - Carbon Monoxide Poisoning
    - Decompression Sickness
    - Acute Necrotizing Infection
    - Gas Embolism
    - Other
13. Demonstrates knowledge of potential for alteration in comfort, fluid, and electrolyte balance related to nausea and vomiting.
14. Demonstrates knowledge of altered health maintenance related to knowledge deficit for:
    - Management of chronic wounds
    - Restrictions following decompression illness
    - Symptoms to report after CO poisoning

Barotrauma Management

1. Know and demonstrate knowledge of the signs and symptoms of barotrauma.
2. Know and demonstrate knowledge of the immediate management of barotrauma.
3. Demonstrate instruction to clear ears (yawning, modified Valsalva, etc.).
4. Demonstrate instruction to patient to clear ears during compression and decompression.

Oxygen Toxicity Management

1. Know and demonstrate knowledge of the signs and symptoms of central nervous system intolerance to hyperbaric doses of oxygen.
2. Know and demonstrate knowledge of the signs and symptoms of pulmonary oxygen Toxicity.
3. Know and demonstrate knowledge of the various methods that serve to reduce the likelihood of immediate management of central nervous system toxicity.
4. List the complicating factors associated with the development of pulmonary oxygen Toxicity.

Hypoglycemic Management

1. Demonstrate obtaining patient blood glucose level.
2. Discuss blood glucose levels required prior to HBO.
3. Discuss how to increase blood glucose levels.
4. Discuss importance of blood glucose levels post HBO treatment.

Pulmonary Barotrauma

1. Know and demonstrate knowledge of risk factors for pulmonary barotraumas on ascent.
2. Know and demonstrate knowledge of immediate management of suspected pulmonary barotrauma on ascent.
3. State the differential diagnosis of:
    a. Cerebral arterial gas embolism
    b. Pneumothorax
    c. Tension pneumothorax
    d. Mediastinal emphysema
    e. Subcutaneous emphysema

Cardiopulmonary Complications

1. Proficiency in obtaining vital signs
2. Knowledge of common clinical signs of severe, acute onset, cardiovascular distress
3. Proficiency in basic CPR

Infection Control – HBO

1. Know and demonstrate knowledge of standard universal precautions.
2. Recognize patient and equipment risk factors for cross-contamination.
3. Demonstrate care and cleaning of HBO chamber.
4. State reasons for cleanliness in HBO area.
5. Inspection of acrylic after each HBO treatment for signs of drainage. If present, clean chamber prior to next treatment.
6. State when chambers are to be cleaned.

Wound Care

1. Appreciate the general principles of wound homeostasis, infection control and treatment and wound healing and non-surgical wound care.
2. Assist in the evaluation of wounds
3. Assist in the limited debridement of wounds, wound dressings and their respective applications.

Marketing and Client Relations

1. Demonstrates knowledge of building relationships with clients and partner facilities.
2. Scope of practice is stated in marketing materials.

Cost-Effectiveness in Hyperbaric Treatment

1. Demonstrates knowledge and practice of cost effectiveness in hyperbaric therapy, obtaining best result with least cost

Safety and quality are the responsibility of each clinical team member in the hyperbaric and wound care centers. Continual processes for ongoing training and competency assessments help to promote the focus of safety, quality care, and optimal outcomes.

References

1. NBDHMT Recommended Guidelines for Clinical Internship in HBO Technology Hyperbaric Technologists – Certification and Recertification Requirements – Resource Manual – Clinical Internship for Hyperbaric Technologists (page 5)
2. BNA Recommended Guidelines for Standard of Practice for the HBO Patient.[1](1988)
3. Undersea and Hyperbaric Medicine Society (UHMS) Accreditation program. http://www.uhms.org
4. Textbook of Hyperbaric Nursing 2002
5. The Competency Continuum: Expanding the Case Manager's Skill Sets and Capabilities, Professional Case Management: May/June 2008-Volume 13-Issue 3-p. 149-150. doi 10.1097/01.PCAMA.0000319967.68981.e9 CE Test

CHAPTER

16

Nursing Research and Evidence-Based Practice

JoAnn Mick, PhD, RN

To anticipate and achieve quality outcomes for patients requiring wound care, healthcare providers must acquire skills for accurate wound assessment, use available systems for wound staging, and demonstrate competencies for a broad range of wound care interventions related to cleansing, debridement, and dressing application. In addition, providers must have knowledge about the unique characteristics of wounds, understand normal wound healing physiologic processes, consider a broad range of variables affecting wound healing (i.e. age, medications, lifestyle), and anticipate any potential complications of wound care, such as wound contamination or drainage management. To add to the complexity of the role of wound management, challenges to remain current with ongoing research findings related to wound care treatments, such as fibrin glue, gene therapy, human skin equivalents, protease inhibitors, oxygen therapy, vacuum assisted therapy, and silver ion dressings provide unique opportunities for providers.[1]

Achieving wound care practice standardization and optimal outcomes has been a major focus of healthcare providers, government regulators, and third party payers for many years. As early as 1991, founders of the Wound Healing Society (WHS) set goals to develop standards and guidelines for wound assessment, care, and treatment. Definitions and standards for wound assessment and evaluation of wound healing were addressed in guidelines published by WHS in 1994.[2]

As the population continues to age, and constraints on healthcare payment mechanisms increase, it becomes increasingly important to prevent the incidence of wounds and to manage wound care by providing cost-effective, efficient interventions that yield high-quality outcomes. A key strategy for improving healthcare quality and patient outcomes, as well as increased professional role satisfaction, is to focus on using available scientific evidence when choosing treatment methods. Healthcare providers can implement best practice recommendations for products and interventions to prevent wound incidence, as well as to follow recommendations to promote wound healing and prevent further complications when wounds occur. Ongoing efforts to contribute to the body of scientific evidence related to wound care by sharing outcome measures that address wound prevention and support natural wound healing are high priorities in healthcare .[1]

EVIDENCE-BASED PRACTICE [EBP] DEFINITION

Sackett, et al. (2000) defined evidence-based practice (EBP) as the conscientious, explicit, and judicious use of current best evidence when making clinical practice and policy decisions. Melnyk and Fineout-Overholt (2005) defined EBP as a problem-solving approach to clinical practice that integrates a systematic search strategy and critical appraisal of the most relevant available evidence to answer a clinical question, while also considering one's own clinical expertise, and patient preferences and values. Therefore, EBP can be described as a problem-solving approach to care delivery that incorporates the best evidence from well-designed studies in combination with clinicians' expertise and patients' unique values, preferences, and circumstances within a context of providing care.[3] EBP promotes the collection, interpretation, and integration of valid evidence, including information that is patient-reported, observed by clinicians, and derived from research. The main aim of EBP is to obtain the best outcomes for patients by selecting interventions that have the greatest chance of success.[4]

EVIDENCE-BASED PRACTICE BELIEFS

An underlying assumption that nurses are professionally obliged to engage in continuing knowledge development and evaluation is implicit in the American Nurses Association Code of Ethics for Nurses.[5] Ongoing professional development includes knowledge and skills acquisition using scientific evidence and best practice recommendations to achieve optimal outcomes. Understanding the reasoning for implemented interventions, and holding values that healthcare outcomes can be improved by employing current evidence based practices, are essential for continuing quality improvement efforts. Melnyk (1994) and Melnyk, et al. (2001, 2006, 2007) tested and published an instrument, The EBP Beliefs Questionnaire, designed to measure clinicians' individual beliefs about the value of EBP and their beliefs/confidence in implementing EBP in practice. Beliefs in EBP were defined by the authors as an endorsement of the premise that EBP improves clinical outcomes and increases confidence in an individual's EBP knowledge/skills. Implementation of EBP was described as a healthcare provider engaging in relevant behaviors, including: seeking and appraising scientific evidence, sharing evidence or data with colleagues or patients, collecting and evaluating outcomes data, and using evidence to change practice.[6]

The EBP Beliefs questionnaire has 2 sections: the first section includes questions about beliefs, and the second section lists questions about use of EBP in practice. The questions are answered using Likert-scale responses from "strongly disagree" to "strongly agree." Examples of belief questions include: I believe that EBP results are the best clinical care for patients; I am sure that evidence based guidelines can improve clinical care; I am sure that implementing EBP will improve the care that I deliver to my patients; and I believe that critically appraising evidence is an important step in the EBP process.[7] Practice questions in the second section of the questionnaire ask clinicians to indicate the number of times during the past 8 weeks that they actually carried out steps of EBP using a Likert-scale range of responses from 0 to >8 times. Examples of practice questions include: Used evidence to change my clinical practice; Critically appraised evidence from a research study; Collected data on a patient problem; and Evaluated the outcomes of practice change.

Evidence from the Melnyk, et al. (2005) research supported the premise that when nurses have stronger beliefs about their ability to implement EBP, implementation of EBP is higher.

FIVE STEPS OF EBP

The evidence-based practice process is underpinned by 5 steps (question framing, database searching, critical appraisal, implementation, and evaluation), which are essential to ensure an evidence-based profession. These skills are considered the cornerstones of evidence-based practice, and when applied effectively, they support healthcare providers to enhance patient care and outcomes.[8] The steps of EBP involve identifying high-level research findings and implementing them in practice, to provide the highest quality and most cost-efficient healthcare care possible.

Best practices in patient care occur when providers continually ask questions about treatments and care, search for and evaluate the evidence to support or refute traditional practices, implement the best evidence, and evaluate the effectiveness of the evidence. Development of skills with asking appropriate clinical questions, searching scientific databases, critically appraising scientific literature, and implementation, evaluation, and dissemination of best practice recommendations are essential to ensure an evidence-based profession.[9]

STEP 1: ASK

IDENTIFYING CLINICAL PROBLEMS

Every day, healthcare providers are challenged with practice questions when deciding the best approach to take to achieve the highest quality outcome. Taking time to make notes as questions arise, such as "Why am I doing this?", "Is there a better way?", or "How can I get a better result?" is a first step to clinical problem identification. With additional thought and consideration, a clinical problem can be more clearly defined, then formatted and used to determine an appropriate methodology to pursue for improving practice and patient outcomes.[3]

DEVELOPING A PICO QUESTION

Healthcare providers are very efficient at problem solving or creating workarounds to practice barriers. One of the challenges of EBP is to overcome the tendency to fix problems without establishing a clear understanding of an issue and its scope and taking the time to search the literature for best practice recommendations that can lead to optimal outcomes. In EBP, Act is the 4th step in the process, so while everyone likes to skip the literature search, encouraging providers to follow the steps of EBP by beginning with development of a clear clinical question is critical to achieve the best possible outcomes. A tool that can help with clinical question development is PICO, a simple mnemonic device that supports inclusion of important elements of a question to help clearly define the question, and to assist in searching the available literature.[10] The components of PICO are:

P- Patient or population: The characteristics of a patient or population of interest.

I- Intervention or event: The prognostic factors, specific therapy, diagnostic tests, or assessments to be considered.

C- Comparison or reference group: Determining if current evidence supports that a proposed intervention is more or less effective than the current practice.

O- Outcome of interest: The criteria to measure effectiveness of a clinical outcome for the patient or population of interest.

To practice with PICO, begin by using the letters P, I, C, and O to create an outline and then brainstorm to identify each component for the topic of interest. As a novice, this step may initially be considered time consuming; however, question development is the most important step in EBP because it will support conduct of more efficient literature searches by retrieving fewer articles that are most associated with the clinical area of interest. After creating the draft of PICO components, a well-constructed clinical question can be easily developed. Next, identify key words or search terms in the PICO question to develop a database search strategy. Keywords use the standard vocabulary of MeSH (Medical Sub-Headings; www.nlm.nih.gov/mesh/meshhome) and the most appropriate electronic databases to locate available literature at the highest available level of evidence.[11] Using appropriate keywords reduces the likelihood of conducting a search that produces either no related material or an abundance of irrelevant information. As the search is conducted, a question can be refined or modified so that it remains focused on the area of interest and to ensure that relevant databases are searched to locate evidence in the literature. A well-developed clinical question will not only direct a literature search, but it will also lead to identification of the correct methodology to achieve the best answer.

CLINICAL QUESTION CATEGORIES

Clinical questions emerge from various sources and for a variety of reasons. Most often, questions are driven by practitioners' intellectual curiosity to assure best practices are being used and that optimal clinical outcomes can be achieved.[8] Examples of types of clinical questions include:

Therapy: Which treatment is most effective, or what is an effective treatment given a particular condition?

Harm/etiology: Are there harmful effects of a particular treatment, or how can harmful effects be avoided?

Prognosis: What is the patient's likely course of disease, or how to screen for or reduce risk?

Prevention: How can the patient's risk factors be adjusted to help reduce the risk of disease?

Experiences or values of patients and caregivers.

Education: Questions regarding best teaching strategies for colleagues, patients, or family members.

STEP 2: GATHER

SEARCHING THE LITERATURE

A primary barrier to EBP is a nurse's skill level with searching, retrieving, and critically appraising research articles. A well-planned literature search that is designed to be comprehensive will underpin the gathering process and enable prompt identification of relevant evidence and finding the most appropriate answers to the posed question. An effective search will support a provider to determine what has already been done and learned from prior studies, and also will assist to identify any gaps in the literature that might justify conducting a research study.[4]

Many libraries offer free classes to learn database searching. Online educational resources are also available. For example, the Evidence-Based Nursing-University of North Carolina, Chapel Hill webpage provides a site with tools and information about literature searches and helpful resources and includes tips for retrieving information (http://www.hsl.unc.edu/services/tutorials/ebn/index.htm). The McGill University Health Centre Research & Clinical Resources for Evidence Based Nursing also provides a webpage with tips on literature searching (http://muhc-ebn.mcgill.ca/). The webpage at http://www.nlm.nih.gov/bsd/pubmed_subsets/sysreviews_sources.html offers several databases for conducting searches and the Evidence-Based Filters for OVID CINAHL site (http://www.urmc.rochester.edu/hslt/miner/digital_library/tip_sheets/Cinahl_eb_filters.pdf) includes information about expert searches with strategies to filter out articles and locate the best evidence.

TYPES OF ARTICLES

When searching the literature, it is always important to search for the highest levels of evidence for clinical decision-making. An initial approach is to be aware of differences between research articles and review articles. Most research articles use the IMRaD-format. IMRaD is the acronym for Introduction, Methods, Results, and Discussion, which is followed by a conclusion and reference list, as the standard structure of a scientific paper.[12] A second step is to determine if the journal is a peer-reviewed journal, and if so, the type of peer review used, such as blinded, non-blinded, or multiple reviewers. Evidence that a journal is peer reviewed can increase confidence that studies have received prepublication review by topic experts. When critical appraisal of a manuscript is done by both editorial review and peer review, both processes can help to increase likelihood that bias and errors in design, methodology, and data analyses have been eliminated. Being aware of the sources of funding the authors received to conduct the study is also important because reputable journals require researchers to disclose funding and any conflicts of interest.[13]

SCIENTIFIC DATABASES

Accessing relevant, scientific, electronic databases is the most efficient way to conduct a literature search whenever seeking information that will be used for patient care and decision making. Examples of commonly used databases in healthcare include MEDLINE, CINAHL, Embase, Cochrane Library Embase, and PsychInfo. PubMed is a resource which provides free access to MEDLINE, the U.S. National Library of Medicine, and the National Institutes of Health database of citations and abstracts in the fields of medicine, nursing, dentistry, veterinary medicine, healthcare systems, and preclinical sciences.[14] PubMed provides a tutorial for efficient search options. The Cumulative Index to Nursing and Allied Health Literature (CINAHL) is a database that provides selected original and full text material for nursing and allied health literature from 1982 to the present.[15] Cochrane Reviews contain published reviews of healthcare interventions and evidence based clinical trials.[16]

SEARCH STRATEGIES

A primary objective in database searching is to use key search terms from the clinical PICO question to find results that yield information on target with the topic of interest. Using a variety of search engines and software to conduct and record a review of the literature helps to assure that relevant information is not overlooked.[10] Using "limits" such as year of publication, type of article, language, gender, and age can help to filter the amount of information retrieved. However, a clinician should never limit a search to "full-text articles only" because important study findings might be omitted if full text is not available in a particular database. Other search strategies include contacting known experts in the field, searching thesis and dissertation databases, and reviewing clinical trial registries, such as the National Institutes of Health CRISP database.[17] Whenever an author's name is identified in reference lists in multiple articles about a specific topic, consider contacting the author as a content expert. Reference lists can also be used to identify other articles for retrieval.

Clinical guidelines are often used to disseminate best practice recommendations. Free, public, online access to registered evidence based guidelines is available through the National Guideline Clearinghouse (NGC), which was established by the Agency for Healthcare Research and Quality (AHRQ) in partnership with the American Medical Association and America's Health Insurance Plans. The NGC site provides access to detailed information on guideline development and how to further the dissemination, implementation, and use of evidence based guidelines.

Using appropriate levels of evidence to answer a clinical question

Searching for the appropriate levels of evidence to address specific types of clinical questions (i.e., therapy, etiology, prevention, experience, etc.) will yield articles that can provide useful practice recommendations. For example, when addressing questions about therapy, it is important to search for randomized control trials (RCTs). For etiology questions, cohort studies will provide the most appropriate information. For questions involving diagnosis or diagnostic test(s), searching for RCTs or cohort studies is the best approach. For prevention topics, RCTs or prospective studies will provide the most relevant information. For questions about prognosis, cohort studies or case control studies are most appropriate; and when searching for meaning, qualitative studies will provide the best sources of information.

Step 3: Appraise

Critical appraisal involves careful assessment of the quality and credibility of the interpretation, rationale, design, methods, presentation, and application of published research findings. The critical appraisal process is essential whenever translating large quantities of research into clinically useful recommendations for practice. The primary purpose of critical appraisal in the EBP process is to determine the relevance of the scientific materials retrieved in relation to the searcher's PICO clinical question by evaluating the accuracy, completeness, and clarity of each article. One efficient way to appraise a scientific article is to use the components of IMRaD to review each section of the article independently.

Appraisal involves using critical thinking to identify if the retrieved evidence provides an answer to the PICO question. Also, critical appraisal assists with decision making related to any identified opportunities for the application of retrieved evidence and practice recommendations in a specific practice setting to make informed decisions about patient care. Developing strong critical appraisal skills enables providers to make judgments about the applicability and appropriateness of incorporating evidence in practice.[18]

Levels of Evidence

Levels of evidence provide an explicit way of ranking evidence by using a hierarchy scale to categorize the strength of the evidence being appraised. Levels of evidence are useful for making clinical practice recommendations.[3] There is no universal hierarchy or leveling system available. A variety of scales exist, however, a common factor of most levels of evidence is that systematic reviews and meta-analysis of randomized control trials are consistently considered the highest level of evidence, and expert opinion or tradition rank as the lowest level of evidence.

Findings in studies at higher levels of evidence are often more readily accepted in a scientific community because most hierarchies are based on the internal validity of the different research methods used. This level of evidence of a study reflects the degree to which the study design was susceptible to bias.[19] Hierarchy of evidence provides important information when evaluating effectiveness of interventions according to impartial standards.[63] Evidence-based clinical practice guidelines based on systematic reviews, meta-analyses, and randomized controlled trials, are considered Level I evidence. Level I evidence should be prioritized when searching for evidence to answer clinical questions about the effectiveness of an intervention.[20] One of the most important EBP practices is to adopt a "levels of evidence" scale and apply it consistently to rank evidence that will be used for decision-making.

Instruments for appraisal

AGREE

The Appraisal of Guidelines for Research & Evaluation (AGREE) instrument is a gold standard guideline appraisal tool that is user-friendly for evaluating clinical practice guidelines. AGREE was developed by an international collaboration in 2004 and has been officially recommended by both the Council of Europe and the World Health Organization (WHO).[21] AGREE has undergone reliability and validity testing and is a useful tool to evaluate guideline development methodologies.[22] The AGREE instrument is available online at http://www.agreecollaboration.org/instrument/.

CASP

Another user-friendly, gold standard tool used for appraisal of systematic reviews is the Critical Appraisal Skills Programme (CASP) available at http://www.phru.nhs.uk/Doc_Links/rct%20appraisal%20tool.pdf. The CASP tool consists of 10 questions designed to assist with critical

Table 1: *Summary Table for Research Critiques*

Use of summary table helps identify commonalities across several studies with regard to study findings and the types of patients to which study findings can be applied.

Citation *	Purpose & Research Questions	Research Design	Sample	Independent Variables & Measures	Dependent Variables & Measures	Statistical Test	Results	Level of Evidence	General Strengths	General Weaknesses	Summary Statements for Practice
Elliot, R., McKinley, S., Fox, V. (2008). Quality Improvement program to reduce the prevalence of pressure ulcers in an intensive care unit. American Journal of Critical Care, 17 (4), 328-333	To improve patients' outcomes by reducing the prevalence of pressure ulcers, identify areas for improvement in pressure ulcer prevention, and increase adoption of preventative strategies in an ICU.	Quazi-experimental	22 audits during a 6-month timeframe, n = 563	One-on-one clinical instruction about preventative strategies; use of study instrument; notification procedures; and skin assessment. Information shared re: audit results	Frequency of pressure ulcers by stage; prevalence; anatomical site; use of pressure-relieving devices. Instrument: Waterlow Pressure Ulcer Risk Assessment Scale: body weight; continence; skin condition; nutritional status; age; sex; mobility; surgery; tissue perfusion; neurological status.	Statistical analysis not performed. Frequencies, raw numbers and percentage rates.	The number of pressure ulcers of all stages, particularly stage 1, showed a downward trend. Prevalence decreased from 50% to 8%. Use of pressure relieving devises for high risk patients increased. Anatomical site remained constant.	III	Inclusion-exclusion criteria defined. Methods led to measurable, improved outcomes. Multi-faceted approach. Timely feedback provided.	Data only collected on weekdays. No information about instrument reliability. Prevalence data are a snapshot in time. Variability in skills of data collectors described.	Quality improvement is a highly effective formula for improving patients' outcomes that is easily implemented using clinical expertise and existing resources.

thinking about a study's validity, results, and implications.[23]

Using Evidence Summary Tables

Creating tables of the evidence identified in a literature search provides an opportunity to examine the entirety of the evidence by arranging it in a format for easy review. As all the evidence is organized into a summary table, the overall quality and applicability of the evidence retrieved can be easily assessed while reviewing the quality and quantity of studies, the consistency of study results, and any identified gaps in the literature.[24]

Patterns of evidence in the literature

Identifying the pattern of information in the literature assists with identification of next steps to be taken by the healthcare provider. Patterns include finding similar results in all published studies, finding a variety of results (positive, negative, inconclusive) or identifying a gap, or lack of information, about the topic of interest.[25]

Step 4: Act

Current practice vs. Evidence Based Practice

An EBP project involves identification of current best practice recommendations and using them to confirm that current practices in a clinical setting are at best practice standards or that a practice change project needs to be implemented. The EBP process can be used for policy and procedure review and to identify studies that can be replicated in the practice setting. Step 4 of the EBP process, Act, involves confirming that current practices include all of the current best practice recommendations. Whenever a deficiency is identified, an action plan incorporating all current recommendations is developed and then implemented in the practice setting. The action plan will include processes for data collection before and after the change is implemented to measure that outcomes are achieved and to assure that all improvements are sustained.

RASCI Model

The RASCI model can be used to provide a responsibility assignment methodology to identify roles and responsibilities during project implementation and/or change management. The RASCI model allows assignment after identifying the persons:

Responsible: The owner of the problem/project.

Accountable: The person to whom "R" is Accountable and is the approval authority for a work plan before it becomes effective

Supportive: The person who will provide resources or play a supporting role in project implementation.

Consulted: The person who will provide information and/or expertise necessary to complete the project.

Informed: The person who needs to be notified of results, but not necessarily be consulted during the project implementation.[26]

Step 5: Evaluate

Evaluation of outcomes involves achieved adherence to processes, as well as the attainment of any planned clinical, fiscal, administrative goals or aims. Evaluation methods can vary, as they are dependent on the specific intervention or change in practice that was implemented. Examples of types of evaluation include: measurement of physiological and psychological measures; functional improvement; decreased costs; decreased length of stay; job retention or satisfaction; and patient satisfaction to determine if aims for improved practice, care, and outcomes are achieved.[8]

EBP Resources

A sampling of available online resources for EBP includes:

1. Netting the Evidence: A ScHARR Introduction to Evidence-Based Practice on the Internet, available at http://ebmh.bmj.com/content/3/2/39.full.html
2. The Joanna Briggs Institute, available at http://www.joannabriggs.edu.au/about/home.php
3. The Academic Center for Evidence Based Nursing (ACE) available at http://acestar.uthscsa.edu/Learn.htm
4. The Evidence-Based Medicine Resource Center available at http://www.nyam.org/fellows/ebhc/index.html
5. The Oncology Nursing Society Evidence-Based Practice Resource Area available at http://onsopcontent.ons.org/toolkits/evidence/index.shtml

EBP Practice Models

A variety of evidence based practice models have been developed to help clinicians translate evidence into practice. A model can support an organized approach to evidence based practice and can maximize time and resources by focusing on key EBP activities. An article by Gawlinski and Rutledge (2008) provides a systematic process that can be used to select a model that best meets the specific needs of a practice setting. Tables assist the reader to evaluate how quickly concepts and steps of each model can be assimilated into a practice setting.

The basic premise of most EBP models is to incorporate four components: scientific evidence, clinical practice expertise, consideration of the situation or environment, and the patients' values and expectations. Barriers to achieving best outcomes occur whenever patient care is driven by only a single component of a model. For example, using only the clinical expertise component of a model may result in care that is provided based on "the way things are always done" within a practice setting or "the way a physician or other provider wants things done." To achieve optimal outcomes, all four components must always be taken into consideration.

Barriers to EBP

Barriers to EBP are wide ranging and include time, lack of EBP mentors, negative attitudes toward research, inadequate resources at the point of care, competing priorities, perceived lack of time to implement best practice recommendations, difficulty reading and understanding research reports, and inadequate critical appraisal or other EBP skills, among others.[27,3,6] In addition, lack of administrative support and lack of resources have been identified as barriers that deter the implementation of evidence based care.[28] It is important to proactively consider and address barriers, such as meeting location, clinician interest and knowledge levels, and the support of managers to sponsor their employees' involvement in EBP projects.

When to conduct QI/PI Projects

Quality Improvement or Performance Improvement should be used when addressing concerns related to internal systems and processes. Usually there are established policies, guidelines, or procedures that should result in a good outcome, but the outcome is not being achieved because of a process or systems issue. A quality improvement project explores the process, and identifies and corrects the system so good outcomes can be consistently sustained. A variety of models and tools are available for quality improvement initiatives.

Quality Improvement/ Process Improvement

A variety of models and tools are available for quality improvement initiatives.

PDCA

The plan-do-check-act (PDCA) cycle is a four-step model to implement change and achieve quality outcomes. The PDCA cycle should be repeated again and again to sustain continuous quality improvement. PDCA can be used when initiating a new improvement project; when developing and implementing an improved process, product or service design; when planning data collection and analysis to verify and prioritize problems or root causes; or when implementing a change project. The steps of PDCA are:

Plan: Recognize an opportunity and plan a ch ange.

Do: Test the change by conducting a small-scale study with data collection.

Check/Study: Review the data, analyze the results, and identify what has been learned by implementing the change.

Act: Take action based on information learned in the study step: If the change did not work, the cycle is repeated with a different plan. If the change was successful,

PDCA is completed on a broader scale with periodic measurements to assure improvements are sustained.[29]

Cause and Effect Diagrams

A Cause-and-Effect Diagram is a tool that helps identify, sort, and display possible causes or characteristics of a specific problem. The diagram is useful to illustrate relationships between a given outcome and all of the factors that can influence the outcome. Constructing a Cause-and-Effect Diagram identifies the possible root causes of a specific concern by sorting and relating interactions among the factors affecting the specific process. The diagram assists with problem analysis so that corrective actions can be taken.[30]

Pareto Charts

A Pareto chart contains both bars and a line graph displaying values in descending order (bars) and the cumulative totals of each category, left to right (line graph). The purpose of a Pareto chart is to identify the most frequent, important factors in a data set.[30]

PROCESS FLOW CHARTS OR MAPS

A flowchart is a diagram that presents process steps as boxes and connects those boxes with directional arrows to identify the process flow. Flowcharts are useful for analyzing, designing, documenting, or managing processes or programs.[30]

RUN CHARTS OR CONTROL CHARTS

Control charts are graphs useful to evaluate how a process changes over time. Using historical data, values are plotted in time order using a central line for the average, an upper line for the upper control limit, and a lower line for the lower control limit. By comparing current data to these lines, conclusions can be drawn about whether a process variation is consistent (in control) or unpredictable (out of control, affected by special causes of variation).[29]

SCATTER CHARTS OR DIAGRAMS

Scatter charts graph pairs of numerical data, one variable on each axis, to look for a relationship. When variables are correlated, the charted values will fall along a line or curve. Points closest to the line reveal the greatest correlation.[29]

SIPOC

SIPOC is a Six Sigma tool acronym for Suppliers, Inputs, Process, Outputs, and Customers. A SIPOC diagram helps to identify process outputs and the customers of each output, so that the input of each customer can be considered when designing a project. During a process, (S) suppliers provide (I) input to the (P) process resulting in (O) output that meets or exceeds (C) customer expectations.[43]

HISTOGRAM

A histogram is a commonly used graph for showing frequency distributions, or how often each different value in a set of data occurs. A common frequency pattern is the bell-shaped curve, or normal distribution. In a normal frequency distribution, values are as likely to occur on one side of the average as on the other. Histograms assist with identification of skewed distributions when a limiting factor prevents a normal outcome pattern on one side of the values distribution.[29]

RESEARCH

There are three basic methods of research: survey, observation, and experiment. Scientific research is a systematic process of building on prior studies and extending findings to gaining valuable new insight. The research process follows organized and sequential steps to collect data to support hypotheses, answer clinical questions, or determine or test outcomes.[31]

STUDY DESIGN

The types of questions to be answered and the best methods for answering those questions will determine the appropriate study design. It is very important to choose the right data collection methodology so data are collected to meet the aims and objectives of conducted research. When a study design is inappropriate, information from data collection will be useless, regardless of data analysis.[32] Methodological designs should reflect diversity and incorporate appropriate scientific, social, and behavioral science approaches. The methods section of a protocol should describe all stages of planning, including the study composition, execution strategies, and the statistical methods that will be used for data analysis. Research is conducted only after obtaining approval of an ethics committee. Study design information should provide enough detail for a reader to be able to comprehend the research plan and procedures for replicating the study in a designated setting.

SAMPLE

Usually a population is too large for a researcher to attempt to collect data on all of its members. Therefore, a sample is used to represent a population by carefully selecting participants with characteristics of the population from which they are selected. The two types of sampling methods are probability sampling, where each member of a population has a known probability of being selected, or non-probability sampling, where members are selected from the population in a nonrandom manner. The sample section of a protocol should provide the inclusion and exclusion criteria and any additional relevant information about the subjects to be selected and recruited for study participation. A justification statement regarding how the sample size was determined should also be included in the protocol.

INSTRUMENTS

It is important to select valid, reliable instruments when conducting research. Whenever conducting a literature review, make notes of possible instruments and their documented reliability measurements. Instruments with a reliability score greater than .70 are considered reliable. Whenever possible, use an existing, tested, reliable instrument rather than designing a new study instrument. When a new instrument is developed, it will require instrument testing prior to using it for data collection in a study. Instrument testing requires IRB approval and can be a lengthy process. If a valid, reliable instrument is available in the literature, it can save time and effort when pursuing improved outcomes for patients.

Validity

Validity refers to the accuracy or truthfulness of a measurement. More specifically, it answers the question: Does the measurement instrument accurately measure exactly what it is supposed to measure?

Reliability

Instruments with measurements that yield consistent results over time are considered to be reliable for data collection. Whenever a measurement is prone to random error, it will lack reliability. The reliability of an instrument places an upper limit on its validity; therefore, a measurement that lacks reliability will also be invalid.[33] Three basic methods to test reliability are test-retest, equivalent form, and internal consistency.

Data Collection Considerations

Data collection techniques support a systematic collection of information about the objects or subjects in a study and the settings in which they occur. When multiple data collectors are involved, consistency of data collection becomes an important concern. A variety of data collection techniques can be employed, including using available information; making observations; conducting interviews, surveys, or focus group discussions; and mapping or scaling. Bias in data collection can create a distortion in the collected data so that it does not represent reality. It is important to implement measures to eliminate potential bias during data collection. Another important factor of data collection is the need to consider whether a research procedure is likely to cause any physical or emotional harm. Harm may be caused in a variety of ways, including violation of a study participant's right to privacy; posing sensitive questions or gaining access to records which may contain personal data; by observing the behavior of participants without their knowledge (concealment); allowing public access to personal information without consent of a participant; and failing to observe or respect any cultural values, traditions or taboos valued by participants.[34]

Data Analysis

A detailed statistical plan should be provided for data analysis, including justification of the appropriateness of each employed test.[13] Data are prepared for analysis by entering data in a computer program or spreadsheet; evaluating data entry for accuracy; transforming the data as required; and developing and documenting a database structure to integrate the various measurements. Descriptive statistics are often used to describe the basic features of study data with summary statements about the sample and the measures. Inferential statistics are used to investigate answers to research questions, models, or hypotheses by making inferences about a population based on the sample data.[55]

Strengths and Weaknesses

Study limitations

Sources of bias can affect study results and even in the best studies, errors cannot be completely excluded. Bias and errors create limitations to the usefulness of study findings. Unexpected high rates of loss to follow-up or study withdrawal may occur during a study or intentional or unintentional, inequitable selection of a study sample may result in misrepresentation of results for the intended population of interest. Possible distortion of the study results resulting from missing values during data collection should also be disclosed. Critical analysis of a study's limitations is important for decision-making and for guiding the direction of future research efforts.[36]

Generalizability

Generalizability refers to the extension of research findings and study conclusions conducted on a sample population to a population at large. Generalizability establishes flexibility for results of a study conducted in a single setting to be similar when the same study is conducted in a new setting. For a result to be considered generalizable outside of a test group, it must produce the same results with different forms of measurement. For maximum ability to generalize study results to a larger population, researchers should ensure that a study sample is relatively large and randomly selected.[37]

Navigating the IRB

Federal regulations pertaining to the Institutional Review Board (IRB) are specified in Title 45 of the Code of Federal Regulations Part 46

(45 CFR 46) and Title 21 Code of Federal Regulations Parts 50 and 56 (21 CFR 50 and 56). When preparing a protocol for IRB submission, it is important to maintain awareness that these federal regulations guide all IRB activities. Ethical foundations for the CFR are contained in The Belmont Report: Ethical Principles and Guidelines for the Protection of Human Subjects of Research (Office for Protection from Research Risks, OPRR, 1979). IRB members will consider a variety of issues when reviewing a protocol, including participant safety, protection of vulnerable subjects, equitable participant selection, freedom from any coercion to participate, and the potential benefits and risks of research. Potential research benefits can include the improvement of physical and mental health, and knowledge that contributes to the welfare of society (OPRR, 1993). Risks can include any physical, psychological, social, or economic harm, the invasion of privacy, and any violation of basic human rights (OPRR, 1979). Writing a protocol with human subjects' protection in mind will assist with meeting the IRB reviewer's expectations. Novice researchers should always seek mentorship of an experienced researcher and pursue educational opportunities to increase research knowledge. Attending an IRB meeting, requesting a copy of an IRB Reviewer's Checklist, and completing a Human Subject's Protection Course are also helpful for learning to navigate the IRB process.

Dissemination of study or EBP project findings

Translation of research findings into sustainable improvements in clinical practice and patient care outcomes remains a substantial obstacle to improving the quality of care. It often takes almost two decades for incorporation of original research findings into clinical practice. The Dissemination Planning Tool was designed with funding provided by the Agency for Health Care Research & Quality (AHRQ) to help researchers create a dissemination plan for research findings that extend beyond traditional methods of peer-reviewed publications and conference presentations. When research efforts yield findings and/or tools that warrant distribution to other researchers or clinicians to improve outcomes, Translating Research Into Practice (TRIP) can be a useful guide for selecting dissemination strategies.[38] Dissemination strategies include hosting or attending seminars or community forums to discuss the research, asking professional agencies to feature the research findings in newsletters and websites, submitting reports to the funding agency, submitting articles to local media sources, distributing flyers, brochures and posters in health centers, clinics, agencies, and neighborhoods, and participation in local healthcare events.

Podium or Poster Presentations

Seminars or conference presentations, abstracts, and posters are traditional methods of information dissemination. The difference between poster and oral presentations is that a poster presents written information in a static, visual medium instead of the verbal information provided by a presenter. Oral and poster communications are often preliminary presentations that provide an author with opportunities to receive feedback on their work before full publication in a peer reviewed journal.[39]

Journal articles

Publication in a peer-reviewed journal remains the most important way of disseminating a complete set of research results. Once results are published, they are available for other researchers to extend knowledge.[39]

Authorship

Authorship should be discussed when initially planning a project's timeline. Decisions can be revisited as the project progresses. It will be important to comply with a journal's established authorship criteria and all scientific publication ethical responsibilities. All authors identified in a manuscript must agree to publication of the material and copyright transfer. All individuals who meet criteria for authorship should be listed as authors on the article when submitting for publication. Individuals who do not meet criteria for authorship should not be included as authors, but may be listed in an acknowledgement statement in the manuscript. Each author listed on a manuscript is individually responsible for the accuracy of all the information and data in the manuscript.[64]

Scientific Publication Ethics

All research must have approval by an Institutional Review Board (IRB) or Ethics Committee, and any studies that appear to involve an element of misconduct must be investigated. Because of the grave concerns about scientific misconduct, the Office of Research Integrity (ORI) was established in 1992 with authority to investigate all allegations of misconduct.[40,35] To avoid concerns about scientific misconduct, clinicians should become familiar with organizational and publication policies that address types of scientific misconduct, such as plagiarism and fabrication or falsification of data. An author's institution may be contacted when they are suspected of scientific misconduct. The original raw data that was collected during a study may be requested for review by ORI when suspicious findings are investigated. A researcher and the researcher's organization may become ineligible for future research funding when scientific misconduct is discovered.

Common ethical issues related to writing and publishing include: authorship, duplicate publications, and failure to disclose any conflicts of interest.[41] To avoid scientific misconduct, researchers should always disclose all information sources and references cited in manuscripts, be sure to acquire the appropriate permission before using information, only submit credible research results for publication, never omit or alter data that did not agree with the original hypothesis, and never commit fraud by submitting the work of other persons.[40]

Journal Clubs

A journal club is a group of individuals who meet regularly to critically evaluate scientific articles. Journal clubs are usually organized around an identified practice topic with a general purpose to facilitate review of research studies and generate discussions about the implications of study findings for clinical practice. Advantages of journal club participation include remaining knowledgeable of current best practice recommendations; increased awareness of current nursing research findings; learning to critique and appraise research articles; becoming familiar with the best current clinical research; and encouraging research utilization. Key factors to promote a successful journal club include selecting relevant topics of interest and encouraging regular attendance and participation. Having a designated session leader to start and facilitate each article discussion can help to ensure that the journal club meetings are productive. Also, scheduling the journal club at a time and location that is convenient for attendance is important. The value of a journal club is that it can promote a better understanding of the research process and improve participants' ability to critically appraise research articles.[42, 57]

Conclusion

Information provided in this chapter may support efforts of wound care practitioners to contribute to the body of scientific evidence related to their specialty. By utilizing the identified steps and strategies to appropriately conduct evidence based practice projects, quality improvement projects, and/or research studies, improvements in cost effective, wound care practices can be identified and optimal patient outcomes can be achieved.

REFERENCES

1. Harvey, C., (2005). Wound healing. Orthopaedic Nursing, Mar-Apr; 24 (2): 143-59.
2. Franz, MG., Robson, MC., Steed, DL., Barbul, A., Brem, H., Cooper, DM., Leaper, D., Milner, SM., Payne, WG., Wachtel, TL., & Wiersema-Bryant, L. (2008). Guidelines to aid healing of acute wounds by decreasing impediments of healing. Wound Repair & Regeneration. Nov-Dec; 16 (6): 723-48.
3. Melnyk, B.M., & Fineout-Overholt, E. (2005). Evidence-based practice in nursing and health care: A guide to best practice.Philadelphia: Lippincott Williams & Wilkins.
4. Craig, J. V., & Smyth, R. L. (2007). The evidence-based practice manual for nurses (2nd ed.). Edinburgh: Churchill Livingston Elsevier.
5. American Nurses Association, (2001). Code of Ethics for Nurses. Retrieved from http://www.nursingworld.org/codeofethics on April 25, 2010.
6. Melnyk, BM., Fineout-Overholt, E., & Mays MZ, (2008). Worldviews on Evidence-Based Nursing. Dec; 5 (4): 208-16.
7. Melnyk, BM. (2007). The evidence-based practice mentor. A promising strategy for implementing and sustaining EBP in healthcare systems. Worldviews on Evidence-Based Nursing, 4(3), 123–125.
8. Cleary-Holdforth, J. & Leufer, T., (2008). Essential elements in developing evidence-based practice. Nursing Standard, Sep 17-23; 23 (2): 42-6.
9. Hockenberry, M., Brown, T., Walden, M. & Barrera. P., (2009). Teaching evidence-based practice skills in a hospital. Journal of Continuing Education in Nursing, Jan; 40 (1): 28-32.
10. Van Cott, A. & Smith, MC., (2009). Nursing research: Tips and tools to simplify the process. Dermatology Nursing, May-Jun; 21 (3): 138-40.
11. Fineout-Overholt, E., Hofstetter, S., Shell, L., Johnston, L. (2005), "Teaching EBP: getting to the gold: how to search for the best evidence", Worldviews on Evidence-based Nursing, Vol. 24, 207-11.
12. Sollaci, LB. & Pereira, MG. (2004). The introduction, methods, results, and discussion (IMRAD) structure: a fifty-year survey. J Med Libr Assoc. July; 92(3): 364–371.
13. Foote, MA. (2007). How to critically review and appraise published clinical literature. Research Practitioner. Retrieved from http://www.accessmylibrary.com/article-1G1-168285600/critically-review-and-appraise.html on April 25, 2010.
14. United States National Library of Medicine and The National Institutes of Health, (2002). PubMed. Retrieved at http://www.ncbi.nlm.nih.gov/sites/entrez?db=pubmed on April 25, 2010.
15. CINAHL Information Systems, (2007). Retrieved at http://www.cinahl.com/library/library.htm on April 25, 2010.
16. The Cochrane Collaboration, (2008). Retrieved at http://www.cochrane.org/ on April 25, 2010.
17. Averis, A. & Pearson, A. (2003). Filling the gaps. Identifying Nursing Research Priorities Through the Analysis of Completed Systematic Reviews." JBI Reports, 1(3):49-126
18. Booth, A. (2006). Critical appraisal of the evidence. In Gerrish, K., Lacey, A. (Eds.) The Research Process in Nursing. Fifth edition. Blackwell Publishing, Oxford, 107-122.
19. Evans D. & Pearson A. (2001). Systematic reviews: gatekeepers of nursing knowledge. J Clin Nurs. 10: 593-9.
20. Atkins, D., Fink, K., & Slutsky, J. (2005). Better information for better health care: The Evidence-Based Practice Center program and the Agency for Healthcare Research and Quality. Annals of Internal Medicine, 142, 1035-1041.
21. Hanson, D., Hoss, BL., & Wesorick, B. (2008). Evaluating the evidence: Guidelines. AORN Journal, Aug; 88 (2): 184, 186, 188-96.
22. Hulshuf, C. & Hoenen, L. (2007). Evidence-based practice guidelines in OHS: Are they agreeable? Irni Healih, 45(l):26-3l.

23. Critical Appraisal Skills Programme, (2007). Retrieved at http://www.phru.nhs.uk/Doc_Links/rct%20appraisal%20tool.pdf on April 25, 2010.
24. Washington State Healthcare Authority, (2010). Evidence Based Review Process. Retrieved at http://www.rx.wa.gov/evidenceprocess.html on April 25,2010.
25. Chapel Hill, (2007). Literature review. Retrieved at http://www.unc.edu/depts/wcweb/handouts/literature_review.html on April 25, 2010.
26. Value Based Management (2010). RASCI Model. Retrieved at http://www.valuebasedmanagement.net/methods_raci.html on April 25, 2010.
27. Hutchinson, AM. & Johnston, L. (2006). Beyond the barriers scale: Commonly reported barriers to research use. Journal of Nursing Administration, 36(4), 189–199.
28. Cooke L. & Grant M. (2002). Support for evidence-based practice. Seminars in Oncology Nursing, 18(1), 71–78.
29. American Society for Quality, (2004). Quality tools. Retrieved at http://www.asq.org/learn-about-quality/project-planning-tools/overview/pdca- cycle.html on April 25, 2010.
30. Handbook for Basic Process Improvement, (2007). Retrieved at http://www.balancedscorecard.org/Portals/0/PDF/c-ediag.pdf on April 25, 2010.
31. LoBiondo-Wood, G., and Haber, J. (2007). Nursing Research : Methods and Critical Appraisal for Evidence-based Practice. 7th ed. St. Louis, Mo.: Mosby/Elsevier.
32. Altman, DG. (1991). Practical statistics for medical research. London: Chapman and Hall.
33. Spector, P. (1981) Research Design. Beverly Hills: Sage.The Academic Center for Evidence Based Nursing (ACE) (2010). Retrieved at http://acestar.uthscsa.edu/Learn.htm on April 25, 2010.
34. International Development Research Centre, (2009). Overview of data collection techniques. Retrieved at http://www.idrc.ca/en/ev-56606-201-1-DO_TOPIC.html on April 25, 2010.
35. Office of Research Integrity, (2010). RCR Points for Disussion. Retrieved at http://ori.hhs.gov/education/point_all.shtml#research_integrity on April 25, 2010.
36. Du Prel, JB., Rohrig, B., & Blettner, M. (2009). Critical appraisal of scientific articles: part 1 of a series on evaluation of scientific publications. Dtsch Arztebl Int. Feb;106(7):100-5.
37. Colorado State University, (2010). Generalizability: Considerations. Retrieved at http://writing.colostate.edu/guides/research/gentrans/com2b2.cfm on April 25, 2010.
38. Carpenter, D., Nieva, V. Albaghal, T. & Sorra, J. (2005). Development of a Planning Tool to Guide Research Dissemination. Published in Advances in Patient Safety: From Research to Implementation. Volumes 1-4, AHRQ Publication Nos. 050021 1-4. Agency for Healthcare Research and Quality, Rockville, MD.
39. The National Academies Press, (2009). On being a Scientist: A guide to responsible conduct in research. 3rd edition. Retrieved at http://www.nap.edu/openbook.php?record_id=12192&page=30 on April 25, 2010.
40. King, CR. (2009). Issues and best practices related to ethical writing and publishing. Journal of the Association for Vascular Access, Spring; 14 (1): 40-5.
41. King, CR., McGuire, DB., Longman, AJ., & Carroll-Johnson, RM. (1997). Peer review, authorship, ethics, and conflict of interest. Image: Journal of Nursing Scholarship, 29, 163-167.
42. Esisi, M. (2007). "Journal clubs." BMJ Careers. 13 Oct 2007. Web. Retrieved at http://careers.bmj.com/careers/advice/view-article.html?id=2631#ref2 on April 25, 2010.
43. Business Knowledge Source, (2009). SIPOC. Retrieved at http://www.businessknowledgesource.com/manufacturing/what_is_a_sipoc_diagram_high_level_process_map_and_how_is_it_used_in_six_sigma_021699.html on April 25, 2010.
44. Edward G. Miner Library at the University of Rochester Medical Center. Evidence-based Filters for Ovid CINAHL. Retrieved from http://www.urmc.rochester.edu/hslt/miner/digital_library/tip_sheets/Cinahl_eb_filters.pdf on April 25, 2010.
45. Fineout-Overholt, E., Johnston, L. (2005), "Teaching EBP: asking searchable, answerable clinical questions", Worldviews on Evidence-based Nursing, Vol. 24, 157-60.

46. Fineout-Overholt, E., Melnyk, BM. & Schultz, A. (2005).Transforming health care from the inside out: Advancing evidence-based practice in the 21st century. Journal of Professional Nursing, 21(6), 335–344.
47. Gawlinski, A. & Rutledge, D. (2008). Selecting a Model for Evidence-Based Practice Changes: A Practical Approach AACN Advanced Critical Care, July/September,19(3), 291-300.
48. Lipman, T. (2000). Netting the Evidence: A ScHARR Introduction to Evidence-Based Practice on the Internet. Evidence Based Mental Health, 3:39.
49. McGill University Health Centre, (2006). Research & Clinical Resources for Evidence based Nursing. Retrieved from http://muhc-ebn.mcgill.ca/ on April 25, 2010.
50. Melnyk, B..& Fineout-Overholt, E. (2002). Putting research into practice. Reflections on Nursing Leadership, 28, 22–25.
51. Melnyk, BM., Fineout-Overholt, E., Feinstein, N., Li, H., Small, L., Wilcox, L. & Kraus, R. (2004b). Nurses' perceived knowledge, beliefs, skills, and needs regarding evidence-based practice: Implications for accelerating the paradigm shift. Worldviews on Evidence-based Nursing, 1, 185–193.
52. National Guideline Clearinghouse, (2010). Retrieved at http://www.guideline.gov/ on April 25, 2010.
53. National Library of Medicine. (2009). MESH: Medical subject headings. Retrieved at http://www.nlm.nih.gov/mesh/ on April 25, 2010.
54. National Library of Medicine, (2009). Related Sources for Searching For Systematic Reviews. Retrieved from http://www.nlm.nih.gov/bsd/pubmed_subsets/sysreviews_sources.html on April 25, 2010.
55.Research Methods Knowledge Base, (2006). Analysis. Retrieved at http://www.socialresearchmethods.net/kb/analysis.php on April 25, 2010.
56. Sackett, DL., Strauss SE, Richardson, WS., Rosenburg, W., & Haynes, RB. (2000). Evidence-based medicine: How to practice and teach EBM (2"" ed.). London, UK: Churchill-Livingstone.
57. Shearer J. (1995). The Nursing Research Journal Club: An ongoing program to promote nursing research in a community hospital. Journal of Nursing Staff Development, 11:104-105.
58. The Evidence-Based Medicine Resource Center, (2010). Retrieved at http://ktclearinghouse.ca/cebm/teaching on April 25, 2010.
59. The Joanna Briggs Institute, (2010). Retrieved at http://www.joannabriggs.edu.au/about/home.php on April 25, 2010.
60. The Oncology Nursing Society Evidence-Based Practice Resource Area (2010). Retrieved at http://onsopcontent.ons.org/toolkits/evidence/index.shtml on April 25, 2010.
61. United States Department of Health and Human Services, (2009). Office for Protection from Research Risks, OPRR, 1979, 1993. Retrieved at http://www.hhs.gov/ohrp/ on April 25, 2010.
62. University of North Carolina, Chapel Hill, (2005). Evidence Based Nursing. Retrieved from http://www.hsl.unc.edu/services/tutorials/ebn/index.htm on April 25, 2010.
63. Akobeng AK. Principles of evidence based medicine. Arch Dis Child. 2005 Aug;90(8):837-40.
64. Katz PP, Yelin EH, Lockshin MD. Journal policies on authorship and disclosures. Arthritis Rheum. 2006 Jun 15;55(33):345-7.

Notes

CHAPTER

17

Performance Improvement and Patient Safety in Hyperbaric Units

SUSAN MELLOTT, PHD, RN AND KATHY BARR, JD, RN

REGARDLESS OF THE TYPE OF ORGANIZATION that you belong to, performance improvement and patient safety must be paramount in the way that you operate. Performance improvement in healthcare has been an ever-changing concept that began to evolve in the early 1950s following the Industrial Revolution after World War II. Industry began adopting quality assurance principles in Japan after the war. Deming, Juran, and others went to Japan in the late 1940s and early 1950s to assist them in revamping their industry and its processes. From there, their concepts were adapted into industry in the United States. In the early 1970s, quality improvement began to evolve into healthcare utilizing the principles from industry.

In the 1970s, Avedis Donabedian defined the concepts of structure, process, and outcomes and how they applied to healthcare. Structure relates to qualifications of staff, and facilities/technology. Structure relates to the things that absolutely must be in place, such as physician and nurse licensure, laboratory controls, and so on. Processes relate to activities in prevention, diagnosis, and treatment. Outcomes relate to results of care or the results of processes. Standards utilized by regulatory and accreditation agencies were developed as structure and processes, rather than outcomes.

Donabedian was one of the first to identify that poor performance was not necessarily related to the lack of knowledge of an individual. He felt that the context in which the process occurs has a major influence on the functioning of a process. For example, individuals know what to do, but for some reason related to the process itself, the individual fails to complete all aspects of the process, resulting in poor performance. We still hold this true today- that the problem is in the process, not the individual, the majority of the time.

Donabedian also established that there is a difference between quality assurance and continuous improvement. Quality assurance consists of monitoring and measurement against a standard, then making adjustments, and therefore, through this process, quality can be "assured." However, no one can "assure" quality. Continuous improvement, in contrast, is continuously monitoring to find improvement opportunities and then making changes. It was in the 1990s that healthcare began the move from quality assurance to continuous improvement.

By the 1990s, Continuous Quality Improvement (CQI) and Total Quality Management (TQM) were adopted by the healthcare sector. The concepts behind CQI and TQM are very similar. Both include the identification of processes that are not functioning well or as expected, finding ways to improve the processes, and to sustain those improvements. Since the inception of these models, different models such as Lean, Six Sigma, Rapid Improvements, and others have evolved. However, all of these still follow the principles of CQI and TQM.

Throughout the 1990s, the term quality assurance continued to be utilized in many organizations, including The Joint Commission (TJC) and the Centers for Medicare and Medicaid Services (CMS). In the 2000s, healthcare facilities have finally dropped the "quality assurance" term and now refer to it as "performance improvement."

Another movement in healthcare in the 1990s was the concept of a quality culture. In 1999, the Institute of Medicine (IOM) published its "To Err is Human" report which defined the lack of patient safety within healthcare organizations. Since that time, the shift has been toward building a patient safety culture. These two types of cultures will be discussed later in this chapter.

Today, as a result of the IOM report, healthcare is focusing on providing high quality of care, high patient satisfaction, and high patient safety. Healthcare is currently being held accountable for their efforts by many governmental and private entities. There is a movement towards transparency, public release of information, and informing consumers to enable them to make knowledgeable decisions regarding their healthcare. The healthcare quality environment is moving to one that utilizes epidemiological and statistical measures to determine the success of their quality improvement efforts. Regulatory agencies and insurers are shifting towards an environment of Pay for Performance, where organizations receive more money for higher quality of care. If the organization is a low quality performer, they receive less money for reimbursement, and so forth.

The Centers for Medicare and Medicaid (CMS) have initiated a list of hospital acquired conditions that the CMS will not pay for. If any of these conditions occur while the patient is in a hospital, the hospital will not receive additional payment for these conditions if they were not present on admission. While the CMS regulations only pertain to Medicare and Medicaid patients, other insurers have followed suit, and will no longer pay for these secondary conditions. Therefore, it is in the hospital's best financial interest to improve the way they give care to minimize the occurrence of these secondary conditions. While CMS does not at this time pay for inpatient hyperbarics, hyperbaric facilities, whether inpatient or outpatient, need to be aware of these secondary conditions and work to prevent them from occurring in their unit. Although it rarely occurs, a secondary condition that can be prevented in the hyperbaric facility is falls, which can result in fractures and head injury.

There is no indication of this trend slowing down or reversing. In fact, it is anticipated that the performance improvement and patient safety initiative will continue to expand as the nation moves into healthcare reform and attempts to decrease the cost of healthcare. The remainder of this chapter is designed to assist hyperbaric facilities with their performance improvement and patient safety efforts. It is through these efforts that an organization will be able to continue offering high quality and safe patient care to its patients.

ESTABLISHING A PERFORMANCE IMPROVEMENT/PATIENT SAFETY CULTURE

Developing and maintaining a culture of quality, performance improvement, and patient safety is a continuous process that will always be evolving. The hyperbaric environment is one that is laden with potential patient safety risks, simply because of the treatment environment itself. However, there is more to a patient safety culture than just the hyperbaric treatment and that environment. Regardless of how intent, well-meaning, and competent individuals are, medical errors will be made.

A culture that consists of continual improvements in performance and patient safety must start with the leadership of the organization. According to the law and accreditation standards, the governing body of the organization is "ultimately responsible" for all that goes on within the organization. The governing body sets the framework under which all the other leaders of the organization function. If the governing body focuses on the finances of the organization, the other leaders will also focus on this. If the governing body focuses on the quality and patient safety within the organization, then the other leaders will follow this path. So, the culture of the organization begins with the governing body.

The leaders of the organization then set the tone for how the organization functions. They utilize the mission, vision, and values of the organization to define the culture of the organization. Culture of an organization is not something that comes about overnight. Instead, it must be developed over a period of time and requires continual reinforcement and support. The leaders of healthcare organizations usually consist of the senior leadership, the medical staff leadership, and the governing body. In larger organizations, a layer of directors, managers, and the like, are also providing leadership at different levels in the organization, and thus influence the culture of the organization.

The leaders of the organization provide the resources of time, money, personnel, and so on, that are needed to be able to implement and maintain a culture of continually improving processes and patient safety. Thus, their leadership and support are crucial to creating such a culture within the organization. Leaders within the organization must be willing to make quality and patient safety a high priority of the organization. They must allocate the appropriate staff, equipment, and other resources that are required. They must analyze processes, implement changes, promote evidence-based practice, and support a non-punitive, error-reporting environment. One example that demonstrates this priority is the placement of quality and patient safety at the top of meeting agendas rather than at the end. This demonstrates that quality and patient safety are top priorities for the organization.

One of the components of a high quality, continual improvement, and patient safety culture is that of systems thinking. Systems thinking involve viewing the organization as being made up of multiple parts that together form the whole. You may have heard the phrase that "the whole is a sum of its parts." If something goes wrong in one part of the whole, it often affects the other parts of the whole. Consider for a moment what happens when you throw a pebble in a pond or lake. It produces ripples over the water that move out from the point where the pebble hit the water. Now, think of two boats passing on the water, leaving a wake of water moving behind the boat. If one of those boats is a sailboat and one is a cruise ship, the cruise ship will leave a much larger wake than the sailboat. If the sail boat is too close to the cruise ship when it passes, the wake may topple the sail boat. If the sailboat is far away from the cruise ship, there may be little, if any, impact as the cruise ship goes by. So, in terms of the culture of the organization, a change in one part of the organization will impact other areas of the organization. However, this can happen rapidly or take time to occur throughout the organization.

Another important component of a high quality, continual improvement and patient safety culture is teamwork. The leaders of the organization must work together to define and implement the culture of the organization. If the senior leadership and the medical staff leadership do not work well together, the culture of the organization will suffer. The managers and directors must also work well with each other and with the leadership of the organization. And, of course, there is the teamwork between the clinical and non-clinical members of the organization.

Eliminating medical errors and improving the processes utilized within the organization for clinical and non-clinical actions, involve being able to identify the processes that are not working as desired or which can potentially result in harm or a medical error. In evaluating whether processes need to be redesigned or not includes determining how complex the process is; how consistently the process is being implemented; if there are time constraints that could result in errors; and what amount of human intervention or lack of automation is required to complete the process. Root Cause Analysis (RCA) and Failure Mode Effectiveness Analysis (FMEA) are just two of the many tools that can assist with these efforts.

Other areas that should be examined as the organization moves towards a culture of continual improvement and patient safety include structure, the environment, equipment, and people. The structure involves the design of the facility to promote safety; that licensure, certification, and the like are present and maintained; that the right supplies are ordered; and that policies and procedures address safety concerns. The environment involves the assessment of lighting, temperature, noise levels, surfaces, storage, and ergonomics. The equipment involves the examination of all patient care equipment and assuring that the staff utilizes the equipment in the correct manner. The people aspects include many complex factors, including employee attitudes, motivation, physical and psychological health, cognitive functioning, education, and training.

The Institute of Medicine (IOM) has undertaken a quality initiative aimed at improving the performance improvement and patient safety culture of healthcare organizations. The IOM quality initiative aims for six components of processes: safe, effective, patient-centered, timely, efficient, and equitable. Their initiative encourages organizations to examine all of their processes to assure that these six aims are met.

The Institute for Healthcare Improvement (IHI) has had several campaigns for patient safety since December, 2004. These include their 100,000 Lives Campaign, the 5 Million Lives Campaign, and they are currently implementing their Improvement Map. Participating in these campaigns has assisted healthcare organizations in the movement towards a continual improvement and patient safety culture.

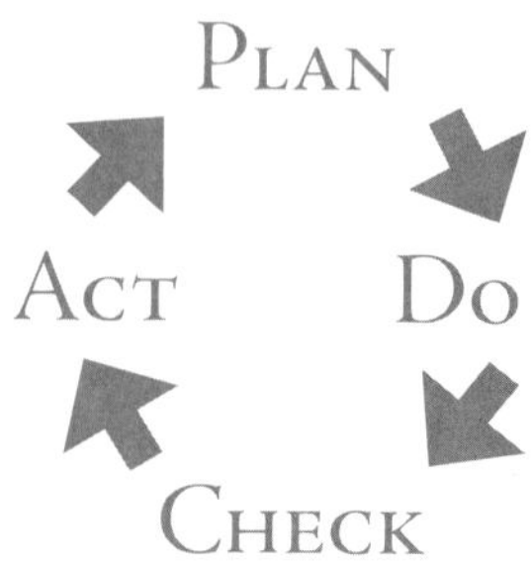

FIGURE 1. ***Plan-Do-Check-Act Cycle.***

PI PROCESS

PLANNING

Planning is the first step in the PI Process. The organization should determine what hyperbaric medicine (and the entire facility, if part of a hospital) will focus on for the year. In order to identify the areas of focus, there are several means to obtaining the information you need. This is a portion of strategic planning that the organization should undertake every year. There may be new legislation or accreditation standards that the facility must now address, or there may have been areas of opportunities for improvement already identified during the previous year. One area that should always be considered is that of patient safety. While clinical aspects of care are the most frequently focused on processes, don't forget to examine other areas of the organization such as equipment management, human resources, etc. In other words, the performance improvement areas must be carried out throughout the organization, not just the clinical areas of the organization. The process of performance improvement is the same, regardless of the processes being studied and/or improved.

UTILIZING A PI MODEL

The choice of a Process Improvement (PI) Model is essential for a successful program. The model must, at the same time, be easy to understand and use, and be effective. It is always best to evaluate what is currently in place when assuming a PI position, as what is not clear to you, may work very well for the incumbent staff. The first question to ask is, "is there a PI model being used?" If there is not, the choice is wide open. If there is, there is a second question to be asked is, "Is it effective?" If it is, you must delve into it and make it yours. If not, you must select a PI model, preferably with the involvement of key staff members, and teach the entire staff the pros and cons of this model. Never ignore the "cons." The staff will find them and your credibility in proposing or selecting the model will be lost.

Model possibilities include, but are not limited to, the PDCA/PDSA (Shewhart-Deming Cycle), FOCUS PDCA, IMPROVE, and Six Sigma. The Plan-Do-Check-Act or Plan-Do-Study-Act (in this chapter we will refer to it by its most commonly known name, PDCA) was developed in the 1950s, and is intended to be a cycle allowing the work to be continuous. PDCA (see Figure 1) represents planning an improvement, doing the improvement on a trial basis (or more broadly, depending on the magnitude of the improvement), checking or studying the results of the test trial, and acting to maintain any gain you may have garnered, or to re-plan and begin the cycle again.

The HCA Corporation decided to utilize a variation of the PDCA model, so they developed FOCUS PDCA. The FOCUS portion of this model represents finding an opportunity for improvement, organizing a team to work on the improvement, clarifying the process as it exists before any improvement, understanding any variability in the process, and selecting the particular improvement the team wants to make. This PI model is based on the fact that every process contains some variability; by eliminating the variability, you can achieve an improvement. The PDCA portion of this model is the same as that explained above.

The IMPROVE model includes Identifying a problem, Measuring its impact on customers, Prioritizing possible causes, Researching and analyzing root causes, Outlining alternative solutions, Validating which solutions might work, and Executing solutions. This PI model is based on finding and correcting the cause of a problem.

Six Sigma is the model proposed by a significant number of industries today. Six Sigma projects follow two methodologies inspired by Deming's Plan-Do-Check-Act Cycle. These methodologies, comprising 5 phases each, are termed DMAIC and DMADV. DMAIC is used for projects aimed at improving an existing business process, while DMADV is used for projects aimed at creating new product or process designs. The DMAIC project methodology has five phases: Define the problem, the voice of the customer, and the project goals, specifically. Measure key aspects of the current process and collect relevant data. Analyze the data to investigate and verify cause-and-effect relationships. Determine what the relationships are, and attempt to ensure that all factors have been considered. Seek out the root cause of the defect under investigation. Improve or optimize the current process based upon data analysis using techniques such as design of experiments, or mistake proofing, and standard work to create a new, future state process. Set up pilot runs to establish process capability. Control the future state process to ensure that any deviations from target are corrected before they result in defects. Control systems are implemented such as statistical process control, production boards, and visual workplaces and the process is continuously monitored. The DMADV project methodology, also known as DFSS (Design For Six Sigma), features 5 phases: Define design goals that are consistent with customer demands and the enterprise strategy. Measure and identify CTQs (characteristics that are Critical To Quality), product capabilities, production process capability, and risks. Analyze to develop and design alternatives, create a high-level design, and evaluate design capability to select the best design. Design details, optimize the design, and plan for design verification. This phase may require simulations. Verify the design, set up pilot runs, implement the production process, and hand it over to the process owners.

Other "homegrown" PI Models are also locally designed and used. Basically, there are as many PI Models as there are PI coordinators out there. The main goal is to select a PI Model that is easy to use and easy to teach. However, it is our recommendation when developing a PI Program that PDCA be used as the PI Model. It is the most easily recognized and, therefore, the easiest to teach. In fact, every process that you do can be expressed as PDCA. For example, you may be thinking about what you want to eat at your next meal. You will plan the meal and buy the products needed to make the meal. (PLAN). You will then prepare the meal (DO). Once everyone has eaten, you will determine if the food was good, if it was easy to prepare, and so on (CHECK). You will then determine if you ever want to make the meal again, or if you want to try something else the next time (ACT). PDCA stresses planning first and foremost, which will save time in the end by avoiding false starts and stumbles.

Data Collection

Data collection is the basis of any good PI program. There is no point to reviewing 1000 medical records every month if your documentation is perfect. Of course, how do you know it's perfect if you are not reviewing the records? There is also no point to observing every patient diving in every chamber if you suspect one staff member is taking "short cuts" in their safety checks. So, you need a focus point. Identify a potential opportunity for improvement, and then attack it until you show you don't need to improve or your potential opportunity is proven a reality. This is the Do portion of the PDCA model. However, having made that last statement, there is always a possibility for improvement; thus, the term "continuous improvement."

It is best to first look in areas you can control easily. Unless you know that you have a safety or clinical opportunity for improvement, Medical Records and documentation is the first place to look. Develop a checklist of what you want to review in the record. For instance, to begin Hyperbaric Oxygen (HBO) treatments, each patient needs a consent, an EKG, and a chest x-ray, as well as a complete legible set of orders with parameters.

The main reason for doing data collection is to improve the process, which the data defines. As an example, in doing record reviews for chest x-ray compliance pre-HBO dives, you discover 25% of the time the chest x-ray is missing. You need to take it a step further and find out if the chest x-ray was done. Going even further, you need to find out if the report was simply not received. When you get all the possible questions answered about the missing chest x-ray, you can begin to develop a process that will ensure the chest x-ray is in the record 100% of the time, not 75% of the time.

A secondary reason for doing data collection

is to prove that you have an opportunity for improvement that you suspect you have. For instance, if you suspect that ear checks are not being done before every HBO dive, you can easily design a process to observe if ear checks are being done. It is always better to have hard numbers when addressing an opportunity for improvement, and not just a gut feeling that improvement is needed. If you don't know where you are before you put an improvement in place, it becomes difficult to evaluate your success or failure.

Once it is determined what is to be monitored, the indicators must be developed and the collection format designed. It is best to utilize data that is easy to record and offers enough choice to allow for variation in the data. How you answer the indicator questions will determine what you can do to analyze the results. If you simply want to know if the item is there or not, then a simple yes/no answer could be selected. For example, "Is the consent for treatment in the medical record?" Yes or no? However, if some of the data to be collected is not required for all records examined, you need to add N/A, as appropriate, to those questions in the tool. It is easiest to enter results into an excel spreadsheet if you equate a "1" to yes and a "0" to no and simply skip the N/A responses. That way, you can calculate and construct graphs with little or no difficulty. If you are looking for more detail than a simple yes or no, you may need to break the question down into multiple parts. For example, you can ask if the consent is present in the record, and then also ask, "Is it completed correctly?" and/or, "Is there a witness to the patient signature for consent?" and/or, "If patient is unable to sign, did the next of kin or Medical Power of Attorney sign for the patient?" It all depends on how much information you are interested in obtaining.

Another type of indicator would have an open-ended answer. For example, "Age of Patient" or "Race of Patient." You could also list the opportunities that you are looking for, and ask the data collector to select one of the available items. For example, with the question regarding age, the answer choices could be: 0-20: ______; 21-40: ________; 41-60: ______; 61-80: ______; 81 and above: ______.

If the data you are collecting involves patient satisfaction, these types of questions require different types of answers. The Likert scale, consisting of choices from 1-5 or 1-10, would be a good scale. You have probably seen this type of scale as a way to measure the patient's level of pain. The scale could also be reworded as Very Dissatisfied to Very Satisfied, with 3 or more choices between these points.

Reviewing records for the items of interest is a good place to start. Each person working in the hyperbaric area can review a few records a week to get everyone involved in the PI process. This is both cost-effective for the unit, and divides the labor for the staff. It provides a learning opportunity for the staff to see first-hand how the documentation may be less than optimal. However, it may not give you optimal results. There is a need for consistency, also called inter-rater reliability, in the data collection that will ultimately make data analysis much easier. If more than one individual is collecting the data, there should be attempts made to assure that all the collectors are doing so in exactly the same manner so that all could produce the same results, regardless of which record they audit. This inter-rater reliability is easily obtained through education of the data collectors and then a simple inter-rater test. Once the checklist or data collection form is developed, there should be training provided for each data collector as to where in the medical record to obtain the data and how to record what is found. Once everyone has been trained, give each data collector the same three records to review independently of each other, utilizing the data collection tool. If there is inter-rater reliability between the data collectors, they should be able to produce the same data from each record. If they are not able to do this, then re-educate them and repeat the testing utilizing 3 new records, until the inter-rater reliability is obtained.

Reliability and Validity

Since this is not intended to be a text on statistical analysis, and you can study every potential safety measure in a hyperbaric facility without conducting pure research, we are including a short overview of these topics for completeness only. More information can be obtained in any statistics book in your local library or online through any search engine. Research requires an association with an Institutional Review Board (IRB) and compliance with all the rules and regulations that Board imposes. NEVER embark on a pure research study without IRB association and approval. If your hyperbaric facility chooses to do actual research, validity and reliability become very important to the process. Together, validity and reliability help us ensure we are studying what we think we are studying, and that the tools we are using are applied consistently.

Reliability is the extent to which an experiment, test, or any measuring procedure yields the same result on repeated trials. Reliability is concerned with the accuracy of the actual measuring instrument or procedure. This also pertains to data collection, as previously described, in terms of inter-rater reliability. You want to be sure that everyone collecting data will be able to get the same answer, regardless of who audits the record. There must be reliability before there can be validity.

Validity refers to the accuracy of a measure to the degree to which a study accurately reflects or assesses the specific concept that the researcher is attempting to measure. There are several types of validity, including external and internal validity. External validity refers to the extent to which the results of a study are generalizable or transferable. A lot of external validity is dependent upon the sampling methodology that is utilized in the study.

Internal validity refers to the study's design and the extent to which the designers of a study have taken into account alternative explanations for any causal relationships. There are several types of internal validity for which we will provide short definitions only and refer you to that ever-looming statistics text. In terms of the quality data collection that hyperbaric facilities undertake, the validity refers to how the data collection tool itself is developed. "Face" validity ensures the study "looks like" it is going to measure what it is supposed to measure. In other words, do the items to be utilized in collecting the data look like they will be able to get the data that is needed? "Criterion" validity measures the relationship between scores on the instrument in question and scores on another instrument. In terms of the items utilized to collect the data, were these indicators developed from criteria relevant to the information required? For example, if collecting data to determine if a procedure was done correctly, do the questions asked directly refer to what the procedure states should be done? "Construct" validity is the most comprehensive form of validity. It includes content validity which refers to the representativeness of the items on the instrument as they relate to the entire content being measured. A construct is not something that can easily be measured or quantified and, therefore, it is difficult to accurately measure. Patient satisfaction is a construct. When attempting to measure constructs, it is best to utilize established a standardized tool such as the Gallup, Press Ganey, or other such tools designed to measure patient satisfaction.

Data Analysis

"In God we trust. All others must use data."

This old quote is from the "Deming Management Method" by Mary Walton. Another adage that applies here is that "the proof is in the pudding" or when paraphrased, the proof is in the data. However, there can always be manipulation of the data to produce the results that someone wants.

It is important to always look at the entire picture when analyzing data. Every data point is trying to tell you something about the process. Gather your data piece by piece and determine the formula that will give a true picture of what the data is trying to tell you. In other words, know how to look at what you are seeing to get a helpful answer. An easy example may help: You're late to work every morning. You instantly think you need to get up earlier, and quickly find that does not help. So, you start to gather data, and look at your morning processes- shower, dress, eat, drive. You time those processes for a few days and discover that selecting clothes to wear as part of your dressing process takes twice as long as any of the other process and that by getting up earlier, it takes even longer. The solution: select your wardrobe the night before.

This example points out an important principle to follow. Frequently the answer to a problem is not what you thought it would be. Examining what the data is telling you will lead to a better solution to the problem. Data is defined as the specific data points that you collect. Combining and examining this data leads you to revealing information. With this information, the best solution can be found.

Knowing what you have uncovered in your data collection is paramount. In order to know how far you have come with your improvements, you must know where you started from. For example, when individuals reach a certain age, probably somewhere around 40, the physician often requests an EKG to utilize as a baseline. The physician will then utilize this baseline EKG in the future to make determinations as to whether there have been any changes. You need this data with your own processes to be able to determine if there is a need for improvements to be made. You then have a baseline (pre-improvement) so that you will ultimately be able to evaluate the effectiveness of any implemented improvement.

When you study a possible area for improvement, you may find uncontrollable issues that impact that area, you may find controllable is-

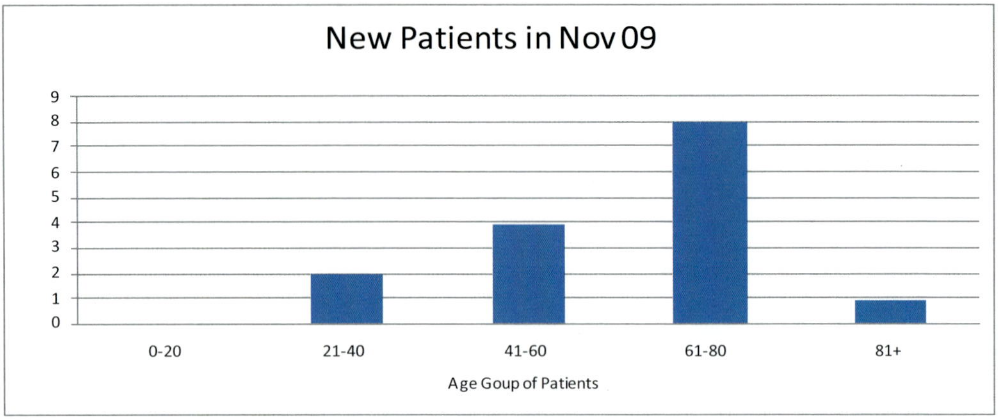

Figure 2: ***Histogram.***

sues that impact that area, and you may find issues that could impact a change in the area. When approaching these issues, you should turn first to the controllable issues and see if that causes an improvement. If there is no improvement, you can turn to the issues that might impact a change and see if changes in those areas cause an improvement. If you still have no improvement, you can look at the uncontrollable issues again to see if they are truly uncontrollable, or if in fact you could cause an improvement by trying to utilize one of those.

In trying to determine what kind of analysis to perform, it is best to start with the type of data that was collected. In the previous section of this chapter, we discussed different types of data to collect and the ways to record that data. Whatever you decide to utilize will be the driver of what you can do with the data to analyze it here. There are 2 different types of data: categorical data and continuous data.

Categorical data is also called count, attribute, or qualitative data. This data falls into categories, or groups, that you can then utilize to count how many are in each group. For example, if you collected the data utilizing the yes and no options, the data then falls into one of these two groups. You can then count how many yes answers and how many no answers are gathered. This can be utilized with data that is examined based on males or females, or one diagnosis or another. You can count how many of your patients need your services due to actual diving problems versus how many need your services because of other indicators for hyperbaric treatment. In the previous section, we looked at the concept of collecting data by age groups. In that example, we stated that the age groups could be 0-20, 21-40, 41-60, 61-80, and then 81 and above. If the data was collected in this manner, you would count how many data points are in each age group.

Categorical data is most often expressed in the percentage of the whole. For example, 56% of our patients are male; or the consent for treatment was present 98% of the time. Focus on the positive as much as possible. If you have 25% non-compliance in an area; report as 75% compliance. If you want to determine if there is a statistical difference between two groups, you would utilize a Chi Squared test. With categorical data, it is best to display the data in a histogram. Each bar in the histogram then represents one of the categories or groups of data (see Figure 2).

A Pareto diagram is also an appropriate tool to utilize. A Pareto takes the categories of data and arranges them from the highest category to the lowest category (see Figure 3). The Pareto diagram is utilized when you have the need to determine where most of the problem lies. It utilizes the 80/20 rule: 80% of the problem is found in 20% of the data. For example, in the Pareto diagram below, each bar represents the problems that were found when the data was collected. This figure shows that the problems range from "Measurements" to "Signatures." This diagram would be utilized to determine the best place to start making improvements to get the biggest bang for your buck. In this case, it would be in the first two columns, as this is where most of the problems lie. If the issues of measurements and goals not being present were resolved, that would leave only the non-compliance areas of pain management

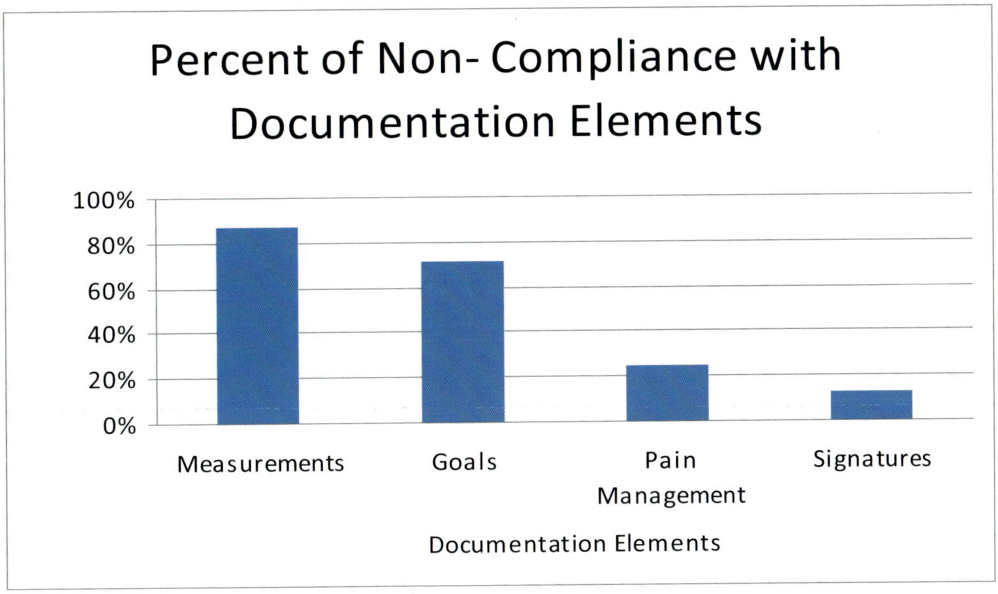

Figure 3: *Pareto Diagram.*

and signatures to be dealt with. You can make the most of your time by tackling the areas with the most non-compliance first.

Continuous data is also known as measurement data, or quantitative data. This is data that has measureable intervals between each number. For example, take a ruler; it has exactly the same distance between 1 inch and 2 inches as the same amount of distance between 2 inches and 3 inches. Other examples would include a thermometer, length of stay, the amount of pressure utilized in the hyperbaric tanks, and so on. Typically, data considered to be continuous data are time, volume, money, and measured data.

Continuous data can be analyzed utilizing mean, medium, and mode tests. These tests will let you know about the spread of the data around the middle of the data. If you have extreme values (data that is very different from the other data) it is best to utilize the median (middle) rather than the mean (average), as the mean is affected by the extreme values but the median is not. The mode is utilized when you have numbers that repeat within the data and it signifies data that is similar to the other data. If you wanted to determine if there is statistical difference between two scores or amounts, you would utilize a t-test. The t-test produces a "p" score that will range between zero (0) and one (1). If the p-score is 0.05 or less, there is statistical difference between the two scores or amounts. This means that the difference is not by chance, but that something is making the two scores so different. With continuous data, it is best to display the data in run or control charts. Each dot on the run or control chart equals a point in time, be it one data point or one mean for a day, month, quarter, etc. (see Figure 4). A control chart is nothing more than a run chart with control limits applied to it (see Figure 5). In healthcare most control charts have the control limits set at the second control limit (95% of the data will be between the control limits) or the third control limit (99% of the data will be between the control limits).

By utilizing a run or control chart, you can further analyze the data to determine the spread of the data around the mean or median. This will help to determine if there is common cause or special cause variation. Common cause variation is considered normal variation that occurs in all processes. Special cause variation occurs when something outside of the process interferes with the process. For example, take the time that patients come for their hyperbaric appointments. You assign a time for each patient to be at your facility or department for their treatment. Some patients will be on time, some will be early, and some will be late. This is an expected or common cause variation. But every once in a while, the patient does not come for the appointment and does not call to cancel. You later find out that the patient was in the hospital having emergency gallbladder

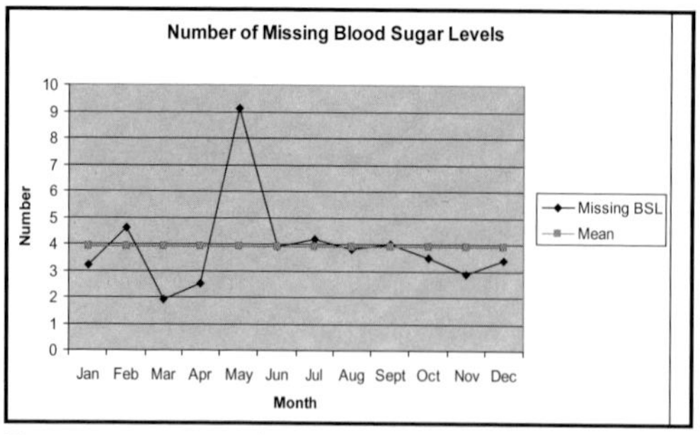

FIGURE 4: ***Run Chart.***

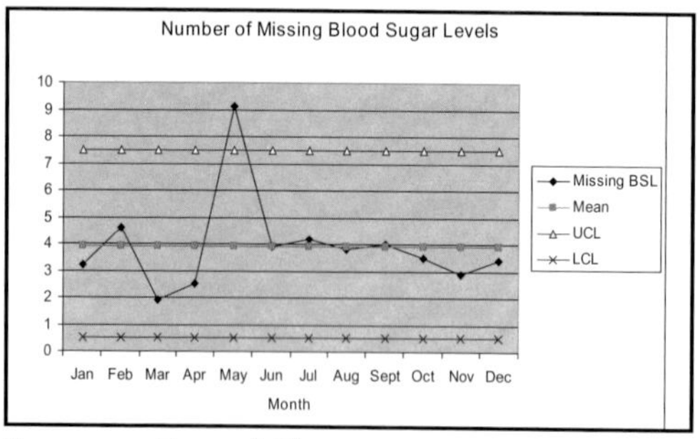

FIGURE5: ***Control Chart.***

removal and did not have time or remember to call and cancel the appointment. This is special cause variation where something outside the process has interfered with the process.

There are many special cause rules as to how to interpret the data in a run or control chart, but really only three are utilized in most healthcare settings. When a special cause is identified, there must be an investigation as to what caused the special cause variation and the actions taken to prevent it from occurring again, or if it is positive, to try and make it occur again. These rules can be utilized with both the run and control charts.

Rule 1: Any data point outside of the upper or lower control limit, or in a run chart, any extreme value

Rule 2: 6 data points in a row going up or going down

Rule 3: 8 data points in a row above or below the mean

Although you can apply all sorts of statistical formulas to your data, it is best to keep it simple. The statistics other than mean, median, mode, and percentages are best calculated utilizing specific software programs. If you are comfortable enough with those statistical formulas to be able to explain them and your results to your peers and supervisors, by all means use them.

REPORTING THE DATA

Data is reported to whoever requested and/or needs the data/information. This may be a committee, your boss, another department, or even the CEO and the governing board of the organization. The data should be reported in a format that will make it easy to read and understand. If you can, display the data as a graph. However, pie graphs are not usually utilized. All of the graphs can be developed by hand, with Excel or other such software. There are several programs that can be utilized with Excel that are capable of making control charts and completing some of these statistical tests.

Graphs often make it easier to see where an improvement might be beneficial. Most adults are somewhat pictorial learners rather than purely verbal learners, so a picture can show more than words. But remember, you always need to be able to explain what you show. Never give someone a graph that needs explaining or one that you cannot explain. There should always be a title for the graph indicating what the learner is observing. The horizontal and vertical axis of the graph should be clearly labeled as to what they represent. It's a good technique to put "better is up" or "better is down" or arrows to describe that on the graph, or in the legend, for ease in interpreting the graph. You can even add text within the graph itself that displays the value of the data point, or which explains what a special cause is, and so forth. Accreditation agencies also expect to see graphic presentation of your data and the explanation of what the graphs mean.

If the data is to be reported in a dashboard or scorecard format, it is best to have pre-established targets that can visually be displayed to the reader. A dashboard may also be called a report card, or a scorecard. Think of the report card that you got while you were in grade school. Every 6 weeks you received a new set of grades displayed to the right of the grades from the preceding grading period. At the end of the year, your report card showed all your grades from the year and what progress you had made. In terms of the scorecard, think of a baseball game scorecard. Each inning indicates who got a hit, who struck out, and who got a run. At the end of the game, you have a record of what happened during the entire game. With a dashboard, think of the dashboard of a car. The car dashboard has all types of indicators on it that monitors how well the car is running. It lets you know when a door is ajar, when you need gas or an oil change, as well as how fast the car is moving. Regardless of what you call it, in healthcare

QUALITY DASHBOARD	Threshold	First Qtr	2nd Qtr	3rd Qtr	4th Qtr
Medical Record Review					
EKG's present	> 95	99	97	98	100
Complete order	100	100	99	100	100
Blood sugar level	100	92	95	100	100
Pain level	>95	95	93	94	96
Equipment Monitoring					
Temperature	≥98	98	99	100	99
Humidity	≥98	98	99	100	99

Figure 6: ***Dashboard.***

we use a dashboard or scorecard to demonstrate the current status of a particular department, service line, or the overall organization. This allows the user an easy way to determine if the information on the dashboard or scorecard demonstrates a need to make improvements in a certain area or to celebrate how well an area is doing. To make this information easier to read at a glance, many organizations have taken to color coding the data based on a typical traffic light, utilizing those pre-established targets mentioned previously. Green indicates that the data is within the excellent range based on the targets; yellow indicates the data is acceptable, but is not best practice; and red indicates that the data is not acceptable (see Figure 6). The goal should always be to have data that is in the green area, thus demonstrating excellence. However, this is often not possible to maintain.

Reporting your data is essential. If you do not convey the information you have learned, nothing can be done with that information to determine where the organization stands or to improve the processes as appropriate. Be prepared to report the criteria used to collect the data, the process utilized to perform the data collection, what the findings are, and finally any additional information pertinent to the report. You must always report exactly what you find. Never hedge because you are concerned about the ramifications. If you have found information through a record review, a database review, or a study of direct patient care, you report that information. If your boss handles a process that is reviewed at his or her request, and results show a low level of compliance, you report it. It might be best to inform your boss of what the data shows before you share it with others, but you do report it. In fact, the individual who is your boss, the chair of a committee, or other individual who will be receiving the report, may have some suggestions for additional ways to present the data or extra data to be collected before it is presented to others.

Patients are a key component in all of your processes and deserve to be included in the reporting of things like clinical outcome data and satisfaction survey results. A PI board (like a posted bulletin board in the department) works well. Posting graphs showing clinical outcome data, satisfaction survey results, and special study results allows patients and staff to see exactly where efforts are being made to improve processes. One facility identified a decrease in patient satisfaction due to timeliness of being seen. A review study was designed which included the patients and the resultant data was posted on their PI board. Many patients commented on the fact that the results were posted. They could see what the problems were and how they could help by arriving on time for their appointments. It was easy to do and garnered the best results they had seen to date.

When the data is reported, one of several actions will occur. This is the Check phase of the PDCA model that we are utilizing for this chapter. There could be a determination made that the data is within the desired target range. If this is the case, move on to study other areas that may identify opportunities for improvement. However, periodically come back and restudy this data to see if it remains at an acceptable level. There could be a determination made that while data is not at an optimal level, the importance of moving forward at this point, and the resources required to do so, prohibit moving towards improving the process at this time. The data should continue to be collected to determine if the process continues to deteriorate or the improvement priorities change. Another action could be to determine that improvements need to be made to the process at this time.

If you determine that no further improvement efforts are needed at this time you Act to sustain the gains you currently have. If you determine that performance improvements are needed at this point in time, you Act by moving back through the PDCA cycle again. Look at your data and determine where you can make an impact. For example, in doing blood sugar reviews of inpatients undergoing hyperbaric treatments, you discover a wide variety of preventative measures for maintaining blood sugar in the chamber. You Plan the improvement you need, a list of possible preventative measures aligned with specific blood sugar levels. You Do or implement the plan by developing a chart of potential preventative measures with the assistance of the hyperbaric staff, and then match the blood sugar levels with the most appropriate preventative measure. You gain approval for this list from your medical staff and post it in the area used to prepare patients for hyperbaric treatment. You now have a more controlled way to select measures intended to maintain blood sugar levels in the hyperbaric chamber and, therefore, potentially improved patient outcomes. You Check to make sure blood sugar levels are better maintained in the chamber with the use of the chart. If they are better maintained, you Act to sustain the gain. Otherwise, you move again back to the Plan phase and try to determine what else needs to be changed to make the process better.

SUSTAINING THE GAIN

Sustaining the gain is very important. Once you have worked to achieve an improvement, you want to be certain you do not lose that gain. If the improvement was based on a pilot, you would want to implement the revised or new process throughout the facility as appropriate. That portion of the "sustain the gain" is really moving back to the Plan, Do, and Check part of the PDCA cycle. However, in doing so, you cannot forget about the areas that have already had successful improvement while working on further implementation in other areas. When taking the pilot organization wide, be sure to alter any associated policy to include the improvement and educate your staff on any changes that you have made. Where clinical skill changes are made, ensure you host a return demonstration inservice of the clinical skill that was improved and document it in the competency assessment files.

When the goal is to sustain the gain, it is not the time to stop keeping your eye on the process, but the organization must continue to Act to keep it there. If there was a team working on the improvements, then they should determine who and what should be monitored on an ongoing basis. The monitoring of the process should continue quarterly for a year to determine if the level of performance is maintained. If the level of performance begins to drop, someone needs to quickly get in there and reinforce the revised process and get it back on course. If the level of performance is maintained for a year, the monitoring of the process could be decreased to two or three times a year. If it is maintained a second year, the process should then be monitored at least once a year for as long as the process results are important to the organization. There will come a time when the organization can determine that they will only monitor the process if they notice a problem or issue arise that might affect the gain that had been maintained previously. However, do not stop the monitoring for at least a year. All change theory suggests that there must be continual reinforcement of the new process for it to truly take root and become a habit rather than a project. Continuing to monitor and report the data to the shareholders will help let everyone know that the process is still being reinforced.

Always let staff and patients know what you have done and why. Staff will be more accepting of changes if they have been involved in the review process and have been kept current on results that were found. Patients will appreciate knowing improvements to their care are being made. There may be other areas of the organization that can benefit from what you have learned and changed in the process that was improved.

EXAMPLES

This section will include a number of examples of areas that have been studied in a wound care environment and several safety-related reviews that can be accomplished in an HBO environment. Some have already been addressed but here will be presented with criteria and review process that will ultimately lead to the results you are seeking.

Many areas that you choose to study as a hyperbaric facility will be related to what the Undersea and Hyperbaric Medicine Society (UHMS) looks at during certification visits. They are most interested in anything to do with the safety of hyperbaric dives. You may choose to study anything from patient satisfaction to staff competency to the UHMS safety items. Here we will look at a variety.

First, we will look at a study generated by a drop in patient satisfaction results attributed to patients being seen more than 15 minutes past their appointment times. Our goal with this study was to see what was causing the delay in being seen. Our criteria included time patient arrived, time patient was taken to a treatment room, and time patient was seen by the physician. Our process included having the patient sign in with the time of their arrival AND the time of their appointment. We also posted a list at each treatment room for the person escorting the patient to the room to annotate the time the patient was placed in the room and the time the patient was seen by the physician. At the end of each day, the sheets from sign-in and doorways were gathered and placed in the PI office. The PI coordinator tallied these sheets and uncovered some uncontrollable issues (patients needing to undress or toilet); some controllable issues (only one RN on duty); and some areas that might impact a change (patients arriving late). These findings were posted and the patients immediately noted they were part of the problem. Complaints about being seen late stopped, satisfaction climbed, and several patients actually asked to continue signing in with appointment and arrival times, saying that it helped them to stay honest- it has worked.

Next we will look at a study generated by a "gut feeling" that leg pressure tests (Ankle Brachial Index, or ABI) were not being accomplished before compression wraps were applied. Criteria used included the patient having a wound on the lower extremity; ABI being complete; lower extremity wrap applied; ABI documented on superbill; and, if ABI was missing, there must be an explanation in the physician and/or nursing section of the record. The process included running a list of all patients evaluated between 1 July and 30 September, and records were pulled and reviewed against the stated criteria in the Medical Records department. Ability to locate records was limited by illness of employees in Medical Records. Therefore, 72% of all evaluation records were located with 99.3% of those being 100% compliant. Only 0.7% (1 record) was problematic. In this case, data proved the "gut" wrong.

Hyperbaric oxygen therapy requires a strong focus on safety. Each hyperbaric facility needs a safety director, and from a PI perspective, each safety item needs to be monitored for any possible opportunity to improve. Several areas to consider include record reviews for the consent for treatment, EKG and CXR, blood sugar changes within the chamber, barotrauma to the ears within the chamber, assessment of the lungs before each chamber dive, and verification of any implants before any chamber dive.

These hyperbaric studies are fairly easy to design and take limited time to observe. Record reviews can be accomplished while any other record review is being done and should be reported in the same manner. A blood sugar study is simply an attempt to see if our patients enter the chamber with enough calories onboard to sustain their blood sugar through the entire treatment. Noting blood sugar pre-treatment, any preventative given, and blood sugar post treatment will tell you if enough calories are being given to sustain the blood sugar. Results of this actual study were discussed earlier in this section under improving performance. Evaluation of process for ear exams is an attempt to prevent ear barotrauma and can easily be assessed. Criteria include technique used to examine the ears, process used to educate the patient on equalizing the ears, documentation of ear exam, and needed follow-up. Process was to observe patients being prepared for treatment and reviewing records after the fact. Evaluation of effectiveness of lung assessments is an attempt to prevent lung problems during a hyperbaric treatment. Criteria include each patient's lungs being assessed, the technique used to assess lungs, and documentation of assessment. Process was to observe lung assessment technique with on-the-spot education as needed and reviewing records after the fact. Before any hyperbaric treatment is started, implanted devices must be verified for compatibility with pressurized oxygen. Criteria include that verification is obtained for each implanted device prior to any treatment. Process was to do review of safety check sheets that we use when preparing patients for beginning a series of hyperbaric treatments.

It is our hope that these few simple examples of hyperbaric studies can assist you in setting up similar studies for your hyperbaric facility and designing others in order for you to be successful in improving patient care and quality, as well as meeting accreditation and certification criteria.

REFERENCES

1. Larson-Lohr V and Norvell H. Editors: Hyperbaric Nursing (2002) Best Publishing Co. Flagstaff, AZ.
2. Undersea & Hyperbaric Medical Society, Inc. Clinical Hyperbaric Facility Accreditation Manual, 2005 edition; Dunkirk, MD
3. http://www.socialresearchmethods.net/tutorial/Colosi/lcolosi2.htm
4. http://www.bc.edu/research/csteep/CTESTWEB/whatistest/Validity.html

CHAPTER

18

Legal Implications in Hyperbaric Nursing

Tricia West, RN, MBA

HEALTHCARE DELIVERY IN THE TWENTY-FIRST CENTURY has posed many areas of concern and interest to healthcare practitioners. With increases in high-tech treatments and advances, so increases the risk of that very improved treatment to the public. As such, a more intimate weaving of the legal and medical systems has been experienced.

In an effort to protect both stakeholders, the public and healthcare providers alike, this chapter will provide a medical legal background and best practices to ensure the delivery of quality healthcare, as well as avoiding medical malpractice. It will focus on the legal implications of documentation and how sound medical record reporting can greatly assist in the defense of medical malpractice claims. It will also outline the legal process in the medical arena.

An area of civil law that includes medical malpractice and negligence is called tort law. A tort is a wrongful act that is committed by an entity or individual (i.e., a hospital or healthcare provider) that causes injury to another person or property. Negligence is a failure to act as an ordinary prudent person or reasonable person would do under similar circumstances. Professional negligence is different from ordinary negligence as professionals are held to a specific standard of care for the area in which they practice. Ordinary negligence is conduct that involves undue risk of harm to someone caused by the failure to act as an ordinary prudent person would have acted.[10] This is important in matters involving dependent adult and elder abuse. We are seeing more pressure ulcer cases filed as adult dependent abuse cases rather than professional negligence. The main reason for this

> "QUALITY IS NEVER AN ACCIDENT; IT IS ALWAYS THE RESULT OF HIGH INTENTION, SINCERE EFFORT, INTELLIGENT DIRECTION, AND SKILLFUL EXECUTION; IT REPRESENTS THE WISE CHOICE OF MANY ALTERNATIVES."
>
> —***William A. Foster***

is that there are no tort limits on adult dependent abuse matters where there are on professional negligence cases.

For example, a nursing assistant puts the meal tray of a patient who needs to be fed on the bedside table across the room from the patient and walks out. The nursing assistant does not return to feed the patient but does remove the untouched tray. There was no special knowledge or skill required and this was an act that an ordinary prudent person would have known would cause harm (not allowing the patient to eat).

The person who sustains injury as the result of tortuous conduct is known as the plaintiff, and the person who is responsible for inflicting the injury and incurs liability for the damage is known as the defendant.

Three elements must be established in every tort action. They include:

1. First, the plaintiff must establish that the defendant was under a legal duty to act in a particular fashion. An example would be a doctor/patient or nurse/patient relationship.
2. Second, the plaintiff must demonstrate that the defendant breached this duty by failing to adhere to the standard of care for the specialty and treatment. That said, these standards must be determined in order to see if there has been an act of omission or commission that has caused the damage/injury to the patient.
3. Third, the plaintiff must prove that he suffered injury or loss as a direct result of the defendant's breach. Damages may present in a variety of different ways, for example: loss of nurturance; pain and suffering; mental anguish; loss of love and affection; emotional distress; loss of chance of survival; past, present, and future medical expenses; loss of earnings; premature death; or loss of enjoyment of life.

Causation

First, a tort must be the cause in fact of a particular injury, which means that a specific act must actually have resulted in injury to another. In its simplest form, cause in fact is established by evidence that shows that a tortfeasor's act or omission was a necessary antecedent to the plaintiff's injury. Courts analyze this issue by determining whether the plaintiff's injury would have occurred "but for" the defendant's conduct. If an injury would have occurred independent of the defendant's conduct, cause in fact has not been established, and no tort has been committed. When multiple factors have led to a particular injury, the plaintiff must demonstrate that the tortfeasor's action played a substantial role in causing the injury.

Second, plaintiffs must establish that a particular tort was the proximate cause of an injury before liability will be imposed. The term proximate cause is somewhat misleading because it has little to do with proximity or causation. Proximate cause limits the scope of liability to those injuries that bear some reasonable relationship to the risk created by the defendant. Proximate cause is evaluated in terms of foresee-ability. If the defendant should have foreseen the tortious injury, he or she will be held liable for the resulting loss. If a given risk could not have been reasonably anticipated, proximate cause has not been established, and liability will not be imposed.

When duty, breach, and proximate cause have been established in a tort action, the plaintiff may recover damages for the pecuniary losses sustained. The measure of damages is determined by the nature of the tort committed and the type of injury suffered. Damages for tortious acts generally fall into one of four categories: damages for injury to person, damages for injury to personal property, damages for injury to real property, and punitive damages.

The law of torts serves four objectives. First, it seeks to compensate victims for injuries suffered by the culpable action or inaction of others. Second, it seeks to shift the cost of such injuries to the person or persons who are legally responsible for inflicting them. Third, it seeks to discourage injurious, careless, and risky behavior in the future. Fourth, it seeks to vindicate legal rights and interests that have been compromised, diminished, or emasculated. In theory, these objectives are served when tort liability is imposed on tortfeasors for intentional wrongdoing, negligence and ultra hazardous activities.

Most injuries that result from tortious behavior are the product of negligence, not intentional wrongdoing. Negligence is the term used by tort law to characterize behavior that creates unreasonable risks of harm to persons and property. A person acts negligently when his behavior departs from the conduct ordinarily expected of a reasonably prudent person under the circumstances. In general, the law requires jurors to use their common sense and life experience in determining the proper degree of care and vigilance with which people must lead their lives to avoid imperiling the safety of others.

Not every accident producing injury gives rise to liability for negligence. Some accidents cannot be avoided even with the exercise of reasonable care. An accident that results from a defendant's sudden and unexpected physical ailment, such as a seizure or a blackout, generally relieves the defendant of liability for harm caused during the period of unconsciousness. However, defendants who have reason to know of such medical problems are expected to take reasonable precautions against the risks the problems create.

Intentional torts include acts such as battery, assault, false imprisonment, and intentional infliction of emotional distress. Medical battery is the touching of a patient associated with the lack of informed consent to perform procedures or treatments. An example of this would be patients who refuse to continue their hyperbaric chamber treatment. They have in essence revoked their consent. Once consent is revoked, as a nurse, you would explain to them and teach them why this is an important part of their care. But if they insist on coming out of the chamber, they have revoked their consent, and one must stop their hyperbaric treatment and notify their physician.

Percipient Witnesses

If you are called to testify, either in a deposition or at trial, you are either the defendant or a percipient witness. A percipient witness is a witness who testifies about things they perceived.[25] The percipient witness most frequently is a co-worker. This would include healthcare professionals or ancillary personnel such as certified nursing assistants, dietary staff, or even a volunteer or patient roommate.

Although possible, it is unusual for a nurse to be named as a defendant in a professional negligence matter wherein the injury caused to the patient was not intentional. It is much more common for the facility (hospital) and/or physician to be named. The reasons for this are multi-fold: first the hospital is responsible for the actions of their employees. This is known as a legal doctrine of respondent superior. Secondly, as a class, nurses are revered in the community. A jury is less likely to find against a nurse. Third, it is always better to go after the deep pockets. Lastly, from a plaintiff position, it is better to create a "system-wide problem" when possible rather than just a specific incident problem. This, if successful, could leave the defense open to punitive damages in some cases.

Depositions

A deposition is sworn testimony. Although conducted in a less formal environment than a courtroom, the deponent is under the same oath as in a formal court of law. A court reporter creates a written record of all that is said – questions and answers. Opposing counsel will use the deposition to discover as much information as possible about you and the instant case. Both attorneys will be evaluating you in terms of your strength as a witness. Opposing counsel will be hoping to gain information that can be used against you at trial, if the case proceeds that far. Interestingly, medical malpractice and adult dependent abuse cases settle far more often than proceeding to trial, along the line of greater than 95% settle. Of the +/- 5% that do not settle and proceed to trial, 80% are defense verdicts.

The deposition will begin with an explanation of the deposition process by the deposing attorney. The attorney will instruct the deponent on the "ground rules." These might include explaining how non-verbal responses such as nodding, saying "uh-huh," or shrugging shoulders are not acceptable as answers. The witness should not interrupt the attorney asking the questions. It is important to listen carefully and answer only the question being asked. Never offer more information or an explanation unless it is specifically requested. If the attorney asks the "wrong question," do not correct the question. Your job, as a deponent, is to listen carefully, and answer only that which is clearly asked. It is the attorney's job – to ask the right questions for the information they need.

Any healthcare provider involved in the care of the plaintiff may be deposed. The plaintiff attorney will ask questions about the percipient witnesses, education, training, experience, and employment. The witness will also be asked questions about the care of the plaintiff. Recollections of the plaintiff will be queried. Most often, the medical record or part thereof will be referenced in the deposition and entered as an exhibit to the deposition. The facility's Policies & Procedures may also be referred to and will, therefore, be entered as exhibits.

In normal speaking, we talk over one another all the time and do not even realize it. We frequently anticipate the end of a question being asked and rush to answer it. However, at a deposition, everything is being taken down by the court reporter and they are not able to hear and report two people talking at the same time. Therefore, it is essential that you refrain from talking when another is speaking and wait until the examining attorney finishes their question before answering.

After hearing the question posed, it is important to take time to 1) allow your attorney to object, and 2) make sure you understand and have "processed" what was asked of you. If the question was unclear or you are not 100% certain of what was asked, do NOT guess at your answer, and do not answer what you think maybe someone wants to hear. Depending upon what state you reside in, you may or may not even be allowed to provide a guess. In California for instance, the witness is not allowed to guess at answers. Yet in other states, guessing or a best guess is considered acceptable. In states where you cannot guess, you can however provide your best estimate. Here is an example of the difference: You are asked how large the conference table is in my conference room. Having never been there, your answer would be a complete guess. However, if we were sitting at that table and I asked you that question, even without a tape measure, you could estimate based upon your prior life experience and visually looking at the table.

You should take what time you need to think about the answer to the question. If you do not understand the question, or if the way in which it was asked is unclear, request that it be repeated or rephrased. If you still do not understand the question, ask - do not worry about again saying you do not understand. You should never attempt to answer a question you do not understand. Once the question is answered, it is assumed that the witness understood the question. Remember, at trial, in front of a jury, you will be held to the answers you provide at your deposition. One loses all credibility if at trial your answers are different than they were at your deposition. If you give an answer at trial that is inconsistent with your deposition testimony, opposing counsel will pull out the transcript of your deposition, and quote from it to the jury and the court. You can only imagine the comment counsel will make about how your answer has materially changed!

If your attorney objects to a question, you will then be told that you can still answer the question. In some instances your attorney might instruct you not to answer. In that case, you will be asked by the examining attorney whether you are going to follow your attorney's instruction. The answer is always yes, you will follow the advice of the attorney defending your deposition.

If the medical record is introduced during your deposition, which is most likely, be certain to ask to review the medical record in question right then and there. Do not rely on your memory or feel bad about asking to see it. A deposition is NOT a memory test. It is an examination of your knowledge of a particular event – an exam that you have no obligation to have every detail committed to memory. And remember, this is usually an event that occurred at least three years earlier, and in many cases, more than that. In the same vein, if the examining attorney reads into the record either at trial or deposition what you had charted and then proceeds to paraphrase it or say what it is you meant by that, listen very carefully. Often, even a word or two is changed or the inflection is changed, which then changes the entire substance of what was written. Should this happen, do not let it go unaddressed! It is important to let the attorney know that was not what was charted. In other words, be sure you speak up and say that is not what it says.

Similarly, you may provide an answer to a question, at a deposition or trial, and a few minutes later, counsel will say, "You just told us that _____. Isn't it true that ________, Nurse X?" Being on the spot, nervous and inexperienced at giving testimony, many will just reply yes when in fact, that is NOT exactly what you said or meant. In fact it totally misstates your testimony. Take time and listen carefully, not allowing anyone to put words in your mouth. It is perfectly acceptable to say that you respectfully disagree with the attorney's characterization of your testimony. You can also correct the attorney by saying that is not what you said, or if it was, that you misspoke. But you need to make the correction immediately, as that information will stick in the jurors mind.

Deposition Tactics

One tactic that is frequently used is to make the deponent physically uncomfortable. Do not let this happen. You have every right to ask for a break. Go to the bathroom, get some water, walk around. If you are uncomfortable, take a break. Another way witnesses are frequently beaten down is to have a deposition go on and on for hours, trying to wear the deponent down just from sheer exhaustion. Getting up for even just five minutes will help this.

The skilled trial lawyer will often ask a question, listen to your answer, and then just be silent, even though it is pretty clear that you have finished answering the question. The lawyer does this hoping you will be uncomfortable with the silence and then continue to just talk. Resist all temptation to fill in the quiet space! Once you have answered the question, stop and just be quiet. Wait patiently for the next question no matter how long counsel waits.

As a percipient witness, it is also not your job to teach opposing counsel. His expert witnesses get to do that, or not, but in no way is it your responsibility. Sometimes counsel will "play dumb," as if they do not know or understand something. You can pretty much bet that is not the case and this is just another tactic.

As a witness, it is important to tell the truth to the questions asked. This includes saying "I don't know" when that is the truthful answer. Do your best to avoid the words "always and never" – they can come back to haunt you. It is too easy for counsel to pin you in a corner about always and never.

At the conclusion of the deposition, you will be told that forthcoming, you will be provided with the transcript of your deposition for your review. You will be asked to review the transcript and complete an errata sheet indicating any changes you would like to make. That said, you will be warned that any substantive changes you make can be commented on at the time of trial. This would be of significance if you were to change "yes" answers to "no" after the fact, or any other changes that materially change your testimony. So it is never in your favor to make significant changes to your deposition transcript, which is why giving an accurate deposition is important. You may also be asked if you will waive your rights to review your deposition transcript. This is never a good idea.

What is the Standard of Care?

Standard of care (SOC) is a term used to designate what a reasonable and prudent healthcare practitioner would do given the same conditions and conduct under the given circumstances. There are many sources that contribute to the standard of care. In nursing for example, state Boards of Registered Nursing, Nurse Practice Acts, facility policies and procedures, professional organizations' position statements, American Nurses Association standards, The Joint Commission standards, federal and state regulations, critical pathways and guidelines, authoritative texts, and professional peer reviewed journals are all examples of what establishes standards of care. The standard of care is NOT what the most experienced, most senior nurse would do.

Documentation

The medical record is THE MOST important evidence in a medical malpractice or elder abuse case. It is a legal document, and as such, healthcare providers must take care to assure its entirety, accuracy, and legibility. It also serves as the main communication tool between healthcare providers.

Simply stated, documentation in the medical record can make or break a legal malpractice case. States have what is called a statute of limitations. The statute of limitations is the maximum amount of time after an event that legal proceedings based upon that event may be initiated. This varies from state to state. In New York, a medical malpractice action must be filed within thirty months of the date of the act of omission that gave rise to the injury. Some states have longer statutes. California, for instance, has a statute of limitations for medical malpractice of one year. As one can see, it can be quite some time before an action is even filed. From that point, the discovery phase begins, which is quite lengthy. The legal system is not known for the speed at which the process progresses; it can and usually is years from the time of the alleged malpractice act until the case goes to trial – or even to deposition. The likelihood that one would remember in detail all facts of the assessment, case, and interventions for a specific patient is most unlikely. BEWARE! The nursing notes, and all of the documentation you create real time are either going to serve you as your best friend or your worst enemy.

When charting, the nurse should be cognizant of the mantra from nursing school: If it wasn't charted, it wasn't done. This always comes up in medical malpractice and/or elder abuse cases almost without exception. When legal nurse consultants or plaintiff attorneys are analyzing the medical records and nurses' charting, they look carefully for documentation deficiencies which will show a breach in the standard of care. Often, what is omitted or not said is just as important or more important than what was charted. Based upon the standards of care, and what is required by regulation, opposing counsel will focus on the breaches that have occurred.

Obviously, not every single thing that is done for a patient and every conversation can be charted, as the nurse would be left with no time to actually care for their patients. It is essential to chart the key care rendered, instructions given, and any patient teaching provided. For example, if a patient is at risk for developing a pressure ulcer it would be critical for the nurses to regularly document the patient's skin assessments, nutritional status, position changes, communication to the physician about any wound development, consultation by a wound care specialist, and care planning to address pressure ulcer prevention, as well as the patient's response to all of the aforementioned. Also included should be notification to the patient and family (when appropriate).

Federal and state regulations mandate charting requirements in healthcare settings. Information specific to each state is available by internet search using a search engine to find the official code of regulation site. For example, the Code of Federal Regulation for charting and documentation in a General Acute Care Hospital is:

CFR 42 §482.24(b) Standard: Form and Retention of Record

The hospital must maintain a medical record for each inpatient and outpatient. Medical records must be accurately written, promptly completed, properly filed and retained, and accessible. The hospital must use a system of author identification and record maintenance that ensures the integrity of the authentication and protects the security of all record entries.

States will have their own code of regulations mandating what is required in the charting. For example, in California, the state regulation for hospitals requires:

§ 70215 (b) The planning and delivery of patient care shall reflect all elements of the nursing process: assessment, nursing diagnosis, planning, intervention, evaluation and, as circumstances require, patient advocacy, and shall be initiated by a registered nurse at the time of admission.

In Rhode Island, the state regulation for hospitals requires:

R23-17-HOSP

§ 27.5 Entries in the medical record shall be made by the responsible person in accordance with hospital policies and procedures.

§ 27.6 The medical record shall contain sufficient information to identify the patient and the problem, to describe the treatment and document the results.

§ 27.7 The content of all medical records (inpatient, outpatient, ambulatory and emergency) shall conform with applicable standards of reference 9. Further, medical records shall document the primary language of the patient; shall document any hospital provision of interpretive services by bilingual clinicians, qualified interpreters, or qualified sign language interpreters; and shall document the inability to provide interpretive services by bilingual clinicians, qualified interpreters, or qualified sign language interpreters as required by the patient.

Regulations for all healthcare facilities can be located by internet search. This is important, as regulations are different depending upon the facility type in which you practice. Regulations at a general acute care hospital (GACH) are not the same as a long term care (LTC) facility or a skilled nursing home (SNF) versus a residential care facility (RCFE). The regulations are often also included in the facility's own policy and procedure manual.

The Legal Process of Medical-Record Review

When a prospective plaintiff retains an attorney for alleged medical malpractice (or elder abuse), the first item on the attorney's agenda is to evaluate whether or not the potential case has any merit. The medical records will be read and analyzed, most likely by a legal nurse consultant (LNC) or if not, by another in the law office very familiar with medical charts. Deciphering what is charted in the medical record is a talent unto itself. Knowing what is expected in the records makes reading the records possible. That is why it is usually a registered nurse, specifically trained as both an RN in that field in which the alleged malpractice occurred, as well as a legal nurse consultant who is familiar with what is needed to substantiate a claim of medical malpractice.

Clear and concise handwriting is of the utmost importance. If a passage in the medical record cannot be read, it does not mean the author (nurse) gets a free pass. Instead, what it is more likely to mean is that they will be asked to read what they wrote out loud into the record at their deposition. Everything said at a deposition is written down by a court reporter. One can only imagine how embarrassing it would be to not even be able to read ones own handwriting three years later, let alone the writing of your colleagues – which you are supposed to be using as a means of communication.

Legal nurse consultants know it is important to NOT ignore charting that cannot be deciphered. Their position will be "this may be my smoking gun" and more, not less, effort will be committed to understanding what was in fact done and charted. It is also wise to be aware that there are frequently inaccuracies or conflicting information in the patients' records. This is due to a healthcare provider making a (honest) mistake and then that information/mistake being carried forward to many other documents. Like the childhood game of telephone, this gets more convoluted as the error is (innocently and unintentionally) carried forward. One needs to pay close attention and then validate or invalidate information on the chart. If inaccuracies are identified, the author of the error should be identified and all efforts to correct it carried out.

What to Remember to Do and Chart

Charting should allow another healthcare provider to be able to "see" your patient. It should give others, who may not know or have never seen or cared for your patient, the sense that they have a clear picture of them. Charting is your picture of your patient. It is important to document what you assessed, what you did, how you did it, what the outcome was and if it was not what was expected, what interventions, and reassessment was done. The medical record is the primary communication tool between healthcare team members. Although as nurses we give report to oncoming shifts, we know that due to time constraints and emergencies, it is not always possible to verbally report off all information. Other healthcare providers do not have the opportunity to hear the nursing report, yet still need to have the information regarding the patients' status. This would include pharmacists, physical therapists, occupational therapists, and the litany of medical specialists on any given case. It is important that all of these disciplines have 24-hour access to accurate and complete information if they are to receive science-based, current information about the patients.

General guidelines for proper documentation, as well as to help defend your care should a lawsuit be filed, include:

Write legibly – illegible writing does nothing to help you and can only potentially hurt you. If necessary, print! Remember, the purpose of charting is for those caring for your patient after you to know your patients' status and what was done for them.

Make sure your charting is thorough. This means to be certain to include the date and time, as well as your signature, for every entry.

- Remember to include: who, what, where, when, and why.
- Keep your charting to objective, factual information. Your colleagues need this for continuity of care.
- Use only facility approved abbreviations. Many times, the fewer abbreviations the better. Abbreviations often have multiple meanings.
- Honest charting is critical! Never misrepresent, exaggerate, misstate, or falsify the medical records. This seems obvious – however, one would be surprised how obvious falsified medical records can be. In order to "successfully falsify" a medical record, all healthcare providers would have to be in cahoots. Obviously, this does not happen. So the misstatements of one provider become a red flag and only serve to worsen any possible error.
- Late entries: Charting should be done contemporaneously, making sure all charting is completed before your shift ends. Follow your facility's policy and procedure for late entries.
- No finger pointing in the medical record. This is not the place to assign blame, or make "CYA" notes – this too is very obvious and only serves as fodder for malpractice actions. This does nothing to advance the care of your patients.

  Example: The nurse calls a physician regarding a change in condition. The nurse should document placing the call. If the nurse spoke to the answering service, she should indicate with whom she spoke and the time. If the physician does not return the call within 5 -30 minutes (depending upon the urgency of the change in condition), document a return call, again with the same notations. If no response, the nurse should go up the chain of command and again document with whom she spoke, their title, and the date and time. Charting of the calls should all be factual. Please leave all and any opinions out of the charting. One should not chart, "Dr. X did not return call, as usual."
- Charting is the basis for care decisions, as well as assisting in a good legal defense. Accurate and complete responses to treatment and patient outcomes are an important part of this process.

Just as what is NOT charted that one could expect, there are other elements of the medical record that raise a red flag for the legal nurse consultant, expert witness, and plaintiff attorney. There are often notations in the medical record that just cannot be reconciled. In fact, entries can be oppositional. For example, when reviewing a medical record and the LNC sees that the CNA reports that patient ate 90% of every meal plus snacks, yet the chart reflects a 10-pound weight loss over the last two weeks, something is not accurate. The charting and the clinical picture do not reconcile, such as when it is charted that the patient needs feeding, yet there are no notes indicating that anyone has fed the patient. The following is an example of an incongruous medical record. This is a patient who had:

- Stage 3 pressure ulcer
- Braden scale was reported as 20 (a low or mild risk)
- Ambulates with minimal assistance
- Eats well
- No complaints of pain

The next day, the same patient's chart indicates:

- Stage 4 pressure ulcer with tunneling
- 60% slough
- 6x7 cm, 3 cm deep, 4 cm tunneling
- Foul smelling drainage

And the third day:

- Sacral ulcer improved 2x2x1 cm
- 100% granulation tissue
- Minimal serous drainage

By the fourth day, the patient is in septic shock with a very low blood pressure, a temperature over 102 degrees F, and tachycardia.

This inconsistency in the medical record allows the plaintiff's attorney to present a very grim picture to the jury regarding the care delivered at this facility.

Just as a physical exam is always conducted from head to toe to decrease the possibility of missing something, charting in a routine manner will also help to avoid gaps in documentation. Assessing patients from head to toe and then documenting head to toe will assure you have not inadvertently omitted anything. After you chart, review what you have written and assure it meets these criteria.

Pressure Ulcers

History

Pressure ulcers have been described as far back as the time of the Egyptian mummies (21st Dynasty, 1070-945 B.C.). Their cause, namely, loss of blood supply to the skin and underlying subcutaneous tissues, was suggested over 400 years ago. However, causation has been debated for several hundred years (denervation versus alterations in the autonomic nervous system versus loss of blood supply). Finally, the etiology became clear from studying those convalescing from wounds during World War I and later scientific studies conducted during World War II.

The National Pressure Ulcer Advisory Panel (NPUAP) serves as the authoritative voice for improved patient outcomes in pressure ulcer prevention and treatment through public policy, education, and research (http://www.npuap.org/). Pressure ulcers have been defined as "localized injury to the skin and/or underlying tissue usually over a bony prominence, as a result of pressure, or pressure in combination with shear and/or friction." Pressure ulcers that reach full thickness, that is stage III or IV, deep tissue injury, or those that are unstageable are considered "never events." That is, they should never happen. That said, it is critical that a distinction is made as to the stage of the ulcers. According to the NPUAP advisory paper on staging pressure ulcers, the pressure ulcer should be inspected and described by licensed vocational nurses. It is important to know your own state's Nurse Practice Act in order to assure compliance. In California, for instance, only registered nurses can assess patients. Licensed vocational nurses can gather data, and report that data to a registered nurse.

Wound Care Documentation

Wound care documentation should be done at least once a week, or as often as needed to ensure an accurate description of the wound is in the medical records. Most often, this should be done with each dressing change. Federal regulations exist to further protect the public in healthcare settings. Two examples of Federal regulations, located in Title 42 of the Code of Federal Regulations (42CFR), that apply to patients with pressure ulcers include:

§483.20(k) Comprehensive Care Plans

(1) The facility must develop a comprehensive care plan for each resident that includes measurable objectives and timetables to meet a resident's medical, nursing, and mental and psychosocial needs that are identified in the comprehensive assessment. The care plan must describe the following:

(i) The services that are to be furnished to attain or maintain the resident's highest practicable physical, mental, and psychosocial well-being as required under §483.25; and

(ii) Any services that would otherwise be required under §483.25, but are not provided due to the resident's exercise of rights under §483.10, including the right to refuse treatment under §483.10(b)(4).

§483.25(c) Pressure Sores

Based on the comprehensive assessment of a resident, the facility must ensure that--

(1) A resident who enters the facility without pressure sores does not develop pressure sores unless the individual's clinical condition demonstrates that they were unavoidable; and

(2) A resident having pressure sores receives necessary treatment and services to promote healing, prevent infection, and prevent new sores from developing.

To assure all state and federal regulations in relation to wound care are met, healthcare providers need to be familiar with what the regulations are in their state. It is also important to realize that there are state and federal regulations that conflict with one another. Which one applies? The regulation that is most strict in terms of protecting the patient is the one that will trump the other.

In general, to assure compliance with regulatory mandates, charting needs to address the following:

- type of wound: surgical, pressure, stasis, diabetic, trauma, etc.
- how it occurred
- locations and staging of the wound(s)
- size which should include the length, width and depth (at its deepest point) in centimeters
- undermining or tunneling/sinus tract
- exudates including the type, color, amount, and odor
- pain, if present: its nature, frequency, and what relieves it
- wound bed: color, type of tissue, and an assessment of evidence of healing
- wound edges and surrounding tissues. For example: rolled edges, redness, hardness, or maceration
- wound status – it is healing, unchanged, or advancing
- a photograph of the wound (please see section below for more information regarding photographs)

When evaluating the charting, the legal nurse consultant and/or plaintiff's attorney will want to know:

- Were appropriate and timely assessments done?
- What were the assessment skills that were used, and were they done when the patient was admitted to establish a baseline?
- What interventions were done to prevent and/or minimize skin breakdown?
- Was documentation of any skin breakdown accurate, timely, and appropriate?
- Was the physician aware and/or notified of the skin beginning to break down?
- Does the nutrition support the needs of the patient?
- Does the documentation verify notification of a change in condition to the physician and the doctor's response?
- If the physician did not respond, did the registered nurse go up the chain of command and advocate for the patient – bottom line: did the nurse get what was needed for the patient?

A well-documented and complete medical record is a critical tool for delivering solid, science-based care. The use of the pressure ulcer scale for healing (PUSH) is an effective tool when assessing the pressure ulcer based upon the length and width, the exudate amount, and the tissue type. The NPUAP developed this effective tool to monitor the change in pressure ulcer status over time. As this tool has been shown to reliably capture key assessments to identify whether a pressure ulcer is improving or getting worse; used properly, it is of great value when defending care against a lawsuit. It is also an important tool in preparing the healthcare providers, attorneys, and expert witnesses to defend a law suit. Conversely, an incomplete, sloppy chart is a huge liability for defense counsel and a potent weapon for the plaintiff's attorney bringing the complaint. Competent, experienced attorneys have a heyday when there are gaps in the medical records. This is especially true when the time around the incident has missing information, or time gaps strongly suggesting negligence. Based upon the untoward outcome, it does not take much for a skilled trial attorney to suggest to a jury what in fact happened to their client during that time period. Add to that the emotional impact to the jury viewing severe pressure ulcers (blown up on to a 5 foot screen) and a plaintiff verdict is not far away.

The facility should be able to show that its treatment protocols are based upon current standards of practice and have met with the medical director's review and approval.

Photographs

Controversy exists around whether or not to document wounds with photographs. The benefits of maintaining photographic documentation outweighs any downside. It assists to establish the rate of healing, as well as any deterioration from changes in measurements, provides a good communication tool, and serves to encourage the patient. The patients often forget how bad their wounds were and can become very discouraged. This is especially true with burn patients. Having photos to document the progress of healing goes far in helping the patient to see how far they really have come.

Photographs should be taken of all abrasions and wounds and documented into the hospital record upon admission. This needs to be done as an adjunct to treatment documentation and should support one another. There should be policies and procedures standardizing the photography process in order to have consistency in the photographs. Same lighting, positions, and distance should be maintained. The unit protocol should be consistent with accepted standards in wound care management. That would include having a means to assure digital images are accurate and not modified. All photos should protect the patients' identity and dignity. Labeling the photos should be done following these guidelines:

- initials only (no full names)
- date and time the photos
- location of the wound
- measurements with a linear measurement scale
- photos should be taken pre and post wound care

Photographic documentation of wounds aids in communication between healthcare providers, as it assists in evaluating nursing care. It also assists in validating the benefits of the care being provided. If there are no improvements, it is easier to see in a photograph, and the treatment plan may need to be re-evaluated with new interventions implemented. Often, insurance companies want verification of the effectiveness of the very costly treatment they are paying for. Photographs are a good way to justify payment for care.

Legally, photographs become part of the historical archive of care delivered to the patient and its outcomes. As every significant event relating to the history and care of the patient is important, photographs help to provide concrete documentation. All documentation is used to determine if the standards of care were met for a particular patient, as well as to memorialize professional responsibility and accountability. That said, with good nursing care being delivered, the charting ,and specifically the photographs, can be used by the nurse as a shield in a legal action; whereas, poor quality nursing care reflected in the records will be used as a sword against the nurse.

A good example of this is the "ambulance pressure ulcer." This is where the patient is being transferred from one facility to another. When the patient leaves facility one, there are no documented photographs or nursing notes indicating a pressure ulcer ever existed; yet, when they arrive at the new facility 8 minutes and 5 miles later, they are identified as having 3 stage 3 pressure ulcers and 1 stage 4 pressure ulcer! Hard to imagine how this can be, but even harder to imagine how the first facility's defense attorney is going to defend the staff!

What if You are Named in a Suit?

"The mistakes are all there, waiting to be made." Savielly Tartkower, chessmaster, 1887-1956

If you are working in a facility and find yourself involved in an adverse event, the first thing you want to do is go to your supervisor. If you feel your supervisor does not provide you with the appropriate response or support, just as you would do for a patient, go up the chain of command – to the Chief Nursing Officer, if necessary. Do not talk to your colleagues about it, or try to explain your side of it. If it was a reportable event wherein the Department of Public Health (DPH) was to be notified, let management handle that. If at a later date you are ever approached by a representative from the DPH, again make no statements without representation from management.

This is not to imply at any level that errors should be hidden – quite the contrary. It is just that you are not functioning alone, and the facility in which you work needs to be involved.

Decreasing the Risk of Medical Malpractice- Apologize

According to Brennan, et al., a Harvard medical practice study indicates that the incidence of adverse events and negligence in hospitalized patients is much greater than once believed. The most recent numbers from the Institute of Medicine suggest over 200,000 lives are lost each year due to medical negligence.

Errors in medication administration account for 770,000 adverse events annually where patients are either killed or injured.

As young children we are all taught to say, "I'm sorry," when we have done wrong. We have been told to "Follow the Golden Rule. Do unto others as you would want done unto you." Apologizing allows emotional fences to mend for both parties. It can be a powerful catalyst in improving communication and relationships.

The power of an apology can truly ward off litigation. It can actually empower the practitioner, while restoring the dignity and respect of the injured party or family. Yet in the arena of medical malpractice, we seem to have manipulated the rules. Counsel, whose job is to protect their clients, advise them, making sure nothing is said that would imply guilt or wrongdoing. If the doctor walks in and stonewalls the patient/family, the victim or his/her family boils, for what comes across as arrogant righteousness from the physician. The stage is set to build walls rather than bridges before legal complaints are even filed.

After an adverse event, a full and honest explanation and an apology should be provided routinely. Studies have shown that after an adverse event, patients expect more detailed information than doctors believe should be given. A physician's hesitation to provide detailed information to patients and/or the family after adverse events have occurred may be multifold fold: 1) it may be a concerned attempt to protect the patient from potentially detrimental anxiety; 2) the physician may avoid telling patients because it is a time consuming, difficult, and an unpleasant task; 3) the physician fears losing a patient's trust; 4) being blamed; and 5) the physician is worried about being sued. In addition, according to Leape (1994), it has been suggested that the current medical culture, in which error is often automatically equated with professional incompetence or inadequacy, makes admission to either patients or colleagues difficult. In a study, Young and Philips report that failure to provide information, an explanation, and an apology increases the risk of litigation and erodes the patient-doctor relationship. Young's findings verify that after an adverse event, patients want disclosure of the event, admission of responsibility, an explanation, an apology, and to know that implementation of prevention of future similar errors is in place. In some cases, the injured party also wants the offender to be punished and to obtain financial compensation. As both a clinician and legal nurse consultant, I can substantiate Young's findings. On many occasions I have had the experience of patients and families saying, if only the physician or nurse or hospital administrator said he/she was sorry; if only (the person) said, "I am so sorry. I truly regret what happened," they would not have sought legal advice and remedy. If the physician walks in and is evasive with the family, the likelihood of legal action increases. In today's world of easy access to information, whether via the internet databases or chat rooms, it is simple for one to obtain information that something substandard has caused the untoward outcome. Although an apology takes some of the bitterness away in litigation, understandably, the practitioner does not want to equate that civility and regret as an admission of liability that could come back to negatively affect him/her. Southern Methodist University law Professor, Daniel Shuman, who has researched apologies in the field of law, said the Indiana Malpractice Bill, in which defendants in lawsuits could not be punished for apologizing to plaintiffs before a trial, is a step in the right direction. "The likelihood of an injured party suing has less to do with the severity of the injury than with the actions of the doctor," Shuman said. "However, if the doctor expresses sympathy or apologizes, the patient or grieving family would heal faster and would harbor less of the negative feelings that can lead to large lawsuits," he said. That being said, we do know that the practice of medicine is not an exact science. It will never be 100% free of errors. What we do need are realistic expectations of the limitations of medicine and its practitioners. We need accurate informed consent (yes, which means the practitioner MUST take the time to provide ALL information, including alternate therapies and second opinions). The public is becoming savvier about what are possible complications and what constitutes malpractice. Failure to acknowledge an adverse event arising during treatment may have serious professional consequences for a practitioner.

The estimate of 100,000 lives lost each year in the United States due to medical errors is just that, an estimate. In fact, updated reports suggest it is closer to double that number! As there is no national reporting mandate of medical mistakes, the seriousness or death as a result, it is difficult to get accurate numbers. The Harvard School of Public Health (2003)[11] reports that physicians document less than 30% of their mistakes. 44% of specialists report that they were discouraged from reporting or encouraged to not report medical mistakes. So why is nothing done about this tremendous loss of life and injury?

After all, as healthcare providers, have we not in one way or another taken the oath to "first do no harm?" Why do these mistakes happen? How can we prevent them? In quality, we look at situations and care in terms of processes and systems. Were we to have a national reporting database, perhaps we could track trends and identify system deficits. But, for the most part, medical malpractice issues happen quietly and one at a time. There is no public outrage. And generally, no one addresses how best to rectify a situation so that the error cannot happen again. Without any other tools at our disposal, the injured party goes after the healthcare provider, and they are sued. One thing that keeps coming to the forefront from injured patients is, will this be prevented from happening to another? "I am not suing for the money, I am suing so that maybe it will make an impression and more caution and care will be exercised the next time with another patient." Cases are held close to the vest, no one talks openly about the mistake. And, no one learns from it either. In practice, we have numerous cases with the same theme: patient was dropped while being transferred from the wheelchair; dialysis patient's access was infected, the wound opened and the patient bled to death; a subclavian was inserted and the catheter was used prior to a chest x-ray confirmation for placement; no one followed up on the diagnostic test results, with the patient dying due to misdiagnosis; acute MI was misdiagnosed due to a lack of communication between healthcare providers. We could all go on and on with one similar example after another. And the message is the same, but for a reporting system and an opportunity for quality assessment with process and system revision, the incidents of medical malpractice resulting in patient death and serious injury continue to rise.

The Institute of Medicine (IOM) study (1999)[18] found that the cost associated with these errors in lost income, disability, and health care costs is more than $29 billion annually. And there are other studies that support the IOM report. The two seminal studies on medical error[4] have shown that adverse events occur in about 34% of patients. Leape, 1994,[13] found in their study that the average intensive care unit (ICU) patient experienced almost two errors per day. This translates to a level of proficiency of approximately 99%. 1 out of 5 of these errors were potentially serious or fatal. If performance levels of 99.9%, which is substantially better than those found in the ICU, applied to the airline and banking industries, it would equate to two dangerous landings per day (at one airport!) and 32,000 checks deducted from the wrong account per Leape, 1994.[13] In these industries, certainly we would see public outrage! It is agreed that to err is human, but there is nothing divine about forgiving repeated medical errors which cost tens of thousands of lives and tens of billions of dollars for nonexistent processes and systems that do not provide preventative protection to those most vulnerable in our community. To resolve the medical malpractice crisis, we, as professionals, need to acquire a system of checks and balances instituting processes and systems that will not allow for the current level of error.

Conclusion

Understanding that nursing documentation is often the beginning step in a medical malpractice action will help one to see what an important role nurses play in preventing legal actions before they begin. Proper documentation that memorializes nursing care and meets the standard of care can deter a potential plaintiff from filing a complaint or provide defense counsel the leverage to stop it in its tracks.

It goes without saying that the proper documentation of all care provided increases the nurses already burdened workload. Yet without it, excellent care cannot be provided, as an important communication and assessment tool would be lost. Defensive documentation will not only assure that the healthcare provider has provided care to the standards, but will also help to protect the healthcare provider should an adverse event occur.

Should a sentinel event occur, we need to give the patients a voice. And in the instance of a human error, we need to humbly say, "I'm sorry," as we rise to do whatever we can to make this tragic event less traumatic to the injured patient and family.

References

1. American Heart Association, Circulation, 102 (Suppl. 1), 140–141, 2000.
2. Ball, D. Theater Tips and Strategies for Jury Trials, 2nd ed., National Institute for Trial Advocacy, Notre Dame, IN, 1997.
3. Babitsky, S. How to Become a Dangerous Expert Witness: Advanced Techniques and Strategies. Massachusetts: Seek, 2005.
4. Brennan TA, Leape LL, Laird NM, Herbert L, Localio R, Lawthers AG, et al. Results of the Harvard medical practice study I. Incidence of adverse events and negligence in hospitalized patients. New England J Med 1991; 324: 370-376
5. Vincent, C., Young, M., Phillips, A., "Why do people sue doctors? A study of patients and relatives taking legal action," The Lancet. 343 (June 25, 1994) 1609-1613.
6. Carter B., Drawing the line: attorney involvement in preparing expert reports, For The Defense, 15–19, 86, August 2001.
7. Cohen, M., Rosen, L.F., & Barbacci, M. (2008). Past, Present, and Future: The Evolution of Nurse Expert Witness. The Journal of Legal Nurse Consulting, 19(4), 3-7.
8. Croke, E. and Fyler, P., Nurse experts: contributing members of today's litigation team, Journal of Legal Nurse Consulting, 13(1), 8–12, 2002.
9. Frey v. United States, 293F.1013 (D.C. Cir. 1923).
10. Garner, B. ed. Black's Law Dictionary. West Publishing Co., St. Paul, MN, 2004.
11. Harvard School of Public Health retrieved online
12. Iyer, P. and Banes-Gerritsen, C., Working with nursing expert witnesses, in Iyer, P., Ed., Nursing Malpractice, 2nd ed., Lawyers and Judges Publishing Company, Tucson, AZ, 2001.
13. Leape, LL (1994) Error in medicine. JAMA (272) (23)
14. Morris, C., Effective communication with deposition witnesses, Trial, 70–75, July 2000.
15. Rosemary Gibson and Janardan Prasad Singh, 2003.
16. Ross, J., How jurors perceive expert witnesses, Trial, 51–57, June 2000.
17. Sullivan v Edward Hosp., 806 N.E. 645 (Ill. 2004).
18. To Err is Human: Building a Safer Healthcare System. Institute of Medicine, November 1999.
19. West, T., "Deciphering medical hieroglyphics: The "how to's" of making the most of your medical discovery documents," Journal of Consumer Attorneys Association of Southern California, The Advocate, July 2006. http://www.theadvocatemagazine.com/West%20article
20. Zimmerman, P. G. (2008). Providing Expert Witness Testimony: Lessons Learned, The Journal of Legal Nurse Consulting, 19(4), 15 -17.
21. Pressure Ulcers: guidelines for Prevention and Management Third Edition 2001 JoAnn Maklebust, Mary Sieggreen
22. Wound Care Essentials Practice Principles 2004. Practice Principles. Sharon Baranoski, Elizabeth A. Ayello.
23. Title 42 Code of Federal Regulations online http://www.gpoaccess.gov/cfr/
24. www.npuap.org
25. Legal Nurse Consulting Practices 2010 Third Edition Chapter 1 The Legal Nurse Consultant as Expert Witness Cosby, M and West, T.

Notes

APPENDIX

1

Sample Job Description Medical Director Comprehensive Wound Center

Competencies

- Team Work
- Business Acumen
- Managing People
- Strategic Thinking
- Communication
- Multi tasking
- Problem solving

1. Qualifications:

Medical degree and three to five years related experience. Prefer specialty practice in the field of hyperbaric medicine or chronic wound management.

2. Supervisory:

The incumbent in the position will informally supervise 8-20 employees. Work in a collaborative environment with senior wound center leadership.

3. Education/Experience:

Doctor of Medicine (MD)
Doctor of Osteopathic Medicine (DO)

Essential Duties and Responsibilities

1. The Medical Director is solely responsible for quality of patient care within the center.
2. Collaborate with Clinical Coordinator, Program Director/Manager, and Safety Director if providing hyperbaric oxygen treatment so that the center meets the requirements of all regulatory and accrediting agencies, including, but not limited to, the State Health Facility Licensing Agency, the U.S. Department of Health and Human Services, the Joint Commission for the Accreditation of Health Care Organizations (JCAHO), and the Undersea and Hyperbaric Medical Society (UHMS).
3. In cooperation with Hospital Administration and Program Director, review and respond to any complaints and grievances and recommend or take corrective action where appropriate, in accordance with the bylaws, rules and regulations of the hospital or hospital's medical staff, as the case may warrant.
4. The Medical Director will serve as liaison with affiliated medical institutions for services such as hospitalization and emergency medical services.
5. The Medical Director will monitor physician documentation to ensure completeness, timeliness, and accuracy of services provided and applicable billing charges.
6. The Medical Director is responsible for overall HBO chamber quality and safety and will work closely with the designated Safety Director and Program Director to maintain all applicable standards of practice and care. He/she must ensure that every treatment is for an approved indication and that there is a physician present for every

treatment in accordance with local rules and regulations. He/she must further ensure that the physician's presence is appropriately documented and there are orders and progress notes for each treatment.

7. The Medical Director shall be responsible for the training and orientation of all wound center physicians. He/she shall be responsible for conducting a new physician orientation program in which all new wound care physicians will demonstrate to the Medical Director an adequate knowledge of the clinical competencies to include: knowledge of any practice guidelines that are in use, debridement techniques, routine, and high tech dressings.
8. The Medical Director shall provide a means for continuing wound care education. The Medical Director shall serve as an educational resource for the entire WCC including the medical, nursing, and administrative staff.
9. Actively schedule and participate in one-on-one discussions about center services with physicians in other medical specialties.
10. Provide regular formal presentations to various audiences (i.e., medical staff meetings, hospital department meetings, grand rounds presentations, local medical and community organizations, service clubs, etc.) to enhance the visibility of the wound center in the local marketplace and surrounding catchment area.
11. Act as spokesperson for wound center services when local media opportunities arise.

APPENDIX

2

Patient Condition Indicators for Determining Individual Acuity

Hyperbaric Oxygen Therapy

Medication other than PO: Refers to patient who needs additional medication either through IM, IV, or Per Tube route(s).

Anxiety/Stress: Refers to patient who requires a great amount of emotional support provided by nursing personnel during dive. Includes communication barriers between patient and personnel.

Mobility Assistance: Refers to the effort required by nursing personnel in giving mobility assistance to patient due to cast, splint, restraints, arthritis, medical or developmental restrictions, etc.

> Medium effort requires less than five minutes of nursing time per occurrence or assistance given with a moderate amount of difficulty.
>
> High effort requires five to ten minutes of nursing time per occurrence or involves an intense degree of effort in giving mobility assistance to the patient.

Frequency of mobility assistance required: Refers to numbers of times assistance is given during the visit.

> Medium is two times or less.
>
> High is three times or more.

Incontinence: Refers to patient who is actively incontinent of urine or feces. Does not need to be marked if patient has indwelling catheter.

Nursing supervision: Refers to the patient who requires nursing personnel at the chamber during the entire dive due to severe psychological distress or a history of unstable, pre-existing medical conditions.

WOUND CARE CENTER

Other: Refers to animal bites, mosquito bites, snake/spider bites, cellulitis, and radiation necrosis.

Mobility Assistance: Refers to the effort required by nursing personnel in giving mobility assistance to patients due to cast, splints, restraints, arthritis, medical or developmental restrictions, etc.

Medium effort requires less than five minutes of nursing time per occurrence or assistance given with a moderate amount of difficulty.

High effort requires five to ten minutes of nursing time per occurrence or involves an intense degree of effort in giving mobility assistance to the patient.

Frequency of mobility assistance required: Refers to numbers of times assistance is given during the visit.

Medium is two times or less.

High is three times or more.

Cognitive/Special Needs: Refers to patient and/or family receiving documented special instructions during the visit. Also refers to patient and/or family requiring a great amount of emotional support by nursing personnel during visit. Includes communication barriers between patient and personnel.

Incontinence: Refers to patient who is actively incontinent of urine or feces. Does not need to be marked if patient has indwelling catheter.

Diabetic Wounds: Use Wagner's scale for grading.

Pressure Ulcer: Staged according to AHCPR guidelines.

Debridements: If multiple debridements, add time for each.

Simple debridements are 11040, 11041, and 11042.

Complex debridements are 11043 and 11044.

Warm Springs Rehabilitation Hospital

Point scale for Classification of Patient Acuity

Class I- 0-30 min
Class II- 31-60 min
Class III- 61-90 min
Class IV- 91-120 min

Patient Classification Tool

HYPERBARICS

		Patients 1	2	3	4	5	6	7	8	9	10
Indicators											
New Admissions	90										
In-patients (Transportation)	20										
Diabetic Patient	5										
HBO prep	20										
Infectious Patient	20										
Medication other then PO	5										
Anxiety/Stress	15										
Unna Boots(each)	20										
Dressing Changes											
Simple	10										
Complex	20										
Total Contact Casting	45										
Mobility Assist											
Med	5										
High	10										
Frequency of Mobility											
Med	5										
High	10										
Incontinence											
Bladder	5										
Bowel	10										
Wound Care Visit	40										
TCp02	60										
Nursing Supervision (Dive)	90										
TOTAL POINTS		**0**	**0**	**0**	**0**	**0**	**0**	**0**	**0**	**0**	**0**
Classification											

CLASS I	0 Pts	X	0.5 Hours	0
CLASS II	0 Pts	X	1 Hours	0
CLASS III	0 Pts	X	2 Hours	0
CLASS IV	0 Pts	X	3 Hours	0
	0 Total Pts			0 Patient hours

Pt hrs/Total pts= #DIV/0! Direct Care Hours

#DIV/0! Direct care hours x 1.10 (non-prod)= #DIV/0! HPPD

#DIV/0! hrs x 0 Pts x 365 days= #DIV/0! Total hrs

#DIV/0! Total hrs / 2080 Hrs= **#DIV/0! FTE's**

Copyright Valerie Larson-Lohr 2002

Center Name:

Point scale for Classification of Patient Acuity

Class I- 0-30 min
Class II- 31-60 min
Class III- 61-90 min
Class IV- 91-120 min

Patient Classification Tool

WOUND CARE CENTER San Antonio

Indicators	**Time**	1	2	3	4	5	6	7	8	9	10
New Admission/Evaluation	90										
Diabetic Wounds (Wagner)											
Class I	5										
Class II	10										
Class III	15										
Class IV	20										
Class V	25										
Venous Stasis Ulcers	15										
Pressure Ulcers											
Stage I	5										
Stage II	10										
Stage III	15										
Stage IV	20										
Tracking/Tunneling Wounds	10										
VRE/MRSA Wounds	8										
Unna Boots (each)	20										
Lymphedema Wraps (ea)	30										
Wound Grafts											
Engineered grafts	60										
Wound Vac											
Simple	15										
Complex	30										
Debridement											
Simple	5										
Complex	15										
Total Contact Casting	45										
TCpO2	60										
Other (anml bite, cellu, etc)	15										
Mobility											
Med	5										
High	10										
Frequency of Mobility											
Med	5										
High	10										
Cognitive/Special Needs	30										
Incontinence											
Bladder	5										
Bowel	10										
TOTAL POINTS		**0**	**0**	**0**	**0**	**0**	**0**	**0**	**0**	**0**	**0**
Classification											

CLASS I	0 Pts	X	0.5 Hours	0
CLASS II	0 Pts	X	.75 Hours	0
CLASS III	0 Pts	X	1 Hours	0
CLASS IV	0 Pts	X	1.5 Hours	0
	0 Total Pts			0 Patient hours

Pt hrs/Total pts= #DIV/0! Direct Care Hours

#DIV/0! Direct care hours x 1.10 (non-prod)= #DIV/0! HPPD

#DIV/0! hrs x 0 Pts x 365 days= #DIV/0! Total hrs

#DIV/0! Total hrs / 2080 Hrs= **#DIV/0! FTE's**

Copyright Valerie Larson-Lohr 2002 Page 1

Index

D

M

N

O

P

Q

R

V

W

LOURDES LIBRARY
0 1225 0107638 6

JAN 24 2012